Understanding the Global Dimensions of Health

S. W. A. Gunn, Chief Editor
P. B. Mansourian, Coordinating Editor
A. M. Davies, Associate Editor
A. Piel, Associate Editor
B. McA. Sayers, Associate Editor

Understanding the Global Dimensions of Health

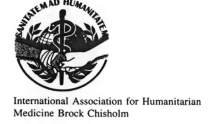

International Association for Humanitarian
Medicine Brock Chisholm

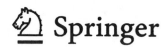 Springer

S. W. A. Gunn
International Association for Humanitarian
    Medicine Brock Chisholm
La Panetiere, Bogis-Bossey 1279
Switzerland

P. B. Mansourian
World Health Organization
Geneva, Switzerland

A. M. Davies
Hebrew University of Jerusalem
Jerusalem, Israel

A. Piel
World Health Organization
Geneva, Switzerland

B. McA. Sayers
Imperial College of Science,
    Technology, and Medicine
London, UK

The *International Association for Humanitarian Medicine Brock Chisholm* (IAHM) is a professional, non-profit, non-governmental organization that promotes and delivers health care on the principles of humanitarian medicine, named after Dr. Brock Chisholm, first Director-General of the World Health Organization. In particular, it provides medical, surgical, nursing, and rehabilitation care to patients in or from developing countries deficient in the necessary specialized expertise; brings relief to victims of disasters where health aid is lacking; mobilizes hospitals and health specialists in developed countries to receive and treat such patients free of charge; promotes the concept of health as a human right and bridge to peace; and advocates humanitarian law and humanitarian principles in the practice of medicine.

Library of Congress Cataloging-in-Publication Data

Understanding the Global Dimensions of Health/[edited by] S. William A. Gunn.
    p.   cm.
    Includes bibliographical references and index.
    ISBN 0-387-24102-7 (hbk.) — ISBN 0-387-24103-5 (eBook)
    1. World health.   1. Gunn, S. William A.

RA441.U42 2005
352.1—dc22

                                          2004065388

ISBN-10: 0-387-24102-7   e-ISBN: 0-387-24103-5   Printed on acid-free paper.
ISBN-13: 978-0387-24102-9

Printed in the United States of America

9 8 7 6 5 4 3 2 1

springeronline.com

Foreword

In today's convulsively changing world, scientific advances, political mutations, profit maximizations, social interventions, and human interpretations are producing new, and often confusing, perceptions of health and disease, to the extent that one wonders if such primary human aspirations as equity, well-being, and freedom from suffering are being forgotten. What *are* often forgotten are the fundamental principles of the World Health Organization. As Milan Kundera has put it so poignantly, "The struggle against human suppression is the struggle between memory and forgetfulness." In this context I believe that the many who over and over again tend to belittle WHO's constitutional definition of health have forgotten its innate significance and continuing pertinence: "Health is a state of complete physical, mental and social well-being and not merely the absence of disease or infirmity." This definition is immediately followed by the following injunction: "The enjoyment of the highest attainable standard of health is one of the fundamental rights of every human being without distinction of race, religion political belief, economic or social condition." Let me also remind the forgetful about the link between the inspirational and practical in that the WHO Constitution in Article 1 states: "The objective of the World Health Organization shall be the attainment by all peoples of the highest possible level of health." Perhaps a vision of ethics, of equity, of happiness and achievable well-being, that one of the authors of this book calls eudaemonia.

I see startling patterns of inequities in the health scores throughout the world. I am not talking of the first or second or third or fourth world — I am talking about ONE WORLD — the only one we have got to share and care for. And I continue to support the resolve to provide levels of health that will allow ALL PEOPLE of this ONE WORLD to lead socially and economically productive lives. For I believe that health can truly form a leading edge for social justice, especially when we are dealing with situations where the basic issue is survival, where people are trapped — as millions indeed are — in the vicious circle of extreme poverty, ignorance, and apathy. WHO's morally binding international contract of Health for All and its integral strategy of Primary Health Care do, I believe, shift health control towards people's own commitment and participation, implying profound social reforms in health, with much more social justice and community empowerment. Health may not be everything, but without health there is very little well-being.

There have been many books and reports in recent years dealing with these and other global problems in health. This book selectively discusses, in the form of scholarly chapters, a few critical issues: the fundamental historical, political, and socio-economic aspects of health in the world at large; the different views about values, systems, and technologies; the dynamics of global health; how to face the human rights challenges; how to cope with epidemics and pandemics; how to interpret the changing age structures; how to remedy food and nutrition problems in most countries. All these, and challenging new analytical methods and tools that confront the scholar. These are personal, social, economic, scientific, and worldwide issues replete with controversy that this book confronts boldly from different — and sometimes heterodox and conflicting — perspectives. It provides valid and mature insights towards understanding much of the global dimensions of health. It is certainly worthwhile reading and digesting.

Halfdan Mahler, MD
Director General Emeritus, World Health Organization

Contents

SECTION III. THE DYNAMICS   157

SECTION IV. THE CONTROVERSIES   229

Introduction

Health and disease, at once humanity's happiness and yoke, have marched with history and marked time with it. They have moulded and, it turn, have been influenced by the degree of social and intellectual development in any given space or time. Yet whatever the flux, humankind has constantly pursued disease as its target and health as its goal.

This dichotomy will never end as the search for health continues and the control of disease becomes increasingly possible. But that equation has been proving ever more complicated as numerous direct and indirect factors interact on being well and being unwell, creating unsuspected dimensions that cannot be ignored and need clearer understanding.

This book is about that understanding, an endeavour to weigh the multifacetted and sometimes contradictory elements that react personally, communally, environmentally and globally to ensure health or threaten disease.

There are few aspects of human activity that do not impact on health, of groups or of individuals. And from agriculture to world peace, climatic change to human rights, economic policy to world travel; all have implications for the health of people. The galloping spread of globalization, the increasing realization that no nation is isolated from another and that health is essential to progress, have led to attempts to engage those factors that influence national and international health. They are many and a detailed analysis of the determinants and the controversies around them fills libraries.

Twenty-one writers, all long involved in their different ways in the various aspects of health—scientific, clinical, social, economic, anthropological or administrative—have come together to discuss their concerns and share their understanding of the interlacing dimensions of health and disease. They have chosen to approach a limited number of outstanding issues in depth, so this can only be a partial coverage of the vast field still untapped, leaving it open to others to join the search and to explore further aspects of the global dimensions of health.

New global forces have eroded national borders facilitating the transfer of goods, services, people, values and lifestyles from one country to another. Socio-cultural, political and even religious influences, as well as economic, ecological and behavioural factors are perceived as shaping the future world order. Globalization of trade, technology and travel are quoted as important new phenomena with direct relevance to world health. Related inquiries are far from eliciting a consensus, triggering arguments between so- called 'globalizers' and 'anti-globalists'. Yet interdependence between sectors and between countries has been under investigation for several decades, including, for example, the 'Club of Rome' studies, over a quarter of a century ago.

The book approaches the difficult problematique in a pragmatic way: the first section,'Fundamentals', discusses basic aspects of health, history, ecology, ethics and international relations. Section II, 'Systems', makes a selective survey of health policies and systems issues, including technology, evidence-based medicine, and specific problems of therapeutic education. Section III, 'Dynamics', looks at individual major issues of global import, humanitarian, scientific, technical and epidemiological. Section IV, 'Controversies', presents original critical essays in various dimensions of our attempt to 'understand' global health. Is there really agreement on what is meant by health and disease? What are the oft-neglected parameters which impact public health? How do politics inter-digitate with health policy? And are there alternative visions of health? A postscript reflects on the many issues involved in global health, how the preceding chapters relate to the whole and suggests what needs to be done in the future.

Faced with the realities of global health, investigators are under an imperative to search for the key factors, the crucial interactions, the more revealing methodologies. The different authors here have been motivated, arising from their personal experiences, to focus attention on a variety of observations and approaches to global health issues, and on the insights that they themselves have gained. Inevitably, vantage points differ. As a result, these presentations have a very wide scope; assembling them together offers an opportunity of allowing fresh ideas to emerge—a desire fully justified by the complexity of interacting issues affecting global health.

We are particularly grateful to the Director General Emeritus of the World Health Organization, Dr. Halfdan Mahler, for having added his thought-provoking views from the world standpoint.

Special thanks are due to the individual authors whose contributions have made this book possible. The collaboration of the International Association for

Humanitarian Medicine Brock Chisholm is graciously acknowledged. We should also like to thank Mr. Bill Tucker, Senior Editor at Springer, New York, for his invaluable professional input.

S.W.A Gunn
P.B. Mansourian
A.M. Davies
A. Piel
B.McA. Sayers

Section I

Fundamentals

Chapter 1

A Brief History of Advances Toward Health

JOHN LAST

Three major discoveries determined the health and history of the human species. The first occurred almost a million years ago, when our hominid precursors discovered how to use fire to cook the meat they had hunted. They found that cooked meat tasted better, it didn't go bad so quickly, and eating it was less likely to make them ill. Our understanding of nutrition, a basic tenet of public health science, and the art of cooking have been improving ever since.

About 12,000 years ago, as the world warmed up after the last Ice Age, two more discoveries transformed human communities forever. Our forebears, perhaps our women ancestors, learned how to domesticate animals for food, milk and clothing. About the same time, they discovered that seed grain could be planted, harvested, and stored from one season to the next, and then used to make flour and thence bread and similar high-density carbohydrate foods. These two great discoveries eliminated dependence on precarious hunting and gathering, and made the founding of permanent human settlements possible. They are the indispensable basis for every human achievement since those ancient times.

The secure food supply led to the first great population surge. Little settlements became villages, which became towns, and towns grew into cities. Before long, civilizations with religions, laws, history, customs, traditions, and sciences arose on fertile plains beside the great rivers in Egypt, the Middle East, India, and China. Our ancestors had begun to climb the long road to health, towards our present situation. (We might ask as we consider the wars, the suffering, the injustices of the world of the early 21st century, "Where did we take a wrong turn?" But that is the story of civilization.)

As humans grew fruitful and multiplied, so did the variety and number of their diseases. Permanent human settlements transformed ecosystems, and abiding by epidemic theory, the probability of respiratory and fecal-oral transmission of infection rose as population density increased. Ecological and evolutionary changes in micro-organisms account for the origins of diarrhea , measles, malaria, small-pox, plague, and many other diseases. Micro-organisms evolve rapidly because of their brief generation time and prolific reproduction rates. Many that previously had lived in symbiosis with animals began to invade humans, where they became pathogenic. Some evolved complex life cycles involving several host species, such as humans and other mammals, humans and arthropods, and humans and fresh-water snails. These evolutionary changes in host-parasite relationships occurred at least several millennia before we had created written histories. Our oldest written records that have a bearing on health date back about 4,000 years. The Code of Hammurabi (c. 2000 BCE) contains ideas indicative of insight into the effects on health of diet and behaviour. It also suggests rewards and punishments for physicians who did their jobs well or poorly.

Information about the impact of diseases, especially of epidemic diseases, from those ancient times has come down to us in myths and biblical accounts of pestilences and plagues, although we cannot reliably identify the nature of the epidemics that afflicted ancient populations. The Greek historian Thucydides provided a meticulously careful description of an epidemic that struck the Athenians in the second year of the Peloponnesian War in 426 BCE, from which the forces of Athens perhaps never fully recovered. Modern infectious disease specialists have puzzled over this epidemic. Was it typhus, a virulent form of epidemic strepto-coccal infection, that is, a variant form of scarlet fever, or something completely different? Similar questions have been raised about other ancient epidemics, for instance the sweating sickness that recurred many times in mediaeval Europe then vanished, never to be seen again, almost 1,000 years ago. There has been debate too about the exact nature of the Black Death, the terrible pandemic that devastated Asia Minor and the whole of Europe in 1347–1350. This is usually attributed to the plague bacillus, *Yersinia pestis*, but revisionist historians and epidemiologists have raised the possibility that other pathogens, for instance, the anthrax bacillus, might have been responsible. Here, as with the plague of the Athenians, the plague of Justinian, the medieval sweating sickness, the accounts of apparent fulminat-ing epidemic syphilis (that may really have been another sexually transmitted disease or may have been caused by a highly virulent variant of the causative organism of syphilis, *Treponema pallidum*, which has slowly lost its extreme vir-ulence and infectivity), and, indeed, as with all other great epidemics of histor-ical times before the rise of modern microbiology, we can only speculate about the exact aetiology and pathogenesis. This is a rather sterile, albeit fascinating, quest.

It is more productive and useful to focus on what we know with reasonable certainty, and it is simplest to describe this knowledge in relation to some of the heroic figures who have contributed to advances in our understanding of epidemics and other diseases that have helped to shape history. This account therefore concentrates on a handful of the heroes of public health through the course of written history.

Hippocrates (460–370 BCE), the father of medicine, was also the father of public health. He practised and taught in a school of medicine at the Temple of Asklepios, near Epidaurus in Greece, and alone or with members of his school, laid the foundations of rational clinical medicine with careful descriptions of diseases and common sense ideas about ways to manage them. The Hippocratic writings contain rich medical wisdom based on careful observation of sick and healthy people and their habits and habitats. *Epidemics* is a series of case records of incidents of diseases, many of which we now know to be caused by infectious agents. The accounts of tetanus, rabies, and mumps, for instance, could have been written by a modern clinician. *Airs, Waters, Places* outlines environmental health as it was understood two-and-a-half thousand years ago. The relationships of environment, social conditions, and behaviours to health and sickness is made explicit in the timeless advice of the opening paragraph:

> Whoever would study medicine must learn of the following. First, consider the effect of each of the seasons... and the differences between them.... Study the warm and cold winds... and the effect of water on health... When a physician comes to a district previously unknown to him he should consider its situation and its aspect to the winds... and the nature of its water supply... Whether the land be bare and waterless or thickly covered with vegetation and well-watered, whether in a hollow and stifling, or exposed and cold. Lastly, consider the life of the inhabitants—are they heavy drinkers and eaters and consequently unable to stand fatigue, or being fond of work and exercise, eat wisely but drink sparely.

In short, study environment and life style, which are very modern concepts.

For well over a thousand years after Hippocrates' lifetime, human communities were afflicted with ever-present respiratory and gastrointestinal infections that cut deeply into the lives of everyone, and most deeply, as a rule, into the lives of young children who all too often died before they reached adolescence, carried off by measles, scarlet fever, diphtheria, bronchitis, croup, pneumonia, gastroenteritis, or typhoid. From time to time, this steady drain on long life and good health was punctuated by great and terrifying epidemics—smallpox, typhus, influenza, and, most terrible of all, the plague, or the "black death." The causes of these periodic devastations, the contributing reasons to why they happened, were a mystery. Many at the time believed they were God's punishment for sin, or the work of evil spirits. Ideas about contagion were rudimentary, even though it had been dimly understood since antiquity that leprosy, perhaps the least contagious of all the infectious diseases, was associated with propinquity and uncleanliness.

The 16th century Italian monk, Fracastorius, recognized some ways infection can spread. His conclusion, that disease could pass by intimate direct contact from one person to others, was easy to draw because he saw the dramatic epidemic of syphilis that was so obviously spread by sexual intercourse. He described this in a mock heroic poem, *Syphilis, sive morbis Gallicus* (1530) about the swineherd Syphilis, and how he got and passed on to others the "French disease" then raging in Europe. His anti-hero, of course, gave us the name of the disease.

Fracastorius's other concepts, contamination by droplet spread and by way of shared contaminated articles, such as clothing and kitchen utensils, were published in *De Contagione* in 1546. Fracastorius is important because he made a conceptual breakthrough—he brought about what Thomas Kuhn calls a paradigm shift in understanding of infection and some ways to control it.

After Fracastorius, the pathfinders on the road to health became numerous, but mention here will be made of only a handful of public health heroes: Paracelsus, John Graunt, Antoni van Leeuwenhoek, Bernardino Ramazzini, James Lind, Edward Jenner, Johann Peter Frank, John Snow, Ignaz Semmelweiss, and Louis Pasteur.

The Swiss alchemist Theophrastus Bombastus von Hohenheim, known as Paracelsus (1493–1541), occupies the junction of medieval alchemy with scientific chemistry, pharmacy, medicine, and environmental health. He was a colourful character, a foul-mouthed drunkard who insulted and sometimes fought those who disagreed with him, whom he considered superstitious nincompoops. He recognized the relationship of goitre to cretinism, the fact that inhaled dusts caused lung disease, and that some common mental disorders were diseases, not caused by witchcraft or 'possession' by evil spirits. He experimented with chemical remedies containing compounds of mercury, lead, and other galenicals, observed their effects, and, thus, could be considered also a founding figure of pharmacology.

John Graunt (1620–1674), a London merchant haberdasher, was an amateur scientist and an early Fellow of the Royal Society. He was interested in the impact of epidemics, especially the plague, and how plague outbreaks caused the numbers of deaths, and the age at death, to vary from one year to another. For over 100 years before his time, parishes had kept records of baptisms and deaths, and what was then understood about causes of death was inscribed in the Bills of Mortality. Graunt collected and analyzed these Bills of Mortality. He demonstrated statistical differences between males and females, between London and rural areas, and the ebb and flow of epidemics of plague. He published his work in *Natural and Political Observations ... upon the Bills of Mortality* (London, 1662). This work was the foundation for the science of vital statistics. John Graunt demonstrated the importance of gathering facts in a systematic manner, to identify, characterize and classify health conditions of public health importance. The diagnostic categories in the Bills of Mortality tell us what was understood 400 years ago about the variety of human ailments and their causes.

The nature of diseases caused by things not visible to the naked eye was long a mystery that began to unravel when Antoni van Leeuwenhoek (1632–1723), a Dutch linen draper and amateur lens-grinder in Delft, perfected the first functioning microscopes, with which he viewed drops of water, vaginal secretions, feces, his own semen, and the detailed structures of plants and insects. He lacked any formal scholarly training but in a series of 165 letters to the Royal Society of London, he described accurately and in detail all that he saw. He did not suggest that the tiny creatures he was the first to see with his microscope were capable of causing diseases, but he is nonetheless regarded as the first of the 'microbe hunters' who sought and identified the pathogenic micro-organisms responsible for many diseases.

Bernardino Ramazzini (1633–1714) was an Italian physician who observed and classified workers in many occupations, and reported his observations and conclusions about the diseases to which workers in each of these were vulnerable in De morbis artificum diatribe (On the diseases of workers, 1713). It is a tour de force, a masterly account in the form of sweeping generalizations, and although the evidence supporting these generalizations was often flimsy, Ramazzini introduced a new way of thinking about ways in which work conditions can affect health.

James Lind (1716–1794) was born and educated in Edinburgh. He was apprenticed to a surgeon when he was 15, and spent nine years as a naval surgeon, during which time he saw many cases of scurvy, a disease that disabled and often killed sailors on long ocean voyages. Lind thought this disease might be caused by a diet lacking fresh fruit and vegetables. He conducted an experiment, giving different diets to each of several pairs of sailors. This was the first clinical trial ever conducted—although the sample sizes were very small, there was no random allocation, and no informed consent was obtained from the sailors. The two sailors who received fresh oranges and lemons recovered rapidly from the scurvy, the others did not, or got worse. Lind also initiated the first effective measures aimed at enhancing hygiene in the British navy, but he is best known for his work on scurvy, reported in A Treatise of the Scurvy (1753). Not only was this the first reported clinical trial, it also was proof that a dietary deficiency can cause disease, that a well-balanced diet is essential for good health. Thus Lind, like Fracastorius, was responsible for an important paradigm shift in the understanding of causes and control of disease.

Johann Peter Frank (1745–1821) studied medicine in Heidelberg and Strasburg, was a professor of medicine at Göttingen and Pavia, and taught in many other centres of learning including St Petersburg, before he ended his career in Vienna where he was professor of medicine at the Allegemeines Krankenhaus. Early in his career he began writing System einer vollständigen medicinischen Polizey, his great work on ways to improve population health. This appeared in a series of nine volumes from 1779 to 1827. It was, as the title indicates, a system dealing with every then-known way to protect and preserve good health, including community hygiene, personal health protection by cleanliness, and a suggested set of laws and regulations to govern the control of conditions in lodging houses and inns, medical inspection of prostitutes, and so on.

Edward Jenner (1749–1823) was an English family doctor who practised throughout his life in the village of Berkeley, Gloucestershire. In his days, smallpox was a ubiquitous threat to life and health. In severe epidemics, it killed up to a quarter of all it attacked. When it did not kill, it often left disfiguring facial pockmarks and if it infected the eyes it caused blindness.

The practice of variolation, inoculation into the skin of dried secretions from a smallpox bleb, was invented in China about 1000 years ago and spread along the silk route, reaching Asia Minor in the 17th century. Lady Mary Wortley Montague, wife of the British ambassador to Constantinople, described the practice in a letter dated April 1, 1717, and imported the idea to England when she came home. By the time Jenner was a child, variolation had become popular among educated English families as a way to provide some protection against smallpox.

Jenner knew the popular belief in Gloucestershire that people who had been infected with cowpox, a mild disease acquired from cattle, did not get smallpox. He reasoned that since smallpox in mild form was transmitted by variolation, it might be possible similarly to transmit cowpox. A smallpox outbreak in 1792 gave him an opportunity to confirm this notion. In 1796 he began a courageous and unprecedented experiment—one that would now be unethical, but that has had incalculable benefit for humankind. He inoculated a boy, James Phipps, with secretions from a cowpox lesion. In succeeding months, until the summer of 1798, he inoculated others, most of them children, to a total of 23. All survived unharmed, and none got smallpox.

Jenner published *An Inquiry into the Causes and Effects of the Variolae Vaccinae* in 1798—perhaps the most influential public health treatise of all time. The importance of Jenner's work was immediately recognized and although there were sceptics and hostile opponents, vaccination programs began at once. The frequency and ferocity of smallpox epidemics began to decline early in the 19th century, but the disease remained a menace until the mid-20th century. In 1949, the American epidemiologist Donald Soper worked out the strategy of containment, in other words, vaccinating all known contacts of every diagnosed case. In 1966, WHO embarked on a global campaign to eradicate smallpox. The last naturally occurring case was a girl in Somalia in 1977. In 1980, the World Health Assembly proclaimed that smallpox, one of the most deadly scourges of mankind, had been eradicated. At the beginning of the new millennium, samples of smallpox virus are preserved in secure biological laboratories in several countries, but, thanks to Edward Jenner, this terrible disease need never again take a human life—unless it is used illegally in biological warfare.

John Snow (1813–1858) was a London physician, and a founding father of modern epidemiology. (He was also a pioneer anesthetist who invented a new kind of mask to administer chloroform, which he gave to Queen Victoria to assist at the births of her two youngest children.)

Snow's work on cholera demonstrated fundamental intellectual steps that must be part of every epidemiological investigation. He began with a logical analysis of the available facts, which proved that cholera could not be caused by a 'miasma' (emanations from rotting organic matter) as proposed in a theory popular at that time, but must be caused by a transmissible agent, most probably in drinking water. He confirmed the proof with two epidemiological investigations into the great cholera epidemic of 1854. He studied a severe localized epidemic in Soho, using analysis of descriptive epidemiological data and spot maps to demonstrate that the cause was polluted water from a pump in Broad Street. His investigation of a more widespread epidemic in South London involved an inquiry into the source of drinking water used in over 700 households. He compared the water source in houses where cholera had occurred with that in others where it had not. His analysis of the information about cases and their sources of drinking water showed beyond doubt that the cause of the cholera outbreak was water that was being supplied to houses by the Southwark and Vauxhall water company, which drew its water from the Thames downriver, where many effluent discharges polluted the water. Very few cases occurred in households supplied with water by the Lambeth company, which collected water upstream from London, where there was little or no pollution. John Snow reasoned correctly that the cholera must be caused by some sort of agent in the contaminated water supply. This was a remarkable feat, completed 30 years before Robert Koch identified the cholera bacillus. Snow published his work in a monograph, On the Mode of Communication of Cholera (1855). This book has been reprinted in modern editions and is still used as a teaching text.

The Hungarian physician Ignaz Semmelweiss (1818–1865) was a great but tragic figure. Working in the obstetric wards of the Allgemeines Krankenhaus in Vienna, he tried to transform traditional but ineffective treatment methods by using logic and statistical analysis to demonstrate the efficacy, or lack of it, when he compared treatment regimens. He believed in the germ theory of disease and was convinced that the terrible death rates from puerperal sepsis must be caused by germs introduced into the raw uterine tissues by birth attendants who did not disinfect their hands. He carried out a meticulous comparative mortality study in his own wards, where he insisted that all birth attendants must cleanse their hands in a disinfectant solution of bleach, and other wards run by senior obstetricians where hand-washing was not routine. His senior colleagues regarded his findings as a gross insult to their professional competence. Semmelweiss's rather abrasive nature and his Jewish origins in the anti-Semitic atmosphere of 19th century Vienna made matters worse for him. He was hounded out of his hospital post, and ended his life in a mental hospital. His belatedly published comparative statistical analyses of the death rates from puerperal sepsis in his own and other wards of the Allgemeines Krankenhaus are a model of how to conduct such studies, but, unfortunately, no one in Vienna heeded him and young women continued to die of childbed fever for another generation.

Medical science advanced rapidly in the second half of the 19th century, applying the exciting discoveries of a new science, bacteriology, which transformed public health. The great bacteriologists of the late 19th century identified many pathogenic bacteria, classified them, developed ways to cultivate them, and, most important, worked out ways to control their harmful effects, using sera, vaccines, and "magic bullets" such as the arsenical preparations that Ehrlich developed to treat syphilis. It would be useful to discuss each of them, but I will focus on just one, Louis Pasteur (1822–1895). This French chemist evolved into a bacteriologist, and was a towering figure of 19th century bacteriology and preventive medicine. In 1854, he had recently been appointed professor of chemistry in Lille, and was invited to solve the problem of aberrant fermentation of beer that caused it to taste bad and made it undrinkable. He showed that the problem was caused by bacteria that were killed by heat. In this way he invented the process for heat treatment to kill harmful bacteria, first applied to fermentation of beer, then to milk—the process known ever since as pasteurization that has saved innumerable children from an untimely death. He went on to study and solve many other bacteriological problems in industry and animal husbandry. He developed attenuated vaccines, first to prevent chicken cholera, then, in 1881, to control anthrax, which was a serious threat to livestock and, as well, occasionally to humans. Before this, in 1880, he began experiments on rabies, seeking a vaccine to control this disease, which without treatment is invariably fatal.

As a result of the success of the anthrax vaccine, he believed that an attenuated rabies vaccine could be made. This, of course, was many decades before the virus was visualized. He prepared and successfully tested his rabies vaccine in 1885 on a boy, Joseph Meister, who had been bitten by a rabid dog. Pasteur became not just a national but an international celebrity.

Born in the same year as Louis Pasteur, the Austro–Hungarian monk Gregor Mendel (1822–1884) was another amateur scientist, a botanist. Experimenting with varieties of garden peas, he cross-pollinated them and observed and recorded the results. Unfortunately, he published his findings in an obscure journal where they remained un-noticed for many years, but when they were unearthed about 15 years after his death, Gregor Mendel was retroactively honoured as the father of a new science, genetics, which soon found many applications in clinical medicine, with the recognition of the fact that many inherited diseases were caused by genetic disorders. Almost 100 years after Mendel's death, other discoveries with great public health relevance include development of genetically modified sterile insect vectors of disease, genetically resistant strains of rice, wheat, and so on, and applications of genetic engineering to limit and even control and prevent some recessive inherited disorders.

Pasteur, Henle, Koch, Virchow, and, soon after, battalions of bacteriologists and pathologists firmly established the fact that micro-organisms caused many diseases—the germ theory was a proven fact, not theory. However, many germ diseases require much more than germs before they can cause their worst damage. Tuberculosis is caused by the tubercle bacillus acting in conjunction with poverty, ignorance, overcrowding, poor nutrition, adverse social and economic circumstances, and other enabling and predisposing factors.

The diarrheal diseases, including cholera, are caused by various micro-organisms, but these get into the gut when ingested with contaminated water or food, that is, they are really caused by poor sanitary and hygienic practices.

By late in the 19th century, many of these factors had been clarified. The stage was set for the health reforms that included the sanitary revolution, the beginnings of a social safety net, provision of immunizations, nutritional supplements for school children, prenatal care for pregnant women, and other essential public health functions we take for granted 100 years later. It required a dedicated army of public health workers to achieve all this.

I have singled out and mentioned a mere handful of the public health pathfinders on the road to good health. Many others could be added, but that would turn this brief chapter into a weighty monograph. Often the physician—pathfinders used their own patients as experimental subjects for their path-finding discoveries. Lind's sailors, Jenner's 23 young friends starting with James Phipps, Pasteur's patient Joseph Meister, and all others known and unknown by name who provided the material for the great discoveries of Robert Koch and other members of the Austrian and German schools of bacteriology, should be remembered and honored too.

Many others belong in their company: The great German pathologist Rudolph Virchow recognized that political action as well as rational science are necessary to initiate effective action to control public health problems; Edwin Chadwick and Lemuel Shattuck reported on the appalling sanitary conditions associated with the unacceptably high infant and child death rates that prevailed in 19th century industrial towns; William Farr established vital statistics in England as a model for other nations to follow. And so the list grows from a handful of public health pathfinders to whole armies.

More was needed than scientific discoveries. Such discoveries had to be applied, and this often required drastic changes in the established social and economic order. So, other pathfinders appear on the road to health. They include politicians, administrators, journalists, creative writers, performing artists, and cartoonists. The journalists, creative writers, and artists who transmit the scientific concepts of public health to the general public and to the politicians are indispensable partners in the team that makes it possible for us to advance up the road to better health. The process continues in modern times with investigative journalism and TV documentaries.

I have identified five essential ingredients of the processes that brought about the public health reforms called the Sanitary Revolution of the late 19th and early 20th century, and have shown that these five features are essential for the control of all public health problems.

1. Awareness that the problem exists. John Graunt began this process with *Natural and Political Observations*. Others consolidated his conceptual breakthrough, and it was applied to great effect after the establishment of formal national vital statistics in England and Wales under the inspired leadership of William Farr. By Farr's time, widespread literacy, the proliferation of daily newspapers, and word of mouth helped to enhance awareness among thoughtful people everywhere that there were massive public health problems in society at that time. Modern computer-based record-keeping and effective health information systems with instantaneous worldwide notification of contagious disease outbreaks with public health significance continue to enhance the process.

2. Understanding the causes. In the second half of the 19th century, understanding rapidly increased, as epidemiology and bacteriology, and nutritional and environmental sciences explored previously unknown landscapes of aetiology and pathogenesis. The new mass media—daily newspapers—propagated this understanding among literate people throughout the country. From the middle of the 20th century, news magazines and TV have ensured that knowledge of causal connections—smoking to cancer, diet and lack of exercise to coronary heart disease, alcohol-impaired driving to traffic fatalities, and many more—are very widely disseminated. This, however, has not necessarily led to effective control measures.

3. Capability to control the causes. With astonishing speed, once the initial breakthroughs had occurred, sera and vaccines were developed to control many of the lethal microbial diseases that had plagued earlier generations. Improved dietary practices, pasteurization of milk, improved personal hygiene and, above all, environmental sanitation to rid drinking water of polluting pathogens, all advanced rapidly in the final quarter of the 19th century and the first few decades of the 20th century. Thus many ancient infectious disease scourges have been controlled, most dramatically being, perhaps , the eradication of smallpox. Unfortunately, new infectious pathogens including the human immunodeficiency virus, viral tropical haemorrhagic fevers, the coronavirus of severe acute respiratory syndrome, and a score or more of others, have emerged to take their place . . .

4. The belief (sense of values) that the problem is important. This is an essential prerequisite to the determination to act upon the problem. It is the most fascinating and challenging aspect of the essential features. This belief is the moral imperative that drives public health reforms. Geoffrey Vickers described the history of public health as a process of redefining the unacceptable—an endless process of identifying conditions, behaviors, and circumstances that individuals, communities, and cultures must no longer tolerate. Throwing the contents of the chamber pot into the street, clearing one's nostrils on the tablecloth, coughing and spitting on the living-room floor, all became unacceptable in the late 19th century. Many people outside the boundaries of traditional medical science and public health practice played a role in this process. In the era of the great reforms of the 19th century, they included social reformers like Edwin Chadwick, journalists like Henry Mayhew and Charles Kingsley, novelists like Charles Dickens, cartoonists in *Punch* and other periodicals—all of whom were aided by the rise of literacy in that period. Collectively, they inspired a mood of public outrage that became an irresistible force for reform. In the second half of the 20th century, this sense of moral outrage found new targets—lighting a cigarette without permission in someone else's home, carrying infant and child passengers in a car without safety equipment, dumping toxic industrial waste where it harms others, and more. Yet, much else remains to be done.

5. Political will. There is always resistance to change, there are always interest groups—often rich and powerful withal—who will do whatever it takes to obstruct necessary improvement. In the era of the sanitary revolution, it was the owners of water companies, factories, and tenement housing who resisted most vigorously. Since the 1950s it has been tobacco companies and a host of manufacturers of toxic petrochemical and other dangerous compounds released into the air and water. Legislation and regulation are almost always necessary, and inevitably generate opposition. Nevertheless, when the other four features—awareness, understanding, capability, and values—are in place, the political will to bring about reforms gathers momentum and usually succeeds eventually.

These five essential ingredients required for public health reforms apply to several public health problems that have waxed and waned over time: tobacco addiction, impaired driving, domestic violence, child abuse, irresponsible domestic and industrial waste disposal, and so on.

Lately, mountainous barriers—of our own making—to maintaining our public health have appeared. The most formidable is a cluster of human-induced changes to global ecosystems and the global commons—the atmosphere, the oceans, wilderness regions, and stocks of biodiversity—that threaten all life and health on earth, not just the life and health of humans.

Another barrier is perhaps an inherent flaw in the human character that leads many individuals and national leaders to believe that disputes can be settled by violent means. Currently, we have so many terrible weapons that violence done by them can and does cause immense suffering, innumerable deaths (80% or more of these deaths, as well as a similar proportion of permanent maiming and disability, are among non-combatants), and appalling damage to ecosystems, the environment, and the fabric of society. Sadly, this is rarely recognized as a public health problem. The very first essential ingredient, awareness of the problem, is lacking. Both these massive public health problems, in my view, are linked to the insatiable human craving for petroleum fuels, an addiction far more pervasive and dangerous to mankind and the earth than addiction to tobacco. So far in our only partially sentient and insightful civilization, this particular addiction is not even recognized as a public health problem.

One public health problem that has been recognized is a worldwide pandemic of tobacco addiction and its many adverse effects on health and long life. Recognition of this problem led the delegates to the World Health Assembly of 2002 to approve the Framework Convention on Tobacco Control. Another universally recognized public health problem is the global pandemic of HIV/AIDS. Tobacco addiction and the HIV/AIDS pandemic are both associated with the values of modern life and social behavior, including the marketing practices of transnational corporations. Surmounting these barriers to health will require social, cultural, and behavioral changes and political action.

I am an optimist. I believe that the pace of scientific advances will be maintained in the future, and that values will continue to shift in favor of essential changes towards global ecosystem sustainability. I do not know whether those who follow us will ever reach the ultimate summit or idealized WHO vision of Halfdan Mahler's "Health for All," but I am confident that they will continue to climb towards it.

REFERENCES

Fracastorii, H. (Fracastorius). (1930). *De contagione et contagiosis morbis et eorum curatione, Libri III.* (W.C. Wright, Trans.) London and New York: Putnams.

Graunt, J. (1662). *Natural and political observations mentioned in a following index and made upon the bills of mortality with reference to the government, religion, trade, growth, air, diseases and the several changes in the said city.* London: John Martyn.

Jenner, E. (1966). *An inquiry into the causes and effects of the variolae vaccinae.* London: Dawsons (Facsimile of the original 1798 edition).

Lind, J. (1753). *A treatise of the scurvy.* Edinburgh: University of Edinburgh Press. (Reprint of the 1753 edition)

Lloyd, G. E. R. (Transl.). (1978). *Hippocratic writings.* Harmondsworth: Penguin.

Ponting, C. (1992). *A green history of the world; the environment and the collapse of great civilizations.* New York: St Martin's Press.

Porter, R. (1997). *The greatest benefit to mankind; a medical history of humanity from antiquity to the present.* London: Harper Collins.

Sigerist, H.E. (1967). *A history of medicine, 1. Primitive and archaic medicine.* New York: Oxford University Press.

Snow, J. (1855). *On the mode of communication of cholera.* London: Churchill.

Chapter 2

The Health, Poverty, and Development Merry-Go-Round
The Tribulations of WHO

SOCRATES LITSIOS

INTRODUCTION

The role of better health in socio-economic development has long been argued, as has the need for getting other development sectors to contribute to health development. However, as illustrated below, considerable tension has existed throughout public health history between those who believe that improving health is the key to pulling people out of their misery, and those who argue the contrary, namely, that people need to be economically and socially better-off before they can aspire to better health.

When the World Health Organization (WHO) came into existence in 1948, it inherited this more than one-century-old argument that divided the world of public health. This did not prevent the organization from seeking to control various diseases, operating under the firm belief that such control would be a positive force for human development. Even the evidence provided by the population explosion that followed the control of malaria did not prevent the global malaria eradication campaign from being launched in 1956. Yet despite the past controversies, no effort was made to make a careful accounting of the impact of malaria control/eradication on socio-economic development during the 1950s and 1960s, when the global eradication campaign dominated WHO's agenda.

There have been calls, here and there, for greater attention to evaluating the socio-economic impact of health programmes, but these have rarely been followed up on with field studies of any significance. More revealingly, policy makers have suppressed opinions not favorable to their own so to not jeopardize confidence in the policies which had been decided upon. Thus, WHO rarely treated seriously those who opposed the decision to seek the eradication of malaria. In such a context, it is not surprising that this and similar policies have been pursued without the benefit of any further evidence to judge whether they yielded the results expected.

Given this long history of shaky evidence and poor evaluation, the issue of health, poverty and development is hardly any better understood today than it was 50 years ago. Instead of keeping a steady focus on the subject, WHO has let it come and go, largely as a reaction to external pressures and funding issues. It is currently again on the agenda of WHO. This time, it can be hoped that serious, in-depth evaluation will take place over the coming decades. The framework for such evaluation should not be driven by any one ideological position or by any central bureaucracy that is not open to opposing views. Conflicting opinions should be used to expand the evaluation criteria examined, so that evidence gathered over time helps resolve differences. In short, it is time to learn from experience rather than hold onto beliefs that may, in fact, be wrong.

SOME HISTORICAL BENCHMARKS

Chadwick and the Sanitary Movement (Litsios, 2005)

Edwin Chadwick is credited with having launched England's sanitary movement in the 1830s. He did so in the belief that effective drainage and sewerage would reduce ill-health; improving the health of the English common man would mean less poverty; and less poverty would mean reduced charges on the Poor Rates. As secretary to the Poor Law Commission, his motivations were largely economic.

In the course of his famous study on the sanitary conditions of the lives of England's working class, Chadwick asked William P. Alison, a Scottish physician, "whether the destitution without the filth, or the filth without the destitution, is more effectual in the production or extension of fever." Alison replied that in Scotland, "we have no destitution without filth; but we have many examples of filth without destitution." From his experience "fever neither makes its way into such (non-destitute) families with the same facility, nor extends through them with the same rapidity and certainty, as in the case of the unemployed, or partially employed, disabled, and destitute poor." In fact:

> As long as the condition and habits of the poorest of the people, and their resources when reduced by any cause of destitution . . . continue as at present . . . removal of various nuisances will be perfectly ineffectual.

Alison had reversed the argument. More government spending was needed to reduce poverty before any benefits from sanitary action could be realized.

It took several years for Chadwick to gather the material that he used in his report on the sanitary conditions of the working class. The report itself is made up largely of testimony he obtained from medical officers throughout Great Britain. Recognizing that Alison's views on the subject directly undermined his faith in the economic benefits to be obtained by sanitary reform, Chadwick chose *not* to make explicit use of Alison's views in his report.

Hermann Biggs and the International Red Cross (Litsios, 2005)

Moving ahead nearly a century, to a meeting held in Cannes, France, in 1919, to consider the establishment of an International Red Cross (IRC), Hermann Biggs, a leading American public health specialist, prepared a "statement of general purpose and scope of work" for the IRC, which included:

- As the prevalence of disease, unsanitary conditions and excessive death rates are almost universally and inseparably connected with poverty and ignorance and as these conditions are interdependent, the IRC ... should also initiate aid and direct measures among less forward nations looking to the promotion of education especially along vocational lines and to the improvement of economic conditions so that the productivity of the soil and the productivity of labor may be increased.
- The IRC should create a bureau for the collection, analysis, publication and distribution of information on public health and sanitation including dietetics and soil pollution. It should also collect and distribute similar information in relation to the cultivation of the soil, agricultural machinery and similar topics and should arrange for and conduct demonstrations in those countries where they are most needed.

Biggs wrote to his wife:

> We have been working hard and with great results, I think ... It (the first draft of our scheme) is really mine and I drew this up. It provides for a great international philanthropic organization to aid in giving health and equality of opportunity to the nations of the world. Perhaps they will discard it at Cannes as being too broad and too Utopian.

Biggs was right; a much watered down program was adopted and, when funding proved difficult to obtain, the resulting organization (the League of Red Cross Societies) performed mostly as an international health education organization.

The Divided Pre-World War II World of Malariology (Litsios, 1997)

The impetus to do something in the field of international health following World War I did lead to the creation of the Health Organization of the League of Nations, which, in turn, established a Malaria Commission, owing to the importance of this disease in Europe at the time (1923).

Despite the discovery by Ronald Ross in 1898 of mosquitoes' role in malaria transmission, many of the Commission's members were convinced that socio-economic development was needed before malaria could be controlled. The leading protagonist for this position was C. Price James, who earlier in his career had crossed swords with Ross. He questioned the value of Ross' discovery, as witness this claim made in 1927:

> When the discovery of the mosquito cycle of the parasite was made it was almost universally believed that a single, simple method had been put within our grasp, capable of application in all malarious districts. Since then three decades have passed, and such a method is still to seek.

Of course it was anti-mosquito methods that had eliminated malaria from the Panama canal, but the cost had been extravagant, well beyond the means of any one country. Even the successes that had been achieved on numerous plantations around the world, where the presence of malaria cut into profits, could not be afforded by the average rural community.

Lacking any 'simple method', James concluded that the "*correct way*" of combating malaria is:

> ... to introduce agricultural schemes which aim primarily at improving the economic prosperity of the people ... accompanied by progressive arrangements for adequate medical attention in sickness, for technical and elementary school education and for simple sanitary measures of housing, water-supply, conservancy and general welfare.

Lewis Hackett, one of the leading Rockefeller Foundation malariologists and proponents for anti-mosquito measures, challenged James' views whenever he could. He believed:

> ... the causes of malaria, at least, are in the main independent of the ignorance and poverty of its victims and can be separately handled. It is easier to believe that release from the burden of malaria will help to bring prosperity and knowledge than that a higher standard of living and education must precede the eradication of malaria.

China's Pre-World War II Rural Reconstruction Program (Litsios, 2005)

Several years later, in a different situation (China), the same organizations, that is, the League's Health Committee and the Rockefeller Foundation, found themselves struggling to assist China to develop the rudiments of a rural health infrastructure. The key advisor from the League's side was Andrija Sampar and from the Foundation side Selskar Gunn, a Vice-President.

This time, the two organizations did not differ in their views. Both cooperated at "raising the educational, social, and economic standards of rural China." The program was interrupted by the 1937 invasion of China by Japan. However, by then, it had become clear that extensive land reform was a prerequisite for success, something the ruling powers refused to carry out.

Gunn built on this experience in his introduction of a report of a League meeting on rural hygiene in 1937 in Bandoeng where he wrote:

- One thing is certain . . . unless the economic and cultural level of the rural populations can be raised, there can be no hope of employing curative or preventive measures with any degree of success.
- If this problem (land reform) is neglected, programmes of rural reconstruction not only will be greatly retarded, but will not be able to rest on a permanent basis.

Stampar brought together the results of his China and earlier Yugoslavia experience in a lecture that he gave in 1938 at Harvard at which he concluded:

- Successful health work is not possible in areas where the standard of living falls below the level of tolerable existence. The removal of social grievances, such as the sense of exploitation by others, is of the greatest importance. For social and health services depend for their success on the cooperation of the people, and this will only be given by a population which is reasonably optimistic concerning the future, and which is willing to give at least qualified acceptance of the social order.
- The social ills of rural areas are concerned with a large group of social problems of a medical kind, such as bad housing, social diseases and malnutrition, which cannot be properly understood until their connection with social conditions is realized. Such investigations cannot be conducted in laboratories alone, but involve probing into every smallest part of the people's life and the closest scrutiny of the habits and customs and of the particular sections of the community.
- Successful health work can be attained only if it is correlated with other activities for the improvement of rural life. This naturally depends on a

successful collaboration of the people and their free participation in public affairs. A rural health worker must therefore be a promoter of a social, political and economic peace. For these factors are fundamental requisites to the success of rural health work.

Gunn died in 1944, leaving it to Stampar alone to bring pre-World War II rural health and development experience to the newly established World Health Organization.

Post-World War II Malaria Control and Rural Development (Litsios, 1997)

Malaria was by far the most important disease affecting rural communities around the world. For this reason Selskar Gunn did not hesitate to write in his introduction to the report of the 1938 Bandoeng conference, referred to above:

> Malaria in badly infected areas forms a considerable barrier to the development of other welfare activities and oftentimes must be checked before other types of work become possible.

At the same time, he added: "Malaria is a health and social problem; it must be attacked simultaneously from both these angles."

The conclusions reached at the Bandoeng conference under the leadership of Paul Russell, the senior malariologist of the Rockefeller Foundation, were confined strictly to the health 'angle', as witness:

> In those areas where malaria is the outstanding social and health problem, the resources of the health administration, specially augmented where necessary, should be directed chiefly towards malaria control, even if this should entail the restriction of other public health activities, until malaria is no longer of major importance.

Yes, malaria was a health and social problem, but rather than proposing that it be addressed from both of these 'angles,' the malariologists believed that it was essentially the job of the health administrators to control the disease, augmenting as necessary the resources available, until malaria was reduced to a level where it no longer interfered with community well-being.

Also, malariologists argued that malaria control could serve as an entry point for other public health activities. Hackett gave the example of how malaria stations in Albania were being transformed into health centers "with general programmes of health protection," while at the same time the malaria field directors were "turned into health officers" by winter training and grants for study provided by the Rockefeller Foundation.

Before the arrival of DDT, the tools available to malariologists to control malaria (by interfering with the life-cycle of the malaria-carrying anophelines), could not be afforded. Nevertheless, sufficient knowledge had been gained concerning the biology of the important malaria vectors to suggest that peasants could themselves undertake small measures to control mosquito breeding. Such measures were 'naturalistic methods' and consisted of a variety of means of controlling two basic factors critical to each mosquito species—the nature of the water used for breeding, for example, free flowing versus stagnant, and whether their eggs need shade or sunlight to hatch.

Although there were several successful experiments using such methods, the arrival of DDT in the early 1940s effectively put a stop to such 'natural' methods. The arrival of DDT, however, did not immediately push malariologists to argue that the only reasonable approach was to seek the eradication of the disease. A decade would pass before the global campaign was launched, and during that decade a serious effort was undertaken to develop a cooperative program between WHO and the Food and Agriculture Organization (FAO) to demonstrate that by controlling malaria, agricultural production would increase.

World War II had led to severe malnutrition in countries where extensive fighting had taken place, so much so that in 1948 the Economic and Social Council (ECOSOC) of the United Nations invited the specialized agencies "to study suitable measures to bring about an increase in food production." The US representative to the World Health Assembly had earlier cited malaria as "a direct and important contributing cause of the current world food shortage." The WHO Expert Committee for Malaria, which had already been established in 1947, agreed that "a mass attack on malaria in selected areas of food-producing countries should be carried out as soon as possible."

A joint FAO-WHO Working Party on Food Production and Malaria Control was established in 1949, with Paul Russell and Fred Soper as members. Soper, who previously was with the Rockefeller Foundation, was now Director of the Pan-American Sanitary Bureau (PASB), a post to which he was elected in early 1947. Various possibilities were discussed and actively pursued, but in a few years' time the whole effort collapsed. Although part of the reason was the financial crisis that WHO was undergoing at the time, owing to the loss of a guaranteed percentage of UN Technical Assistance funds, the major reason for the collapse was because the FAO wished to develop projects on a scale far greater than WHO was prepared to participate in, and, more importantly, their (FAO) claim that malaria was just one small element in a complex mesh of factors that needed to be addressed to improve agricultural production in the developing world.

One measure of this complexity can be seen in the design of a Health Demonstration Area in El Salvador, one of the countries chosen for joint action. Milton Roemer visited this country in late 1950 to help design a program for improving "health services as well as activities in related fields." He highlighted the importance of the agricultural sector, noting that the FAO had concluded "that the first need for the Area was a complete Agricultural Survey which would require a number of personnel working for about one year." Only after the survey would they be in a position to develop "an extension educational program."

The survey envisaged by the FAO touched on all aspects of rural welfare: forestation, grazing, family farming, road systems, agricultural marketing and supply facilities, electric power facilities, extension service, and agricultural research. The expertise needed for the project included a forester, a specialist in land utilization and classification, a rural sociologist, an agricultural engineer, several experts in soil and water conservation, an extension agronomist, an extension specialist in animal husbandry, an extension specialist in economic entomology, an agricultural librarian, an agronomist (cereals and row crops), and an agricultural economist.

One can easily imagine the malariologists involved in negotiating joint action with the FAO coming quickly to the conclusion that 'going it alone' made more sense, especially when the FAO began to question whether the population explosion following the control of malaria, as was witnessed in Ceylon and India in the late 1940s and early 50s, didn't exacerbate their task rather than ease it. As Sir Herbert Broadley, Deputy Director General of the FAO, bluntly put it in 1952 to the WHA: "The more successful you are in reaching your goal, the more difficult FAO's task becomes."

It was the dramatic success of DDT that pushed the issue of family planning to the forefront in the late 1940s. The alarming population situation led many public health leaders to call upon WHO to enter this field. However, the Vatican was so opposed to family planning that it was successful in mobilizing countries (Italy, Ireland, and Belgium taking the lead) to oppose WHO taking any action. So fierce was their opposition that in 1952 they even prevented the establishment of an Expert Panel to study the health aspects of the population problem.

Milton Siegel, who was an Assistant Director General under Brock Chisholm, the first WHO Director General, advised Chisholm not to back down when in 1952 the Assembly approached the point where it was being asked to vote on two resolutions, one in favor of the Expert Panel, the other against. Instead, after a 'coffee break' called by the chairman, both resolutions were withdrawn and the matter was closed. According to Siegel, this prevented WHO from doing anything about family planning for somewhere between seven and nine years, thereby forcing the United Nations division of social affairs to take action in a field that they felt was more appropriate for WHO to provide the leadership.

Rural Health

Stampar has been called the 'father of WHO' by some. In any case, it was a WHO event that provided him with perhaps his last major opportunity to plead the case for a broad developmental approach to improving the health of the rural poor. This was at the World Health Assembly Technical Discussions on the subject of rural health, which took place over two years—1954 and 1955.

In a background paper that he prepared in 1954, Stampar reminded his readers how the experts at the League of Nations by the end of the 1930s, "felt more and more strongly that the questions of rural hygiene should be examined in their natural setting because any real amelioration of the standard of health in the rural environment must depend, in the first place, upon the improvement of living conditions generally." However, in the ensuing two decades, the situation of the rural population had gotten "increasingly worse." Paradoxically, this could in part be blamed on the rapidly increasing rural population brought about by the dramatic reduction of disease. He described this development in the following revealing terms:

> The rural population is enjoying the first fruits of social medicine. This cannot stop at the first step. The responsibility of social medicine is to carry on and improve their lives. It cannot let die from hunger people whose lives have been saved from disease. (Stampar, 1954)

One can imagine Stampar's frustration in the technical discussions of 1954 and 1955 concerning rural health in which no debate of the impact of population on health could take place. Nevertheless, the discussions did indicate that a "multi-purpose programme for the community development and for the integrated programmes for the general improvement of the community offers the best approach," and that "health matters should be a part of the welfare community services." (WHO, 1955)

The Launching of the Global Malaria Eradication Campaign

Ironically enough, the 1955 WHA that called for "integrated programmes" was the same Assembly that launched the highly vertical global malaria eradication campaign. Paul Russell was brought on board as a consultant by WHO to convince the WHA to launch a global program, Fred Soper having already done so for the region of the Americas. So confident was Russell that eradication was at hand that he literally threatened WHO by noting that "whatever WHO decided to do, a campaign for world-wide malaria eradication was already under way." WHO should "not be left behind."

The rationale for launching the campaign was based on several assumptions, the most important of which was that the prolonged use of DDT could be expected to lead to mosquito resistance. So it was very important, as Russell put it, "to eradicate the disease before the vector anophelines became resistant to the insecticide." Ideally, spraying could stop after three or four years to be followed by "systematic surveillance and use of antimalaria drugs for four or five more years." (WHO, 1955)

Once launched, all thoughts of linking malaria control/eradication with the goals of agriculture or any other non-health interest were pushed aside. Only within the last 10 or 15 years has it again become fashionable to argue the case for malaria control on economic grounds.

To what degree 'eradication' was in the air when WHO was finally established in 1948 is difficult to judge. Soper, having moved quickly in his capacity as Director of PASB to develop campaigns against diseases including malaria in the American region, was claiming by 1951 that "one cannot doubt that malaria eradication is imminent in Venezuela," and that "it is not too much to anticipate that the rest of the job (eradication of malaria in the Americas) can be done during the next five years." Despite this claim, malaria was never eradicated in Venezuela. Nevertheless, it was added to the list of countries in which eradication was announced to have occurred!

The leader of the Venezuela eradication campaign, Arnoldo Gabaldón, one of the most important malariologists at the time, proposed in 1959 to the PASB Directing Council that an official register be created that listed areas where malaria eradication had been achieved. This was accepted by the WHA in 1960. The criteria of success proposed by Venezuela were those that had been developed in 1950 by the National Malaria Society of the U.S.A. However, the criteria defined by the WHO Malaria Expert Committee, which met in 1961, differed to such a degree that Venezuela no longer qualified. Rather than make an issue of the whole matter, the certification of eradication in "areas of Venezuela" was recognized as a "special case," justified by the fact that the evaluation had been made at the end of 1959, in other words, more than one year before the Expert Committee on Malaria, and WHO instructions to the Governments, had become available. (Litsios, 1998)

There were malariologists who believed that eradication was an impossible goal. To prevent their voices from being heard, they were simply never chosen to participate in the meeting of the Malaria Expert Committee that provided technical guidance to WHO between 1956 and 1969, the year the Assembly chose to bring the global campaign to an end. Lacking a voice in the Expert Committee, opponents were forced to find other ways to make their concerns known, for example, meetings organized outside the WHO context.

A potentially more divisive development was Soper concluding that WHO's revised approach to eradication would not work (Litsios, 2000). Having retired as Director of the PASB in early 1959, Soper embarked on a two-month tour of Asia as a consultant for the Rockefeller Foundation to determine if they might have a useful role to play "to help define the problems that do exist as the final stages of eradication are reached." During this visit he examined the eradication programmes in Taiwan, the Philippines, Ceylon, and India. There he had found that "there had been a shift in technique," a shift that he believed made it impossible for the global goal of eradication to be achieved. The shift involved a "switch from an attack on the malaria parasite in the mosquito with residual insecticides to a campaign against the plasmodium in the human host based on searching out and treating all infected persons," a shift which in no uncertain terms he said "may well be disastrous in its effect on the eradication program."

Essentially, Soper believed that developing countries did not have sufficient resources to develop *both* a spraying program that covered all areas where any malaria risk was present and a surveillance program that checked on the parasite status in the population at risk. He believed that the resources that were available had to concentrate on spraying continuously increasing areas until whole regions were freed of malaria. In his mind, relying on surveillance was admittance of defeat.

As late as 1964 Soper was hoping that matters would be corrected. In May of that year he wrote:

> I refuse to be pessimistic regarding the future... the measures which are building up will eventually force the World Health Organization to abandon the Alvarado, Gonzales proposal for rural health infrastructures and will lead to the development of more highly specialized malaria eradication efforts with adequate technical and administrative support for efficient and honest services.

Alvarado was Director of WHO's Division of Malaria Eradication, having taken over that responsibility in November 1958. Gonzalez was a consultant who prepared the background paper for the 9th Expert Committee meeting in 1962, which laid out the importance of a rural health infrastructure to fulfil the surveillance requirements of the eradication program, especially in Africa.

Whereas the voices of malariologists who opposed the eradication program were denied access to WHO–run meetings, Soper found himself in the awkward position of having launched the campaign and now disagreeing with the approach that WHO had taken. Rather than risk having his opinion used by opponents of the program, he kept most of his criticism confined to his diary notes, from which all of his quotes have been taken. One consequence was the global campaign lasted longer than it probably would have, had his opposing ideas been made public.

When voices calling for an end to the eradication campaign began to dominate the WHA discussions in the second half of the 1960s, WHO temporised with a 2-year study to evaluate the socio-economic benefits that had been achieved by the campaign. Nine countries were studied—Cuba, West Malaysia, Nicaragua, Niger, East Pakistan, Philippines, Syria, Thailand, and Venezuela. Four types of social and economic benefits were identified:

- Increased volume and quality of the working population
- Increased incentive to save
- It rendered the population more receptive to modern technology and the changes involved and
- It had a substantial beneficial effect on all economic development, particularly agricultural development, land settlement, mining, and forestry programmes.

However, "it was extremely difficult to quantify these results due to the absence of the necessary economic studies." The group urged "unceasing efforts to be made in this direction" with WHO stimulating such studies. It was recognized that the evaluation of the socio-economic benefits deriving from antimalaria activities "requires an appropriate methodology, which has yet to be developed." (WHO, 1974) These benefits "need to be studied in the field, and appropriate methods of assessment should be developed." (WHO, 1979) However, as malaria control methods shifted from area-wide anti-mosquito measures to making better use of individual preventive and treatment methods, the call to evaluate the socio-economic benefits of malaria control disappeared, only to be revived in the last decade, as discussed below.

Primary Health Care (Litsios 2002, 2004)

As it became more and more evident that malaria eradication would not be achieved, priority again returned to the question of how to develop rural health services. In 1967, the then–Director-General of WHO, Dr. Marcolino Candau, noted that WHO "was able to make disappointingly little headway in assisting developing countries to establish or strengthen even basic national health services. Yet, in the final analysis, the success of practically all the Organization's activities depends upon the effectiveness of these very services." (WHO, 1967) In 1968, Candau again highlighted the importance of the essential basic health services and called for a comprehensive health plan, within which an integrated approach to preventive and curative services could be developed.

In January 1971, the Executive Board chose as the its next organisational study the subject of methods of promoting the development of basic health services. To facilitate this study, the WHO secretariat prepared in 1972 a background document for the Board's deliberations. In introducing this document, Halfdan Mahler, who in July 1973 took over the position of Director-General from Candau, noted that "there were sufficient financial and intellectual resources available in the world to meet the basic health aspirations of all peoples," and suggested that "there was a need for an aggressive plan for worldwide action to improve this unsatisfactory situation."

The Board's report, prepared for the January 1973 session, concluded that no single or best pattern existed for developing a health services structure capable of providing wide coverage and meeting the varying needs of the population being served—"Each country will have to possess the national ability to consider its own position (problems and resources), assess the alternatives available to it, decide upon its resource allocation and priorities, and implement its own decisions." (WHO, official Records No. 206)

WHO should serve as a "world health conscience" thereby providing a forum where new ideas could be discussed as well as a "mechanism which can point to directions in which Member States should go." To fulfil this role, WHO needed to make better use of the resources available to it and should concentrate on those projects that were likely to "show major returns and . . . result in a long-term national capability for dealing with primary problems."

In May 1973, the 26th World Health Assembly, after a long discussion of the report of the Board, adopted resolution WHA26.35 (Organizational study on methods of promoting the development of basic health services), which, *inter alia*, confirmed the high priority to be given to the development of health services that were "both accessible and acceptable to the total population, suited to its needs and to the socio-economic conditions of the country, and at the level of health technology considered necessary to meet the problems of that country at a given time." (WHO, 1973–1984)

Shortly after Mahler assumed the post of Director-General, a WHO/UNICEF inter-secretariat discussion decided that a document should be prepared under the title "Alternative Approaches to Meeting Basic Health Needs of Populations in Developing Countries." Efforts were initiated to seek out "promising approaches to meeting basic health needs," and among the characteristics that might be considered one finds specific mention of "community involvement in financing and controlling health services, in projects to solve local health problems, in health-related development work, or other relevant ways." (Dorolle, 1973)

The search for new approaches led to two important WHO publications: "Alternative Approaches to Meeting Basic Health Needs of Populations in Developing Countries" and "Health by the People." (Djukanovic & Mach, 1975) Both were published in early 1975. Both highlighted developments in various countries, for example, China, Cuba, Tanzania, and Venezuela, including one community-based project in India. But Newell extended his analysis by including two additional community-based projects.

All three community-based projects undertook activities that Stampar, no doubt, would have whole-heartily approved. One project featured goat and chicken farming to increase the income available to the poorest members of the community. In another project, a community where farmers had lost their cows was aided in finding funds for introducing tractors and for installing deep tube-wells. In the third project, community health promoters were trained as community catalysts, working in areas other than curative medicine, for instance, literacy programmes, family planning, the organization of men's and women's clubs, agricultural extension, the introduction of new fertilizers, new crops and better seeds, chicken projects, and improving animal husbandry.

While Dr. Kenneth Newell, editor of *Health by the People* and Director of WHO's Division of Strengthening of Health Services, expressed excitement at what had been demonstrated in all of these projects, he was particularly enthusiastic about what had been achieved related to community development. He contrasted issues such as improving productivity of resources to enable people to eat and be educated, and the sense of community responsibility, pride, and dignity obtained by such action with the more traditional public health activities of malaria control and the provision of water supplies. The challenge for people in the health field was to accept these wider developmental goals as legitimate ones for them to pursue, even going so far as to admit *that "without them there must be failure."* (Emphasis added.)

Resolution WHA27.44, adopted by the 27th World Health Assembly in July 1974, called upon WHO to report to the 55th session of the Executive Board in January 1975 on steps undertaken by WHO "to assist governments to direct their health service programmes towards their major health objectives, with priority being given to the rapid and effective development of the health delivery system.... " (WHO, 1973–1984) This provided Mahler and Newell with the opportunity of introducing primary health care (PHC) in a comprehensive manner drawing upon the work of the previous two years.

The paper presented to the Board argued that what was needed was that the "resources available to the community" be brought into "harmony" with "the resources available to the health services." For this to happen "a radical departure from conventional health services approach is required," one that builds new services "out of a series of peripheral structures that are designed for the context they are to serve." Such design efforts should: (a) shape PHC "around the life patterns of the population"; (b) involve the local population; (c) place a "maximum reliance on available community resources" while remaining within cost limitations; (d) provide for an "integrated approach of preventive, curative and promotive services for both the community and the individual"; (e) provide for all interventions to be undertaken "at the most peripheral practicable level of the health services by the worker most simply trained for this activity"; (f) provide for other echelons of services to be designed in support of the needs of the peripheral level; and (g) be "fully integrated with the services of the other sectors involved in community development."

Four general courses of national action were outlined with the expectation that each country would respond to its need in a unique manner. These were:

1. The development of a new tier of primary health care;
2. The rapid expansion of existing health services with priority being given to primary health care;
3. The reorientation of existing health services so as to establish a unified approach to primary health care;
4. Making maximum use of ongoing community activities, especially developmental ones, for the promotion of primary health care. (WHO, 1975)

First presented in 1975 to the World Health Assembly, a more ambitious direction was outlined in 1976, when the Assembly was asked to consider a Secretariat paper on Primary Health Care and Rural Development. The 1976 WHA discussion focussed on two issues together, "promotion of national health services relating to primary health care and rural development" and "health technology relating to primary health care and rural development. The resolution adopted (WHA29.74) requested the Director-General, *inter alia*, "to take appropriate steps to ensure that WHO takes an active part, jointly with other international agencies, in supporting national planning of rural development aimed at the relief of poverty and the improvement of the quality of life." On the surface, it would seem that the organization had returned to the position that Stampar had outlined some 20 years earlier. But this was not to be the case; this policy direction never materialized.

Despite the strong advocacy of the new Director-General, Halfdan Mahler, the political and technical leaders of the world strongly resisted moving in the direction indicated. The words were there, but not the commitment. Two episodes illustrate this. First, the position paper presented by the Secretariat to the 1976 WHA on rural development and primary health care elicited no interest whatsoever; there was no discussion of the issues presented. Instead, most delegates chose to inform the Assembly of progress in their countries and indicate their support of the upcoming Alma-Ata conference on primary health care. Secondly, at Alma-Ata itself, where the discussion was divided among three parallel sessions, the session that addressed 'health and development' was very poorly attended. There were literally only a handful of participants who chose to attend that session as opposed to the hundreds who followed the other two. Nevertheless, PHC was identified as the "key" to achieving Health for All by the Year 2000, a social target defined as the attainment by all peoples of the world of a "level of health that will permit them to lead a socially and economically productive life."

Developments which followed Alma-Ata confirmed that the political will supposedly demonstrated by the unanimous adoption of the Declaration of Alma-Ata was not present. Primary health care rapidly gave way to selective PHC with its much narrower focus.

MORE RECENT DEVELOPMENTS

The rapid ascendancy of selective PHC over comprehensive PHC coincided with a shift from an evaluation framework that featured socio-economic gains (as formulated at Alma-Ata) to one that focussed more on traditional health benefits (reduced morbidity, mortality, and disability). This shift, which took place in the 1980s, favored the emergence of the concept of 'burden of disease,' which seeks to measure, in a quantitative and context-free manner, the relative importance of different diseases, chronic illnesses, and disability conditions throughout the world. This has no doubt led to a more complete listing, from a biological perspective, of what constitutes 'ill-health.' In the process, conditions that normally have been associated with the developed world, for example, smoking and mental illness, have been shown to have world-wide importance.

The more complete listing and global accounting of disease burden has led to strong competition among the various public health programmes with which international organizations deal. Much of this effort has been directed to generating numbers that satisfy the 'analytic' criteria that have been adopted. Although this approach has been criticized by many, the numbers generated have attracted the attention of a new generation of economists who, in turn, have explored the question of to what degree investing in health can contribute to economic development.

In January 2000, WHO established a Commission on Macroeconomics and Health to assess the place of health in global economic development. Its report was published in December 2001. Its key findings included:

- The role of health in economic growth has been greatly undervalued.
- A few health conditions account for a high proportion of avoidable deaths.
- Poverty will be more effectively reduced if investment in other sectors is increased as well.
- To achieve an impact on health of the poor will require increased investment in global public goods.
- The recommended increase in spending is large, but so is the potential return. (WHO, 2002)

Malaria control again finds itself at the center of the debate of whether investing in health can be justified on economic grounds. Jeffrey Sachs, who chaired the WHO Commission, has been the leading proponent for this position. His arguments resemble many of those used back in the 1950s but, in the modern context, they may have a greater relevance than ever before. To begin with, burden of disease studies demonstrate what has long been believed, namely, that "where malaria prospers most, human societies have prospered least." (Sachs & Malancy, 2002) Going one step further, Sachs argues that the "causal link from malaria to underdevelopment (is) much more powerful than is generally appreciated." If this is the case, then investing in malaria control should provide economic benefits.

At the household level, reducing childhood deaths in highly endemic countries should translate into greater human capital development. At the macroeconomic level, less malaria risk should have favorable repercussions on trade, tourism, and foreign direct investment. Sachs goes so far as to argue, "Suppressing malaria in poor, highly malarious regions, especially in sub-Saharan Africa, offers the potential to initiate a virtuous cycle in which improved health spurs economic growth, and rising income furthers benefits human health."

The work of this Commission has attracted considerable attention, not all favorable. Some of the criticism reflects the earlier battle lines of public health, for example, the focus on individual diseases, as reflected in the example of malaria, "revives the vertical approach" that has characterized the pre–as well as post–PHC era. (Waitkin, 2003) Of greater importance is the question of to what degree investing in health can lead to more equitable development on both health and economic grounds. When malaria was controlled in the tea and rubber plantations in the early decades of the 20th century, it is true that the plantation workers were healthier, but the economic benefits went to the plantation owners; no "virtuous cycle" was initiated by such investments.

There is considerable concern among some critics of the WHO Commission that its recommendations will further undermine the principles of self-reliance and community participation that were hammered out at Alma-Ata, and in the process create a "new version of colonialism and imperialism." Making available the needed drugs, vaccines, and even bednets, on terms that are economically acceptable to global investors, risks the "imposition on the world's poor of prefabricated, selectively chosen, market- and technology-driven, externally monitored, and dependence-producing programmes." (Banerji, 2002)

A WAY AHEAD

Of the eight Millennium Development Goals set at the United Nations Millennium Summit in September 2000, four relate to health. The work of the WHO Commission on Macroeconomics will no doubt help shape WHO's contribution to the achievement of those goals. If history is any guide, however, the year 2015 will come and few, if any, of the goals will have been achieved. Today, for example, despite the Roll Back Malaria program launched by WHO in 1998, malaria is again on the rise.

History also has taught us, as suggested by the brief overview provided above, that we have not yet learned how to gain a greater understanding and knowledge of the complex dynamics involved wherein better health serves as a lever for development, especially among the world's poorest people. The ideological gap that divides the public health community, which is as great today as it has ever been, has not facilitated matters.

WHO cannot afford to take sides, as it has unfortunately often done in the past. When malaria eradication was on top, the advocates of comprehensive-holistic approaches to health development were largely left out. When the tide turned, and PHC took command (on paper at least), the advocates of sharply defined health programmes (vertical or otherwise) were kept at abeyance (for a very brief time). Today, WHO is trying to keep its options open, but since the vast bulk of international funding lies outside its control, its options are operationally very constrained.

In this context, WHO should seek to develop a global program of evaluation specifically geared to shedding light on the issues that have been covered in this paper and that have divided the public health community for so long. WHO should be in the position of ensuring that all programmes that have human development as their focus, whether specifically geared to gains in health, contribute to a collective global health learning experience. Opposing voices or results that contradict strongly held views should not be silenced as they have so often been in the past. Instead, means need to be found that channel competing energies into constructive work in countries and lead to a better understanding of the merits and faults of different sides of any argument. Only in this way, when the next round of international development goals is initiated, will there be a more solid empirical base to argue the case for investing in human health.

REFERENCES

Banerji, B. (2002). Report of the WHO commission on macroeconomics and health: A critique. *International Journal of Health Services*, 32(4).

Djukanovic, V., & Mach, E. P. (Eds.). (1975). Alternative approaches to meeting basic health needs in developing countries. In N. K.W. (Ed.), *Health by the people*. Geneva, WHO.

Litsios, S. (2005). *Plague legends II: In search of public health (1830–1940)*. Chesterfield, MO: Science & Humanities Press.

Litsios, S. (1997). *The tomorrow of malaria*. Wellington: Pacific Press.

Litsios, S. (2005). Selskar Gunn and China: The Rockefeller Foundation's 'other' approach to public health, *Bull Hist Med*, 79, 295–318.

Litsios, S. (1997). Malaria control, the Cold War, and the postwar reorganization of international assistance. *Medical Anthropology*, 17, 255–78.

Litsios, S. (1998). Arnoldo Gabaldón's independent path for malaria control and public health in the tropics: A lost "paradigm" for WHO. *Parassitologia*, 40, 231–38.

Litsios, S. (2000). Criticism OF WHO'S revised malaria eradication strategy. *Parassitologia*, 42, 167–72.

Litsios, S. (2002). The long and difficult road to Alma Ata: A personal reflection. *International Journal of Health Services*, 32(4), 709–32.

Litsios, S. (2004). The Christian Medical Commission and the development of WHO's Primary Heath Care approach. *Amer J Pub Hlth*, 94(11), 1884–1893.

Memorandum from P. Dorolle (outgoing WHO Deputy Director-General) to all regional directors, July 25, 1973.

Sachs, J., & Malaney, P. (2002, February 7). The economic and social burden of malaria. *Nature*, 415, (6872).

Stampar, A. (1954, March 1). Background to rural health. *A7/Technical Discussions/1*.

WHO. (1955, May 20). Report of the Technical Discussions at the Eighth World Health Assembly. *A8/Technical Discussions/3*.

WHO. (1955). Eighth World Health Assembly. Off Rec WHO No. 63.

WHO. (1974). Malaria control in countries where time-limited eradication is impracticable at present. WHO TRS No. 537.

WHO. (1979). Expert committee on malaria seventeenth session. WHO TRS No. 640.

WHO. (1967). The work of WHO 1966. *Official Records No. 156, Geneva, 1967: vii*.

WHO. *Official Records No. 206, Annex 11*.

WHO. (1973–1984). *Handbook of resolutions and decisions of the World Health Assembly and Executive Board*. (Vol. 2).

WHO. (1973–1984). *Handbook of resolutions and decisions of the World Health Assembly and Executive Board.* (Vol. 2).

WHO. (1975, January). *Documents for 55th session of the EB.* EB55/9.

WHO. (2002, April 23) *Report of the WHO commission on macroeconomics and health.* A55/5.

Waitkin, H. (2003, February 8). Report of the WHO commission on macroeconomics and health: A summary and critique. *The Lancet, 361.*

Chapter 3

Old and New Pestilences

Andrew A. Arata

INTRODUCTION

There has been much popular interest in, as well as technical concern over, newly emerging diseases, and there is a fear that heretofore unknown virulent pathogens will create new, global epidemics. At the time of this writing, two such pathogens are active, warranting such concern: a) cases of SARS (Severe Acute Respiratory Syndrome, caused by a coronavirus) appeared in China in November, 2002, and has spread to Western and Central Europe and North America; b) a strain of Avian Influenza Virus (N5H1), first identified in Hong Kong in 1997, reemerged in 2002 in Southeast Asia. Other avian flu strains found simultaneously in poultry in North America have underscored the concern of local and international health authorities. Both SARS and avian flu demonstrate high mortality rates, but, to date, the number of cases has been only in the hundreds. So, are these pestilences? What constitutes a pestilence? Is the term synonymous with newly emerging diseases? Two definitions of pestilence have near unanimity, but are not very specific:

a) *"Any fatal epidemic disease, affecting man or beast, and destroying many victims."* The Oxford Universal Dictionary, 3rd edition, 1955, Oxford Press, 2515 pp.
b) *"A contagious or infectious epidemic disease that is virulent and devastating."* Webster's Seventh New Collegiate Dictionary, 1965. G. & C. Merriam Co., Springfield, Mass., 1221 pp.

Accordingly, a pestilence should be an infectious disease, devastating (killing) a large number of people (or animals).

The truly epidemic diseases are usually of viral or bacterial origin (although we will make a case for some other types of pestilences). The classification of 'old' and 'new' pestilences requires us to take a brief historical tour of the bio-epidemiological sciences.

- Reports of epidemics of many of the pestilent diseases are found in Greek, Egyptian, and Chinese literatures, and go back as far as 2,500 years, but most are hard to identify as currently known diseases, except for those with very characteristic symptoms (e.g., plague, measles, smallpox, cholera, etc.). These are the classic 'old' pestilences, some of which have been controlled, in part; others remain active today.
- There was no science of infectious diseases, no germ theory, until Louis Pasteur, Koch, and Lister (among others) began their work in the late 1800s—only 125–130 years ago.
- The cycles of vector-borne diseases (malaria, plague, yellow fever, dengue, and filariasis, to name a few) were only elucidated around 1900, which clarified the etiology of some 'old' pestilences while describing the first of those we might consider 'new' (e.g., arenavirus or filovirus outbreaks). The first virus, foot and mouth disease, was isolated in 1898 by Loeffler and Frosch.
- Immunological diagnostic tools used to identify, describe, and classify pathogens and 'new' diseases have become more specific and widely available in the past 50–60 years.
- More specific and effective preventive and treatment measures (vector and environmental control, vaccines, antibiotics, et al.) have been developed and made available in the past 50–60 years since World War II.
- The past half-century, in which most 'new' pestilences have occurred, is marked by large human population increases and densities, changes in natural habitats, and encroachment of human populations into sylvatic areas with their natural populations of active and potentially active pathogens and their vectors, or other routes of transmission.
- There has been a development of local, regional, and global surveillance systems to facilitate rapid response measures.

OLD PESTILENCES (TABLE 1)

Plague

Plague, in both its bubonic and pneumonic forms, is the quintessential pestilence. A myriad of books have been written on the classical plagues, from the Decameron to Camus' La Peste. Although earlier epidemics around the Mediterranean may have actually been plague, the first epidemic historically accepted as the plague was the Plague of Justinian (A.D. 542–43, with intermittent outbreaks

Table 1. **Old Pestilences:** Examples of some of the pestilences that fit into this category are shown below: This is not a comprehensive list and some were known and reported on before others, but all were known prior to, or about, the time of the development of microbiology.

Disease	Etiology	Comments
Plague	Bacterial, flea-borne	Global, but focal; reservoirs in sylvatic rodents
Yellow Fever	Arbovirus, mosquito-borne	Africa and South America, focal; primate reservoirs
Malaria	Protozoal parasite, mosquito-borne	Global; most severe in Africa
Smallpox	Virus, personal contact	Previously global, eradicated by intensive vaccination program: last naturally occurring case, 1977.
Measles	Virus; air-borne, personal contact	Global; number of cases reduced by vaccination; most severe in developing countries
Polio	Virus; personal contact, oral-fecal route common	Formerly global; continued reduction by ongoing vaccination programs in developing countries
Influenza	Virus; air-borne	Global; immunization available annually, virus highly variable
Cholera	Bacterial (vibrio) food/water, fecal contamination	Potentially global; SE Asia remains high risk, often associated with civil strife and/or in disaster areas

that may have been bubonic plague continuing until A.D. 750). The "Black Death" of the fourteenth century, which continued to appear in chronic pockets of Europe and the Middle and Near East for centuries thereafter, is by far the best-known plague, and the one that produced the greatest mortality and social impact on the affected populations. Consider that as a conservative estimate, 25–33% of the European population died, and maybe more. This death rate reduced the available work force so that, for the first time, peasants and landless people could sell their labor, which introduced freedom of movement and resulted in economic changes that eventually contributed to the decline of the feudal system.

The 3rd pandemic of plague began in the 1850s and continues to this date, although reduced in more recent years. A major characteristic of this epidemic has been the dissemination of plague from its traditional homes in Africa and Asia into areas previously plague free, especially North and South America, by the inadvertent transport of rats and their fleas by boat. The infection is now well established in Africa (gerbils); Central Asia (gerbils, ground squirrels or "susliks," and marmots); Southeast Asia (various *Rattus* species); North America (ground squirrels and some native field mice); and South America (introduced *Rattus*). The last major urban outbreak was in Surat, India in 1994: More than 6,500 cases and 56 deaths were reported. However, the impact of this outbreak was also seen in the number of people who fled the plague zone, and the over two billion dollar loss that ensued.

Only a few outbreaks are reported to WHO each year. Indochina and Burma frequently report, as well as sites in Africa (Ovamboland on the frontier between Namibia and Angola); the United States has a vast infected area in the west of the country, but only 8–10 cases per year are reported, with 1–2 deaths on average every 10 years. Many other sites of infection are known and should be monitored, as some rodent species are highly susceptible to serving as effective amplifying reservoirs, whereas others maintain low-level infections for long periods of time, allowing much time to pass between outbreaks. Environmental measures (rat-proofing, rodent and flea control, etc.,) are the first measures of control. Surveillance, prompt diagnosis, and treatment with antibiotics (e.g., streptomycin and tetracycline) are recommended.

Yellow Fever (YF)

Yellow fever is the best known of the arboviral (arthropod-borne virus) diseases. There are some 500 known arboviruses, of which about 100, produce disease in man. Both the yellow fever virus and the primary mosquito vector, *Aedes aegypt*, are of African origin - the species name, '*aegypti,*' refers to classical Africa in general, not, specifically, modern Egypt. Most cases in Africa occur East to West along the transition zone (ecotone) between the savannas and the rain forests inhabited by numerous aedine vectors as well as A. *aegypti*. The disease has two cycles: a 'jungle' cycle involving various tree dwelling mosquitoes and non-human primates as reservoirs, and an 'urban' cycle, with A. aegypti as the vector and humans as reservoirs. The last reported major African outbreak vectored by A. *aegypti* occurred in Nigeria and involved some 20,000 cases and over 4,000 deaths between 1986 and 1991.

Yellow fever was introduced into the Americas one or more times most likely during the age of sail: The virus can be transmitted vertically (transovarian passage) in A. *aegypti*. The mosquito's eggs can easily be laid in water barrels and withstand desiccation for months, only to hatch and develop when submersed at a later date. Epidemics of YF raged throughout the Caribbean and tropical America until the end of the 1800s, when the transmission cycle was elucidated by the team led by Walter Reed, confirming the role of A. *aegypti* which had been proposed by, but not confirmed by, Carlos Finlay. Epidemics occurred as far north as Philadelphia in the United States and the last epidemic in North America occurred in New Orleans as late as 1905, with over 3,000 deaths. Cases (with 25–50%) mortality continue to occur sporadically in Brazil and in the foothills of several Andean countries (Bolivia, Peru, Ecuador, and Colombia). Often the victims are young, indigenous males from the highlands who were temporarily working in the coca processing plants in the forests. These infected areas are only kilometers from large cities (with populations of more than 1 million people) such as Santa Cruz, Bolivia, which are accessible by public transportation and are heavily infested with *A. aegypti*.

Although the YF vaccine is one of the oldest, safest, and most effective available, and immunological protection is rated for at least 10 years, vaccination coverage in many of the affected areas of Africa and South America is low.

Cholera

The Cholera pathogen, *Vibrio cholera*, originally described by Robert Koch, was one of the first human pathogens (along with anthrax and tuberculosis) to be identified, in the late 1800s, shortly after Pasteur's publication of the "germ theory." Koch and his students studied material they collected in Alexandria, Egypt, during an 1883 outbreak. It was difficult to determine the origin of cholera and/or to distinguish it historically from other diarrhetic diseases except by the severity and rapidity of onset. Health historians such as McNeill suggest an origin on the Indian sub-continent, associated with dense populations, poor hygiene, and certain religious practices such as communal bathing; thus the term "Asiatic cholera," by which the disease became known in Europe in the 1800s. The disease's appearance in Europe and the Americas (London and New York in 1832, and again in 1854) were clearly associated with intercontinental traffic. It was during the 1854 epidemic in London that a physician, John Snow, noted the clustering of cases and deaths in people using the same water source, and proposed what turned out to be the correct action to stop the epidemic ("Take the handle off the Broad Street pump!!"), although he had no idea of the actual cause of the disease. However, it was such observations, along with structural, hygienic, and administrative changes in major cities, particularly in Europe and North America, that established the public health measures that we tend to take for granted in this early part of the 21st century.

Cholera is still with us: various serotypes of the vibrio have spread since the early 1960s, affecting over 25 countries in Asia, 21 in the Americas, and into the West Pacific. In 1993, approximately 400,000 cases and 6,800 deaths from cholera were reported. In 1991, the El Tor strain of cholera was reported in Lima, Peru; by 1994, almost a million cases had been reported in the Western Hemisphere.

Measles

Measles is one of the oldest known and most widespread infections of man: Epidemics ascribed to measles appear in the oldest literature, although they are often confused with smallpox. However, in 622 A.D., Ad Ahrun, a Christian priest living in Alexandria, Egypt, described the pox lesion, and in 910 A.D. the Arab physician Al-Razi distinguished between the two diseases. Prior to widespread immunization, measles was common in childhood—more than 90% of people were infected by age 20. Although endemic in large communities, measles became epidemic every several years, with the severity of infection decreasing with the frequency of the epidemics. In his study of the history of plagues, McNeill makes mention of the importance of animal husbandry and zoonotic diseases in the area. Measles, he claims is probably related to both rinderpest (in hoofed-mammals) and canine distemper. Because dogs, sheep, and goats have been domesticated for at least 10,000 years, measles may have been among the first viral diseases to have "jumped the species barrier." As we will see, most, if not all, of the new pestilences are, or may be, derived from animal wild or domesticated reservoirs. To support this thesis, McNeill lists as follows the number of diseases human populations share with domestic animals, with numerous overlaps between the species:

Poultry	26
Rats and mice	32
Horse	35
Pig	42
Sheep and goats	46
Cattle	50
Dog	65

Measles was responsible for (or contributed to, along with smallpox) the decimation of the indigenous Amerindian populations, first in Central and South America at the time of the Spanish conquest (1500s), and later (1700s and 1800s), in North America. Amerindian populations lacked immunological protection from these and other imported infectious diseases. Some attribute this immunological naïveté to the comparatively small number of domesticated animal species—dogs, ducks and turkeys, guinea pigs, and cameloids (llamas and relatives) in the Andes, and few, if any, in large number prior to the European invasion. In any case, the attack and mortality rates were staggering. By one estimate, a pre-conquest Amerindian population of perhaps thirty million by 1556 was reduced by 90%, down to only 3 million. This catastrophe occurred in less than 50 years after the Spanish entered the American mainland.

Influenza

Influenza is another viral disease that has many unstable varieties infecting a host of mammalian and avian species, both wild (sylvatic) and domestic. Epidemics with symptoms similar to modern influenza were noted by Hippocrates as early as 412 B.C., and later, in Rome, by Livy. Various medieval and Renaissance writings describe influenza-like illnesses. Robert Johnson of Philadelphia is credited with the first "modern" description of an influenza epidemic, which occurred in that city in 1793. His description was applied to subsequent epidemics in 1833, 1837, 1847, 1889–90, and 1918.

Antigenic shifts in the structure of the influenza virus may change the virulence of the strains, increasing the likelihood of epidemics. The most severe flu epidemic ever recorded (1918–1919)—also known as the Spanish flu (although it did not originate there)—first struck World War I troops of all combatant nations while in northern France, and it continued on to become a global pandemic. Conservative estimates of mortality range between twenty and forty million persons, and other estimates more than double these figures.

The ease with which the various influenza strains infect domestic mammals, pigs, and poultry (chickens and ducks) producing huge reservoirs of potentially infectious material, often proximate to human habitations, is a major public health concern. Especially worrisome are the conditions under which millions of such animals are raised and brought to market.

Other Pestilent Diseases

The 'old' diseases examined above are only a few of those which might be used as examples of the old pestilences: others might prefer to include schistosomiasis, typhus (murine and/or louse-borne), and several of the classic childhood diseases (diptheria, pertussis, tetanus, rubella), as well as leprosy, yaws, the leishmaniases, and, certainly, smallpox. Fortunately many of those mentioned here (schisto and others) are being controlled rather well in some areas by vaccines, specific drugs, and/or antibiotics when applicable, at least in the more developed countries. Even polio, which had been a major epidemic threat for centuries, has been virtually eliminated as a threat in areas where the politics and health infrastructure allow the efficient application of this very effective vaccine.

Much of the fear engendered by specific diseases depends on the time, place, and severity of the local outbreaks, as well as the knowledge and perception of the community. For example, I was raised in New Orleans, in the Southeast of the United States, during the 1930s. Although I and my brothers were normal, well nourished children, our parents were fearful of dogs (rabies), cuts on unshod feet (tetanus), and any summer colds or stiffness/weakness of the extremities (polio), and they preached cleanliness as a means to prevent anything bad happening.

Special "Old–New" Pestilences (Malaria, Dengue, and Tuberculosis)

These diseases are old, but at present each has developed certain new characteristics that make their modern expression different from their historic ones, and decreases our ability to control them.

In the last 50 years, malaria parasites have developed resistance to chloroquine, the most common, globally used anti-malarial drug; at the same time, the
anopheline mosquito vectors of malaria have progressively developed a parallel
resistance to the insecticides used to control them. Dengue, and Dengue Hemorrhagic Fever (DHF), have spread globally, infecting vast new areas, especially urban
areas where the human living conditions are substandard, but readily suited for
vector breeding. Finally, tuberculosis, whose incidence was slowly reduced in the
late 1800s and early 1900s by improved public health, housing conditions, and
nutrition, has again surfaced as a secondary infection to immuno-compromised
persons, especially those suffering from HIV infections. At the same time, the
causative agent, *Mycobacterium tuberculosis,* continues to develop resistance to the
most economic and readily available antibiotics.

Malaria

Malaria is caused by blood parasites of the genus *Plasmodium* and vectored
by anopheline mosquitoes. There are four species of human malaria parasites:
P. falciparum, P. malariae, P. vivax, and P. ovale, as well as a number of related species
infecting other mammals (non-human primates, rodents, etc.). Historians note that
malaria-like symptoms were discussed in the Chinese Canon of Medicine (2700
B.C.) and malaria-like illnesses were described in 6th-century B.C. cuneiform literature from Nineveh (now part of Iraq). Hippocrates made a connection between
stagnant water and fevers in the local population. It is estimated that there are
still several hundred million unreported cases each year resulting in 1–2 million
deaths per annum, mostly children. Although malaria is still endemic in Asia, Latin
America, and Africa, 90% of the cases are found in Africa, where *P. falciparum* is
the most common malaria parasite.

Such huge figures mask the focal, and sometimes epidemic, nature of malaria,
which may be brought about by natural or man-made environmental conditions.
Some of the human activities that may enhance malaria transmission may be
development projects for agriculture (e.g., irrigation schemes), other water and
land use projects (as in the Amazon basin, converting forest areas through resource
extraction such as mining and logging) into marginal livestock and farming areas.
Often such environmental changes bring about changes in malaria transmission
from 'stable' (endemic) to 'unstable' (epidemic). In highly endemic areas, severe
malaria and death is concentrated in the younger age groups, whereas in the areas
of unstable (epidemic) transmission, severe malaria and death is more evenly
distributed throughout all age groups. Needless to say, prevention and /or case
control strategies must be different for each transmission type.

In many parts of the world the anopheline vectors of malaria have developed
resistance to the insecticides used for their control. Frequently, this is due to the use,
often excessive, of the same or similar insecticides for control of agricultural pests

in the same geographic areas. Such resistance not only hinders control operations directly, but also indirectly, by increasing the need for greater quantities and/or more costly insecticides. Broadscale usage of insecticides has also become limited on environmental grounds, because some donors have reduced funding insecticide purchases.

By far the most serious setback to malaria control in recent decades has been the emergence and spread of chloroquine-resistant strains of *P. falciparum*, the causative agent of the most severe form of malaria, and the most common in Africa. Emerging in the 1950s in Southeast Asia and South America, resistance spread rapidly from these focal points. It was not noted in Africa until 1979–80 but spread rapidly in the ensuing ten–fifteen years. Chloroquine-resistant strains of *P. vivax* have been identified in some areas of Southeast Asia, New Guinea, and Indonesia.

Efforts to produce a malaria vaccine(s) have been under way for over 25 years. A number of candidate vaccines have been produced, but none are operational in humans as yet.

Dengue and Dengue Hemorrhagic Fever (DHF)

Like yellow fever, described earlier, dengue and dengue hemorrhagic fever are vector-borne diseases transmitted (primarily but not exclusively) by the mosquito *Aedes aegypti*. "Classical" dengue is caused by infection with one of the four serotypes of the dengue virus. DHF may occur following a subsequent infection with a different serotype. The following quotation is from an article written by the author in 1999 (R. Lennox and A. Arata, Dengue Fever: An Environmental Plague for the New Millennium. Capsule Report, Environmental Health Project/USAID. 8 pp.):

> With 2.5 billion people at risk and estimated cases in the tens of milllions, dengue is considered by many to be the second most important vector-borne disease in the world (surpassed only by malaria). Classical dengue and its more lethal form, dengue hemorrhagic fever (DHF), now circle the world with endemic illness and continuing threats of epidemics.
>
> Dengue is very much an environmental disease, affecting urban and peri-urban settlements in more than 100 countries. It is characterized by seasonal outbreaks of illness carried by mosquitoes that thrive in household containers which collect water (such as flowerpots and washtubs) and in the detritus of human consumption, such as bottles, tin cans, and old bottles. Children, specially in Asia, are most frequently and seriously affected by the severe form of the infection, DHF.
>
> Mosquito control is the only effective approach to prevention, although effective case management will reduce mortality. Insecticides targeted at larval mosquitoes are effective, but resistance of mosquitoes to affordable and

environmentally safe chemicals as well as declining will and infrastructure have all but eliminated this approach in most countries. Vaccines are in the pipeline, but a system which could deliver them to half the world's population is probably at least a decade away. Community action—to protect containers from becoming havens for mosquito breeding and to dispose of empty containers and trash, along with surveillance and personal protection—is the best hope for transmission risk reduction.

Tuberculosis (TB)

Tuberculosis is another ancient disease that has bridged the old to new definition: The TB bacillus, *Mycobacterium tuberculosis,* was among the first to be scientifically identified and described (by Robert Koch, in 1882). The disease is transmitted by airborne droplets from people with pulmonary or laryngeal tuberculosis. This mode of transmission is most effective in dense populations, and hence TB became widespread with the development of urban centers in the Middle Ages (Europe), and was very common from the 14th century until recently in Europe. With improvements in housing and nutrition TB rates continued to decline (except for periods of war) until the first half of the 20th century. At that time, two conditions emerged: the development of Multiple Drug Resistant TB (MDRTB) and the emergence and spread of Acquired Immune Deficiency Syndrome (AIDS) upon which TB is an opportunistic infection.

Prior to 1984, about 10% of TB bacilli isolated from patients in the U.S. were resistant to even one antibacterial drug: in 1984, 52% were resistant to at least one drug, and 32% were resistant to more than one drug. In the U.S. the cost of treatment of ten cases of MDRTB in Texas in 1990 was US$ 950,443. WHO lists TB as one of the major causes of mortality in the world. A new major funding effort (WHO and World Bank and various bilateral donor groups) is focusing on HIV/AIDS, TB, and malaria as the most serious, and intractable, causes of death.

Other forms of TB, including non-pulmonary cases and those associated with other species of *Mycobacterium* sp. (e.g. *M. bovis*), are sporadic, but suggest the possible very early animal origin of the pathogen group.

Chronic, Non-epidemic Pestilences

Diseases such as Chagas disease and schistosomiasis are examples of diseases that do not easily fit the epidemic definitions of a pestilence mentioned earlier in this chapter, but they do heavily impact the affected populations, not only through mortality rates, but especially through morbidity/disability.

There are several forms of schistosomiasis caused by different species of *Schistosoma,* a blood fluke (trematode)—this is an ancient illness, known from Egyptian antiquity. Infections occur in fresh water where people work and/or wash and children play. Larval worms, known as cercaria, developed in a snail intermediate host, pass through the skin and penetrate diverse organs according to species. The most important effects are those that arise from chronic, and cumulative, infection.

Chagas disease has a very different etiology, mode of transmission, and pathology than does schistosomiasis. By definition it could be new because it was first described in 1907 by the Brazilian Carlos Chagas, who subsequently described the pathogen, a flagellate protozoan, *Trypanosoma cruzi,* and the vectors, blood-feeding triatomine bugs. The disease is also know as American Trypanosomiasis, and occurs only in the Western Hemisphere, from Mexico to Argentina—a few cases have been reported in North America. This form is very different from African Trypanosomiasis (sleeping sickness).

The initial (acute) phase of the disease usually occurs in children; there is then a long latent phase (~20 years or more), culminating later in life in a chronic phase which may include irreversible cardiac and/or intestinal manifestations and shortened life spans in the victims. PAHO and WHO consider Chagas disease to be the most serious parasitic disease in Latin America and the main cause of heart disease in the Region. There is no adequate medical intervention. The infection can be transmitted by vectors, congenitally, or by transfusion of blood or blood products. An estimated 100 million persons in the Region are at risk, and in some countries (e.g., Bolivia) 25% of the 8 million inhabitants have been shown to be seropositive. In addition, in Bolivia, one study demonstrated that the burden of Chagas disease, in terms of Disability Adjusted Life Years (DALYS), was 4 million DALYS, or estimated loss of 494 million Bolivianos: equal to more than 100 million US dollars at the time of the report (1994).

The purpose of this brief segment is to emphasize that pestilences need not carry with them only high mortality. Very high morbidity and sustained disability with all the concurrent social and economic implications can be a tremendous burden on a population—or a nation.

Puerperal Fever

Puerperal fever, a forgotten pestilence, is caused by a streptococcal infection and is an iatrogenic disease (induced by a physician) that was once the scourge of pregnant women, before physicians learned to wash their hands before examining pregnant women and/or assisting at childbirth. Improved hygiene in hospitals was concurrent with the development of the germ theory and mortality rates dropped quickly. This disease, also called childbirth fever, was never reported as one of the great pestilences, however a few figures reveal the state of scientific knowledge regarding any infectious diseases, both endemic and epidemic.

1833–1842 London Lying-in Hospital (no hand-washing): average mortality per year = 587/10,000.

1830–1840 Paris Maternitée (no hand-washing): average mortality per year = 547/10,000.
1825–1834 Dresden Maternity Hospital (no hand-washing): average mortality per year = 305/10,000.

Same general period: home delivery with midwife : estimated mortality per year = 40–50/10,000.
1831–1843 London's Royal Maternity Charity (home delivery): estimated mortality = 10/10,000.

It is frightening that not only was the incidence of puerperal fever higher in the hospitals, but so was the associated mortality: 35 % of the patients died if the disease occurred after a home delivery, but 80–90 % died if the disease was contracted in a hospital.

POTENTIAL NEW PESTILENCES (TABLE 2)

Although we have no crystal ball to predict what, if any, new pestilences are in store for mankind in the future, several groups of zoonotic viruses include likely candidates (Table 2). Also included is HIV/AIDS, truly a new pestilence that already, in a relatively brief period, has taken its place among the worst pestilences ever known to man.

Arboviruses

As mentioned above, there are over 500 **arboviruses** isolated and characterized—about 100 are capable of infecting humans, from nonapparent infections to very severe ones. Two of these have already been mentioned above (dengue and DHF and yellow fever), but the arboviruses as a group represent the source of many potentially new diseases—or, put more correctly, existing zoonotic diseases that emerge when humans accidentally become involved in their cycles. A good example is the recent outbreak of **West Nile encephilitis** in the U.S. In 1999 and 2000, the virus was isolated from/around New York City from large numbers of dead birds (especially crows and jays): 21 human cases and two deaths were confirmed. By 2001, the disease moved west toward the Mississippi River, infecting 55 people and killing nine. In 2002, there were over 2,400 cases (117 fatal); by 2003, the virus, and human cases, were found in all 48 contiguous states (excepting Alaska and Hawaii). The virus has been found in mammals, birds, and mosquitoes throughout the U.S.

But is this a new disease, or just a disease new to us? West Nile virus has been found in over 50 countries since its discovery in 1937 in Uganda, and has been

Table 2. **New Pestilences:** Examples, not comprehensive, of diseases that have become pestilent since the early 1900s, or the beginning of microbiology. This does not mean that all these diseases did not exist earlier but, rather, were not described at that time. Note that the first four listed are groups of related pathogens/diseases: the fifth (SARS/Asian flu) are placed together for convenience rather than etiology.

Disease	Etiology	Comments
Arbovirus Dengue, W. Nile, YF	Arthropod-borne mosquitoes, ticks, etc.	Any of over 500 viruses of several families that are transmitted by arthropods: approx. 100 implicated in human illness: global
Arenavirus Lassa, AHF, BHF	Rodent-borne: aerosol inhalation of rodent excreta	A family of rodent-borne viruses, (*Arenaviridae*) one each from Asia (LCM); Africa (Lassa) and several ($\sim$ 10) from the W. Hemisphere, 4 of which have been implicated in severe human illnesses.
Hantavirus	Rodent-borne: aerosol inhalation of rodent excreta	A series of viruses producing pneumonic (New World) or hemorrhagic symptoms (Old World)
Filovirus Marburg Ebola	No reservoir or vector identified to date: secretions, contaminated syringes	"Natural" cases found only in Africa; first two outbreaks were in 1976 in southwestern part of Sudan and central Zaire (Democratic Republic of the Congo)
SARS/avian flu	SARS—coronavirus; and, influenza strain H5N1: both aerosol, respiratory secretions	These two listed together only because of synchrony (2002) and location (SE Asia) of their initial occurrences
HIV/AIDS	HIV, a retrovirus: sexual contact and/or contact with other infected body fluids	Syndrome first reported in 1981, but cases in the 1970s in various parts of the world: Worldwide, WHO estimates that 4.2–5.8 people were infected with HIV in 2003: overall, Between 34–46 million are living with HIV/AIDS, of which more than 50% live in Africa, south of the Sahara

isolated from horses, bats, birds, and mosquitoes. Human disease is reported from the former USSR, the Near East, India, Indonesia, and parts of Europe.

Using North America as an example (because we have relatively good information from this area), we find numerous other arboviral—related diseases, for example:

Eastern and Western equine encephalitides,
St. Louis encephalitis,

La Crosse encephalitis,
Venezuelan equine encephalitis,
California virus encephalitis,
Colorado tick-borne fever,
and others.

Most of the above are mosquito-borne, and the major mosquito vector genera, *Culex, Aedes,* and *Anopheles,* have global representatives from which a competent vector might be found. The same is true of ticks, sandflies, and other potential vectors. Rodents, or other local vertebrates, may serve as reservoir hosts while infected migratory birds may provide distribution of the infection. Although many arboviral infections have broadly similar transmission cycles, the ecology and dynamics of each may differ widely. Arboviruses do not belong to a single viral family, but rather, to several,which increases their diversification.

Although the potential for increased arboviral epizootics or epidemics is high, the most recent episodes have not been high on the pestilence scale; rather, the most severe arboviral epidemics have been **YF** and **dengue/DHF,** the oldest of the group.

Arenaviruses

The **arenaviruses** were thought for years to be monotypic, a single species, *lymphocytic choriomeningitis (LCM),* occurring primarily in the house mouse/ laboratory mouse, *Mus musculus.* The virus (first described in 1933) has been isolated in numerous locations, but human disease is known only from Europe and the Americas. A second arenavirus was isolated from a phyllostomatid (fruit-eating) bat from Trinidad, but there was no associated human disease. Severe hemorrhagic cases in Argentina and later in Bolivia in the 1950s and 1960s resulted in the discovery of new viruses and diseases in these countries—Junin virus/**Argentine Hemorrhagic Fever** (AHF) and Machupo virus/**Bolivian Hemorrhagic Fever** (BHF). More recently, additional arenaviruses found in **Brazil (Sabia virus) and Venezuela (Guanarito virus)** produce similar hemorrhagic symptoms. AHF is the most common, 200—4,000 recorded annually between 1958 and 1995—the others are only sporadic, but mortality rates are high in all these diseases. In each of these, transmission is by contact with infected rodent excreta, dust, and other substances associated with grain harvesting and storage.

There are another five arenaviruses in the Americas that are not known to cause any illness in humans or their rodent hosts. All of the rodents associated with these viruses belong to only one of the 13 rodent families currently inhabiting South America. These rodent genera (*Calomys, Sigmodon, Oryzomys, et al*), are very closely related, and share a common ancestry. Paleontological evidence indicates that the Isthmus of Panama was a bridge connecting North and South America more than 2–3 million years ago, allowing a faunal interchange. The sigmodont rodent progenitors entered South America at that time, and rapidly evolved into the modern genera and species. Presumably the "ancestor virus" tagged along, co-evolving into the situation that now exists.

By far the most important arenaviral disease is **Lassa Fever:** discovered in Nigeria in 1970, it is known from 15 African countries, mostly in West and Central Africa, but also Zimbabwe and Mozambique. The natural host of Lassa virus is the multi-mammate rat, *Mastomys natalensis,* one of the most common and widely distributed African field rats. Like their South American counterparts, the AHF and BHF hosts, *Mastomys,* is basically a grassland species, easily adapting to the man-made grasslands of maize, sorghum, millet, sugarcane, and other cultivated grasses. Cases of Lassa are generally associated with agricultural activities and food storage: transmission is by contact with excreta of infected rodents.

Without laboratory facilities for confirmation, it is difficult to distinguish Lassa fever from Ebola, YF, or even severe cases of malaria. There are an estimated 500,000 cases a year, with more than 15% mortality rate in hospitalized cases. The disease is more severe in pregnancy, with fetal mortality reported at more than 80%. In the early 1970s (and before Ebola outbreaks occurred), Lassa caused great consternation in Europe and the Americas over the possibility of introduction of this disease. These concerns still exist and have been heightened after the appearance of these other groups of viral hemorrhagic diseases.

Hantaviruses

The **hantaviruses** are comprised of two large groups of viruses, all transmitted by rodents and producing a range of hemorrhagic, renal, and/or pulmonary complications. The **Old World Hantaviruses** are comprised of over 20 different viruses, several known for some time under a different classification (e.g., Hanta virus is the cause of Korean hemorrhagic fever with renal syndrome, an important military disease in the 1950s). Most cases still occur in agrarian and military populations and occur in over 50 countries in Asia, Africa, and Europe: each year approximately 200,000 cases occcur in Eurasia, with more than 50% of these reported in China. Case fatalities range from 0.1% to 10.0% depending on the virus. The 15 or so **New World Hantaviruses** produce a pulmonary, rather than a renal, syndrome. Since being described as a group in 1993, approximately 1,000 cases have been reported in the Americas, with a high case fatality rate (45–50 %).

The natural hosts/reservoirs for the hantavirus groups are mostly muroid rodents (Old World Group), and cricetid rodents (New World Group). This is not surprising, as these two are amongst the largest and most widely distributed mammalian families. However, the manner and zones of transmission are similar— rodent contamination of grain crops in the field and storage where people come in contact with rodent excreta.

Filoviruses

The two closely related **Filoviruses (Marburg and Ebola)** are among the most virulent viruses yet described with an overall fatality rate of more than 75%, and higher in several outbreaks (possibly augmented by use of dirty syringes and needles to give injectable chloroquine (an anti-malarial drug) to the patient's friends who carried him/her to the hospital. **Marburg virus** was first described (1967) among monkeys sent from East Africa to European laboratories, there killing laboratory technicians. Subsequent outbreaks have occurred in Africa. **Ebola virus** appeared in 1976 in simultaneous outbreaks in Zaire (Democratic Republic of Congo). (Barry, 2004) One Ebola strain was implicated in an outbreak in an animal holding facility in Reston, Virginia, U.S.A. Several humans seroconverted but showed no disease symptoms.

The repeated outbreaks of Ebola and Marburg virus, mostly in Central Africa, have been described as commencing with "rapidity and devastation." During an epidemic, transmission is generally by contact with contaminated blood or other tissues from infected persons. Most outbreaks have been in rather remote areas with poor health care facilities, so that patients are seen only with advanced symptoms. We have not been able to find reservoir organisms (there have been subsequent, better equipped expeditions than the one described in the footnote, but none have been successful), nor do we know the mechanism(s) of transmission in the wild. One distinct Ebola virus strain from Ivory Coast was isolated from a chimpanzee: primates are hunted and eaten by humans in parts of Africa and this may serve as the 'link' at which the virus(es) are able to "cross the species barrier" and enter the human population.

(Barry, 2004) The Government of Sudan requested WHO assistance, and the Government of Zaire requested the same from the U.S. Government (CDC). Representatives of WHO and CDC met in the next few days at the London School of Hygiene and Tropical Medicine to work out details and coordination (WHO was represented by Dr. Paul Bres and the author, and CDC by Dr. Karl Johnson). We had all thought of Lassa and Marburg viral fevers, and were surprised when Dr. Johnson said it was neither: He then showed us electron photomicrographs of tissue taken from an early case—the stringlike "6 and 9" figures were just like Marburg. But, he explained, this one was serologically distinct from Marburg, and they proposed to name it after a river in the area, the 'Ebola'.

We agreed that I (AAA) and a virologist (Dr. Bruce Johnson) from the LSHTM would go to the site in Sudan to sample potential reservoirs and/or vectors. Bruce would bring the supplies needed for taking tissue samples and the liquid nitrogen containers needed to return the samples to the UK. I was to gather the animal collecting materials. WHO had no such equipment in Geneva, of course, so I borrowed 'mist' nets for collecting bats from the British Musum (Natural History) and the Museé d' Histoire Naturelle in Geneva and borrowed sample rodent traps from the Swiss Agricultural Research Station in Nyon, near Geneva. We had the traps made in Nzara, one of the sites of the outbreak in Sudan. To autoclave the dissecting instruments we purchased two household 'pressure cookers' at the local super market (Migros) in Geneva. Placed on stones over an open fire, they served well.

An experimental Ebola vaccine has been reported to be successful in trials with non-human primates. Human trials will be conducted soon.

SARS and AAI

Two previously unknown and unrelated human viral infections, **Severe Acute Respiratory Syndrome** (SARS) and an **Asian Avian Influenza (strain H5N1),** originating in Southeast Asia, have received a great deal of popular attention and public health concern. In November 2002, cases of a respiratory illness, subsequently labeled **SARS**, appeared in China. A delay in timely reporting of the initial cases allowed it to spread to other Southeast Asian countries, Australia, the Americas, and at least 10 European countries. Reports of the actual number of persons infected varied, but cases numbered in the thousands, and mortality rates of up to 15% were indicated. Surveys of wild animals captured for human consumption quickly showed that ferrets, civets (related to mongooses), and raccoon dogs (shaggy fox-like carnivores) were positive for harboring the virus, but it is not known if any of these are the true reservoir in nature. The WHO has reported that the chain of transmission may have been broken (no new cases reported in a period of time equal to two consecutive 10 day incubation periods). This is clearly a case of a virus "species jumping". In the world's largest, most densely populated country this could spell disaster, especially if the reporting network is compromised.

The **Asian Avian Influenza** strain initially appeared in poultry in Hong Kong in 1997, when it jumped the species barrier and killed 6 out of 18 infected persons. This recent outbreak spread to Korea (December, 2003), then Japan and Vietnam (January 2004). Hong Kong reportedly slaughtered 1.4 million chickens and ducks, and as many as three million slaughtered through the Southeast Asia region, but other reports indicate that there are nonspecific wild variants of this strain in wild birds that serve as natural reservoirs.

Of major concern is that outbreaks of highly pathogenic avian influenza are increasing in frequency and severity. Reportedly, in the 40 years from 1959 to 1998, there were only 17 outbreaks, but in the past six years, from 1997 to 2003, there have been six, not including the most recent incidents.

HIV/AIDS

If bubonic plague was the quintessential pestilence of the ancient and medieval worlds, **Acquired Immunodeficiency Syndrome,** caused by the **Human Immunodeficiency Virus (AIDS/HIV)** is the chief pestilence of the modern world; and it is still growing, not receding. There is also a vast literature that will not be reviewed here, but the following 2003 data points describe the severity of the pandemic pestilence:

- AIDS is gaining a firmer foothold in the large populations of India and China;
- World wide, 40 million people are infected with HIV;
- 25–28 million of these infected people live in sub-Saharan Africa;
- 5 million persons became infected this year, 700,000 are children;
- 3 million persons died of AIDS this year, 500,000 of them less than 15 years old;
- Existence of Simian Immunodeficiency Virus (SIV) suggests animal origin.

The social damage accompanying this pandemic is not reflected in the bare figures given above; especially the orphaned children, destroyed family structures, and so forth. It has been estimated that 10 billion dollars US, per annum, is required to provide the prevention and treatment facilities and services needed: To date, less than one-half ($4.7 billion per annum) has been made available.

CLOSING OBSERVATIONS

Some of the old category diseases are still strongly with us (e.g., malaria, TB, influenza), and, by adapting traits such as drug-resistance and crossing or jumping species, they expand their reservoir-host base. As such, they could be considered new. Some other old diseases are rather well controlled in the developed countries where the surveillance systems are efficient and vaccination and other preventive services are readily available and properly used. These would include smallpox (eradicated), polio (eradicated in some areas), and childhood illnesses such as pertussis, diptheria, tetanus, measles, and so on. Even bubonic plague could be characterized as being under control—it is widespread, but also well understood, and with vector control and appropriate antibiotics, outbreaks are not severe and mortality is low.

On the other hand, some of the new (most recently discovered) diseases like Ebola and HIV/AIDS are hard to handle. We know little about the natural history of Ebola, Lassa, or the South American hemorrhagic fevers, and our knowledge of HIV/AIDS in the laboratory probably exceeds our understanding of the socio-economic impacts it is having on whole cultures.

When Lassa virus "jumped" from the field rat, *Mastomys*, to humans it was dreadfully virulent, and it seemed to come from nowhere. But, after a few years, we know that (with one exception from a bat) all arenaviruses are well adapted to particular rodent groups; most rodents are grass eaters, and lots of crops are grasses (wheat, maize, sugarcane, rice, etc.); therefore, the arenaviral fevers are seen primarily in agricultural settings and with stored grain. Yet, for the more recently known Hantavirus group, or even less with the multiferous arboviruses, we do not have good data on ecological determinents, or even host-reservoir relationships.

At the same time, people are modifying environmental conditions rapidly and extensively, and we have little information indicating whether such changes will eliminate potential disease cycles or exacerbate them. This may be even more important for diseases like influenza. If they have obligate or opportunistic vertebrate hosts and these are coincidentily reduced in number or eliminated, what selection pressures are set in action on the virus population to select new hosts? And when it comes to modifying environments, man has no equal. Yet we know that this microbial evolution is going on at a rapid pace—just look at how fast drug-resistance develops and spreads!

In reading articles and researching references for this document, I was amazed to discover again how many human illnesses have their direct animal (zoonotic) counterparts, or were vectored/hosted by arthropods, rodents, or snails, and how an avian influenza can become a mammalian influenza very quickly, and how a bat or an oppossum can do the same for the Chagas disease trypanosome. It is in this context that I feel that we know very little of the natural history or the ecological dynamics of the disease transmission cycles we teach.

Especially disturbing is to read of a new strain of Asian avian influenza and the necessity, around the world, to kill millions of birds. If one was to dream up a model pathogen incubator and dissemination engine, the perfect model would be a modern chicken farm of 500,000 birds, defecating as birds do, and that at a constant temperature and with residues of organic chicken feed all about. And we wonder why new diseases emerge? Any farmer worth his/her salt knows that monoculture breeds pests.

This is a good place to bring up one other difficult subject—bioterrorism. It is difficult for one dedicated to public health principles to imagine why anyone would even consider using infectious diseases as a weapon, but it is being done, and we need to be able to distinguish between a natural epidemic and one orchestrated by man. Again, knowledge of the natural history of the organisms, their natural hosts and reservoirs, will help.

Already the U.S.A. is stockpiling smallpox and anthrax vaccines in large quantities.

One final point; most people concerned with new versus old pestilences work as epidemiologists, infectious disease specialists, hospital officials, and so forth. But public health work is broader than the study and treatment of infectious diseases, and the study *The Global Burden of Disease,* sponsored by the WHO, World Bank, and Harvard University, based on measuring DALYS, predicts that fewer infectious disease will be as important in the future as they are at present. For example, "The next two decades will see dramatic changes in the health needs of the world's populations, and non-communicable diseases such as depression and heart disease . . . are replacing the traditional enemies, such as infectious diseases and malnutrition."

Maybe toxic smog and non-communicable diseases will replace pestilences, both old and new!

REFERENCES

Barry, J.M. (2004). *The great influenza* (Vol. 547). Viking Press.

Benenson, A.S. (Ed.). (1995). *Control of communicable diseases manual* (16th ed., p. 577). American Public Health Association.

Berger, S.A., Calisher, C.H., & Keystone, J.S. (2003). *Exotic viral diseases* (p. 252). B.C. Decker.

Cartwright, F.C. (1972). *Disease and history* (p. 248). T.Y. Crowell.

Curtin, P.D. (1989). *Death by migration* (p. 251). Cambridge University Press.

Gregg, C.T. (1985). *Plague: An ancient disease in the twentieth century* (rev. ed., p. 373) University New Mexico Press.

Lederberg, J., Shope, R.E., & Oaks, S.C. (Eds.). (1992). *Emerging infections* (p. 294). U.S. Institute of Medicine National Academy of Sciences.

McNeill, W.H. (1977). *Plagues and people* (p. 340). Anchor Books, Doubleday.

Murray, C.J., & Lopez, A.D. (Eds.). (1995). *The global burden of disease* (p. 46). WHO/Harvard/World Bank. Harvard University Press.

Nuland, S. B. (2003). *The doctor's plague* (p. 191). W. W. Norton, N.Y.

Oldstone, M.B. (1998). *Viruses, plagues, and history* (p. 227). Oxford University Press.

Rosenberg, C.E. (1962). *The cholera years* (p. 256). University of Chicago Press.

Wills, C. (1996). *Yellow fever/black goddess.* Addison—Wesley.

Centers for Disease Control (CDC). Emerging infectious diseases (vol. 1–10). www.cdc.gov/eid or hard copy from CDC, Atlanta GA, U.S.A.

Chapter 4

Value Systems and Healthcare Ethics

BERNARD M. DICKENS

INTRODUCTION

The term value system refers to the personal and societal qualities that individuals and communities consider worthy of holding within themselves and in contrast to the lesser worth of alternative qualities. For instance, those inspired by religious or spiritual values find them more worthy than secular or worldly values, and those who find religious teachings unconvincing or too doctrinaire may favor secular or pragmatic considerations to guide their behavior toward others. The term ethics is understood in several different ways, but in regard, for instance, to health, it is increasingly understood to be concerned with an analysis of the arguments and conclusions which find that a particular conduct affecting health is either right or wrong to undertake. Ethics concerned with human biology is often described as bioethics, which now transcends healthcare of individuals to encompass health interests of groups, societies, and national populations.

Ethical analysis of the application of value systems can be pitched at different levels. The traditional level in, for instance, the healthcare setting, addresses the relationship between service providers, such as doctors, and service recipients, such as patients. This relationship is often described as the person-to-person, or microethical, level. Ethical analysis requires that each person respect the dignity and right to self-determination, or autonomy, of the other. At the level of group or societal interactions, ethics addresses how different groups treat one another and how they treat individuals, including members and non-members of the group or society itself. This is the macroethical level. Transcending individual societies is the level sometimes described as megaethics. At this level are environmental and ecological concerns, and the imbalance evident in a proportionally small segment of the world's population that lives in economically developed countries and consumes a vastly disproportionate volume of the world's resources, including non-renewable resources, and a sizeable number of the world's residents who live in economically developing or under-developed countries and live in poverty, hunger, and deprivation. This inequity is reflected by less than 10 percent of global spending on health research being devoted to diseases or conditions that account for 90 percent of the global disease burden (Global Forum for Health Research, 2000).

Individuals and societies frequently adhere at the same time to different and even conflicting value systems. We want to apply values that embody virtuous, generalizable principles, and we want to behave, and our societies to operate, in ways that achieve desired economic and efficient results. However, pursuit at the same time of virtuous principles and the most effective practices may not be possible. What appears right in principle, such as preservation of human life, may lead to distressing results, such as the imposition on vulnerable, dependent individuals of the agonizing prolongation of their death. What works best in practice, such as women's access to a medically safe, voluntary termination of life- or health-endangering pregnancy, may seem to compromise important principles, such as respect for the value of unborn human life, which is often expressed in religious terms as its sanctity.

CONTRASTING VALUE SYSTEMS

The human instinct for supernatural or religious beliefs underlies the principles of many prevalent value systems. Such beliefs give priority to duties human beings are considered to owe to divine creators, embodied in monotheistic religions as a single god. The duties humans owe to other humans are then only an instrumental or secondary means to serve a god or gods. Service of a god or gods may take a form from which other humans benefit, but may also justify doing immense harm. There are also non-religious or secular value systems, the principles of which are also considered to be morally imperative. In modern western cultures, the teachings of the German philosopher Immanuel Kant (1724–1804) are influential. Kantian principles or values include that, to be ethical, every action should be universally generalizable, so that perpetrators of acts should be liable to be affected by the same acts done to them by others. This principle is consistent with such religious teachings as "to do unto others only what you would have them do unto you." The principle rejects any claims to be exceptional or superior, such as were expressed in practices of colonialism and forced religious conversion. Another Kantian principle is that human beings should never be treated only as objects or instruments, but should be accorded respect for their individual value and dignity. This principle governs, for instance, research undertaken with human subjects, particularly when investigators from one country or culture propose research with persons from other countries or cultures.

Religious and secular principle-based value systems may be consistent with each other in the priority they accord to key principles of their own convictions. They may agree that "right must be done, though the heavens may fall," meaning that their principles must prevail whatever the cost. Accordingly, for instance, the Roman Catholic Church maintains its condemnation and prohibition in principle of artificial contraception involving the use of condoms, including their use to contain the spread of HIV/AIDS by means of safer sex. It urges that the health and lives of many thousands of people that condom use would probably save be saved by sexual abstinence or other religiously acceptable means. Principle-based value systems do not necessarily accommodate each other, however. For instance, the Roman Catholic Church prohibited adherents from reading the non-religious reasoning of Immanuel Kant, by including his writing in its *Index Librorum Prohibitorum* (Index of Forbidden Books).

In contrast to principle-based value systems are pragmatic systems, often described as utilitarian or consequentialist systems. These gauge the value of practices by how well they promote human satisfaction, sometimes expressed as "the greatest happiness of the greatest number," and define happiness by popular or democratic criteria. Principle-based value systems condemn utilitarianism and consequentialism by considering them wrongly to allow the desirable ends of immoral or expedient means or methods to absolve the immorality, and to be manipulative and Machiavellian. Adherents to pragmatic or utilitarian values condemn principle-based policies that disregard or discount the consequences they cause, particularly avoidable human death, disease, distress, and misery. Such adherents do not want "the heavens to fall," and will do what is needed to prevent that consequence, even if their acts may offend abstract principles, such as may be invoked in the name of religion.

A modern contrast in value systems is apparent in considering the provision of healthcare services in different countries. The United States' culture and political system regards provision of health services as being like that of other services, based on the principle of free market enterprise and private initiatives of supply and demand for services. There are limited publicly supported services for the exceptionally poor, and some provision for elderly persons, but the significant majority of citizens depend for provision of care on their own resources or on their employment healthcare service plan. The result is that the finest of healthcare services are available to those with the direct or indirect means to pay, but, of a US population approximating 300 million, an estimated 43 million or more have no reasonably affordable access to medical or related healthcare services, except through often under-funded municipal hospitals. Further, many employees are locked into low-paying jobs, for fear of losing healthcare services for their families provided by their employers. Both employer-provided and privately purchased services are liable to leave many people under-insured. It has been observed that, by adhering to the economic free market value system, the USA has the least affordable and most inequitable health system among the economically developed or industrialized countries of the world (Pollack, 2003).

The US is hostile to "socialized medicine," as provided under slightly different government schemes such as in Scandinavia and Western Europe (Flood, 2000). These schemes reflect utilitarian social planning, by which taxes levied on those with the means to pay provide healthcare services to those who require them regardless of their means. US politicians tend to associate the provision of services by the principle "from each according to his means, to each according to his needs," with objectionable Marxist-inspired communism or socialism. Socialized medicine often displays inefficiencies and some diseconomies in practice, for instance in requiring waiting time for non-emergency care such as surgery. However, rational use of public healthcare resources can be promoted by implementation of evidence-based medicine, and the system appears closer in its consequences to the ethical values of maximizing good (beneficence), social justice, and social solidarity than systems that follow US market principles.

ETHICAL FAILURES AND RESPONSES OF VALUE SYSTEMS

Both principle-based and utility-based value systems often operate in ways that present contradictions. Philosophers tend to fault value systems for errors of inconsistency which show the systems to be incoherent, and political commentators may criticize contradictions in value systems as hypocrisy.

An ethical failure of principle-based policies and practices is that proponents frequently accept no responsibility for the consequences of their actions . Particularly, proponents of religiously based ethics believe they are giving effect to divine wishes specially revealed to them, for instance through divinely inspired leaders or sacred texts. Invoking the mystery and majesty of divine authority, they may look beyond worldly effects to divine salvation and eternal life, and not only their own afterlife but also that of those who innocently suffer according to an adherence to a divine plan. This is an explanation offered by religiously driven terrorists, and also by individual and institutional opponents, for instance, of lawful therapeutic abortion and artificial contraception. They interpret principles of Natural Law to condemn these practices as "unnatural," rejecting evidence of their good effects in reducing the incidence of maternal mortality and morbidity, particularly in resource-poor countries, on the basis that good cannot come from wrongdoing and evil. Similarly, the Roman Catholic leadership appears indifferent to human lives prematurely lost to HIV/AIDS that could be saved by condom distribution programs (Mann, 1992).

Perhaps the most glaring failure of utilitarian values was shown in National Socialist (Nationalsozialist, shortened to Nazi) Germany, where the government democratically elected in 1933 later suppressed all opposition and enacted laws that deprived individuals, notably Jews but also Gypsies and homosexual men, of civil liberties. Jews, for instance, were subject to laws that often deprived them of the right to practice their profession, for instance as doctors or lawyers, of their property, their privacy (by being required in public to wear visibly identifying badges), their right to marry and parent children with non-Jews, their right to live outside concentration camps, to decline sterilization and participation in medical experiments, and to laws that ultimately deprived them of their lives. These discriminatory laws, endorsing concepts of "racial hygiene" (O'Reilly, 1993), received the support of the German population in general, and of many doctors, lawyers, and judges in particular.

A post-1945 reaction to the atrocities associated with the Nazi-influenced governments in Europe, and comparable atrocities committed in Japanese-controlled Southeast Asia, were the international human rights·initiatives taken by the newly formed United Nations organization. The movement developed a principle-based value system, drawn from the best ideals in member-countries' legal systems and constitutional documents, expressed in 1948 in the Universal Declaration of Human Rights.

This was called a "declaration" because it claimed only to declare principles to which member states were already committed, but it was subsequently given legal effect in countries that ratified related international treaties, notably the International Covenant on Civil and Political Rights, and the International Covenant on Economic, Social, and Cultural Rights. These treaties protect in general, among other rights, the right to marry and found a family, the rights to life, liberty, and personal security, to private and family life, and to be free from inhuman and degrading treatment, including involuntary sterilization. Such rights touch on preservation of personal health, but the Covenant on Economic, Social, and Cultural Rights specifically addresses rights to enjoy the highest attainable standard of physical and mental health, and the Covenant on Civil and Political Rights allows people freely to decline participation in medical experimentation.

Reinforcing the two general covenants are universal human rights conventions against racial discrimination, on the rights of refugees, against discrimination against women, and on the rights of the child, as well as regional human rights conventions specific to Europe, the Americas, and Africa. All of these covenants and conventions are in legal effect because enough countries have ratified them to bring them into international and national force. Accordingly, at universal, regional, and national levels, the value system based on respect for the principles of human rights has been widely adopted.

HUMAN RIGHTS VALUES AND HEALTHCARE ETHICS

From the earliest times, healthcare services have been recognized to have two equal aspects, namely clinical care and public healthcare. In classical Greek mythology, the god of medicine whose name the Hippocratic Oath invokes, Asklepios, had two daughters, Hygiea and Panacea. The former was the goddess of preventive health and wellness, or hygiene, and the latter the goddess of treatment and curing. In modern times, the societal ascendancy of medical professionalism has caused treatment of sick patients to overshadow those preventive healthcare services provided by the less heroic figures of sanitary engineers, biologists, and governmental public health officers. Nevertheless, the quality of health that human populations enjoy is attributable less to surgical dexterity, innovative pharmaceutical products, and bioengineered devices than to the availability of public sanitation, sewage management, and services which control the pollution of the air, drinking water, urban noise, and food for human consumption. The human right to the highest attainable standard of health depends on public healthcare services no less than on the skills and armamentarium of doctors and hospitals (Gostin, 2000).

Healthcare ethics also have an ancient history, traceable to the spirit, although not the original details, of the Hippocratic Oath, which has been successively modernized over time. Care for the sick has long been inspired by religious faith. Faith-based institutions and charities of many religious traditions have devoted themselves to tending to the sick and needy in many parts of the world. However, because the primary motivation of such care is duty to perceptions of divine authority rather than to care for sick people for their own sake, care is often denied that would contradict interpretations of divine will. It was Roman Catholic intransigence on matters of tolerating artificial means of birth control to which the modern evolution of bioethics has been attributed. One of the earliest pioneers and observers of bioethics has written of proposals for reconsideration of its position on birth control that the Roman Catholic church invited, but then rejected in the 1960s, that:

> Fertility control was the major issue that spawned bioethics, more than any other single issue—certainly more than any high-technology-related issue in medicine. It was an issue that directly affected hundreds of millions of people; it dealt with quintessentially human suffering and fulfillment ... The theologians, who were the first ethicists working in bioethics, cut their teeth on contraception/sterilization and abortion debates; and in a very real sense, much of

the great energy that was turned toward bioethics around 1970/71 was energy
that was diverted from the then-increasingly futile [Roman Catholic] church
debates on fertility control (Reich, 1999).

In modern times, at first in North America, then in the westernized world, and
eventually almost universally, the area of medical ethics has become dominated by
so-called bioethics. This is so to such an extent that proponents, for instance, of
conventional Roman Catholic religious ethics applicable to healthcare now tend
to be described, and to describe themselves, as bioethicists.

While healthcare ethics in this modern context of bioethics has made advances
in structuring debates about relations between healthcare providers and patients
and for instance, medical investigators and the human subjects of their research,
bioethics has not made comparable advances considering public health services.
Similarly, in the United States, where healthcare ethicists have enthusiastically
addressed such new issues as reproductive technologies, gene therapy, cloning,
and embryo stem cell research—which directly affect the lives of relatively few
individuals—they have failed to address the ethics of a society and political system
in which, amid relative social affluence and national wealth, an estimated 43 million
out of 300 million people lack reasonable access to healthcare services (Lane,
2000). The inequity of this deprivation raises issues of human rights, including
the right to the highest attainable standard of physical and mental health, addressed
in the International Covenant on Economic, Social, and Cultural Rights, which
the United States has signed but refused to ratify.

The relationship between healthcare ethics and human rights has been
explained by Jonathan Mann, a physician who achieved international prominence
in tackling the medical, ethical, and public health responses to contain and reverse
the mounting international HIV/AIDS pandemic. He observed that what ethics is
to clinical medicine addressing individuals' health, human rights are to public
health, addressing the health of populations. He noted that:

> [E]thics and human rights derive from a set of quite similar, if not identical,
> core values. As with medicare and public health, rather than seeing human
> rights and ethics as conflicting domains, it seems more appropriate to consider
> a continuum, in which human rights is a language most useful for guiding
> societal level analysis and work, while ethics is a language most useful for
> guiding individual behavior. From this perspective, and precisely because
> public health must be centrally concerned with the structure and function
> of society, the language of human rights is extremely useful for expressing,
> considering and incorporating values into public health analysis and response
> (Mann, 1997).

He concluded that public health work requires both ethics applicable to the
individual public health practitioner and a human rights framework to guide public health in its societal analysis and response. The value system of principle-based

human rights accordingly is consistent with and embraces the modern understanding of healthcare ethics.

THE RISE OF FEMINIST VALUE SYSTEMS AND ETHICS

Both principle-based value systems applicable to health services and utilitarian healthcare ethics have emerged from traditional centers of knowledge and social authority, such as religious hierarchies, university and comparable institutions that explore and expound on moral philosophy, learned professions such as medicine and law, courts of law, and legislative assemblies. These are all agencies that did not include and often deliberately excluded women from having authority and even a voice in their deliberations and decisions. Several of them, particularly some religious hierarchies, still do. At a time when women serve with distinction in positions of religious leadership, academic leadership in university departments, and as university presidents, professional leaders in medicine and law, chief justices of several national judicial systems, and prime ministers of prominent national governments, the deliberate exclusion of people because they are women discredits the moral authority of institutions that maintain value systems of discrimination against women.

Feminism is not an exclusive commitment of women. Not all women are feminists, and not all feminists are women. Rather, this area of concern attracts those committed to the ending of discrimination on grounds of gender that preclude women's experiences and viewpoints from consideration in decisionmaking. This preclusion has been, and in many regions remains, significantly oppressive regarding women's health, particularly their reproductive health. The World Health Organization has estimated that each year about 515,000 women die from causes related to pregnancy and childbirth, largely in the world's developing countries. This is a rate of over 1,400 maternal deaths every day of the year, amounting to one death almost every minute, and four jet airplanes full of pregnant women crashing each day with no survivors. This number is only the tip of an iceberg of maternal morbidity and acute or chronic suffering from pregnancy-related ill health (Cook, 2003). The indifference of many national and international leaders, in political, economic, religious, and other realms of authority, to these realities casts a shadow over the ethical virtues they profess for their value systems. Indeed, many continue to oppose the concept of reproductive health, advanced at the United Nations International Conference on Population and Development, held in Cairo in 1994, and reaffirmed in 1995 at the United Nations Fourth World Conference on Women, held in Beijing.

Feminist bioethics, philosophy, and jurisprudence have generated an extensive modern literature, but feminist healthcare ethics can be distilled into the simple strategy, developed in the area of assessment of laws, of "asking the woman question" (Bartlett, 1990); that is, asking what effect actual or proposed policies, laws, and practices have on women in contrast to men. In many centers of traditional authority on key values, such as legislatures, courts of law, and religious hierarchies, the question has been not only unanswered, but unasked, in part because no women have authority to ask it.

An historical assumption regarding human reproduction, for instance, has been that decisions on whether and when individuals and families had children were social, legal, and religious matters, to be determined by social, legal, and religious authorities and leaders who were almost invariably, and sometimes exclusively, men. A woman's childbearing was her husband's right and responsibility. Women were not free to determine whether, when, and with whom to have their children, and were condemned for pregnancy outside marriage, for which some societies and legal systems still consider stoning to death an appropriate sanction. When women's sexual flirtations result in family members murdering them, some countries' legal systems and cultures allow reduced punishment, and tolerate nonprosecution. Their societies recognize such murders as " honor killings," because women's sexuality outside marriage taints their "family honor." Women are still similarly "given in marriage" by their fathers or other male family figureheads, in some cultures not uncommonly without the brides' voluntary consent, and killing them for suspected adultery is considered an understandable "crime of passion" that reduces husbands' liability to punishment, although husbands' infidelities do not allow wives an equally "passionate" response.

Contraception by chemical and other artificial means, voluntary contraceptive sterilization, and abortion are condemned by conservative social and religious institutions, including those that remain silent in the presence of evidence of the rates of death, ill-health, and devastation to their lives that women can suffer from pregnancy, particularly when it comes too early, too late, too often, or too closely spaced in their fertile life span. These conservative institutions also condemn women for resorting to medically assisted reproduction, and are indifferent to the multiple disadvantages women can suffer from remaining childless in marriage. However, some feminist advocates are also cautious about the application of some of the reproductive technologies, not only because they may characterize women primarily as childbearers, but also because they can be unnecessarily invasive, and expose women to family pressure to comply involuntarily with treatment regimens.

To redress women's vulnerability to oppressive value systems that regard their fertility as a social asset, or risk, amenable to the decisive regulation of family members, strangers, societies, or political or religious ideologies, the concept of "reproductive health" has been developed (Cook, 2003). This builds on the description of health in the World Health Organization's constitution as a "state of complete physical, mental, and social well-being, and not merely the absence of disease or infirmity." As shaped by the United Nations International Conference on Population and Development in 1994, and the Fourth World Conference on Women in 1995, the definition is that:

> Reproductive health is a state of complete physical, mental and social well-being and not merely the absence of disease or infirmity, in all matters relating to the reproductive system and to its functions and processes. Reproductive health therefore implies that people are able to have a satisfying and safe sex life and that they have the capability to reproduce and the freedom to decide if, when and how often to do so. Implicit in this last condition are the right of men and women to be informed and to have access to safe, effective, affordable and acceptable methods of family planning of their choice, as well as other methods of their choice for regulation of fertility which are not against the law, and the right of access to appropriate health-care services that will enable women to go safely through pregnancy and childbirth and provide couples with their best chance of having a healthy infant.

The value system that this definition reflects recognizes the central position of women in human reproduction, and aims to create equality of choice and reproductive self-determination for women and men. The definition remains fiercely opposed, however, by fundamentalist religious and political administrations, whose ideologies place women's interests at the margins of what they consider relevant. At the 1995 U.N. World Conference on Women, for instance, the numerous representatives of The Holy See, acting on behalf of the Vatican and the Roman Catholic Church, actively courted the support of delegates from the more conservative Islamic countries to reject this expression of women's equal rights to reproductive self-determination and health. Setting aside historical rivalry for people's religious allegiance, they accepted that their enemy's enemy could be their friend in opposing a principle of reproductive health. Their opposition is not to women's health itself, of course, but to women's access to family planning methods that conservative religious interpretations render doctrinally unacceptable, and to women's option of being independent from the decisive control of men. They seek to impose exclusively male-derived principles without regard to the frequently devastating, and even fatal, impact on women. The modern bioethical principles of minimizing harm (non-maleficence), of justice, and of respect for persons of both sexes (Beauchamp, 2001) are subordinated to a value system that gives priority to obedience to divine will, as interpreted by exclusively male religious leaders. However, this resistance to an emerging feminist value system is more a hindrance than a defeat of that system, and does more to discredit than empower its proponents in modern bioethical assessment.

GLOBALIZATION OF VALUE SYSTEMS AND HEALTHCARE ETHICS

The modern context of "globalization" is principally economic and commercial, based on the success in the Cold War of western capitalist countries, led by the US, against communist countries, led by the former Soviet Union. Though initially expressed in military and nuclear terms, the basis of US success was economic, and the US has subsequently urged its market economy model on developing countries and on former Soviet and other countries whose economies are in transition, so that these countries can join those of the democratic, economically developed world. The US has been slow to recognize the inequities and dysfunctions of the provision of healthcare services in its own domestic marketplace, however. The US method of provision scarcely warrants the description of a "system," since it depends so largely on employers' arbitrary and unsystematic choices of employees' health insurance coverage and individuals' personal choices and means of bargaining with private healthcare insurers. The often disastrous and inequitable provision of services in the US medical marketplace (Pollack, 2003) makes it arguably the worst model for developing countries and those in economic transition to follow.

The value system of the US-driven "free" market ideology has, however, permeated such significant international agencies as the International Monetary Fund (IMF), the World Trade Organization, and the World Bank, due in part to the influence of US funding support. Accordingly, the IMF, World Bank, and comparable agencies direct the economies of countries that request their assistance toward market principles, including for provision of domestic healthcare services. In the same way that the US method of healthcare provision pays little regard to the ethical principles of spreading good, minimizing harm, and achieving social justice, however, countries that choose or are obliged to base their health service provision on free market principles such as reliance on commercial health insurance, encouraging moves toward for-profit hospitals and clinics and toward user-fees for patients, are at risk of offending central principles of bioethics.

The US has furnished a valuable global model of an economically developed country facilitating access to healthcare services in resource-poor countries by governmental funding of the US Agency for International Development (USAID). For instance, governmental and non-governmental organizations in resource-poor countries have been able to reduce domestic rates of maternal mortality and morbidity through USAID support of contraceptive and related family planning services. Since the so-called Mexico City policy of 1984, however, conservative US governmental administrations have corrupted the virtuous goals of USAID by making funding support of recipient overseas agencies subject to the US domestic anti-abortion ideology, as urged by fundamentalist religious groups. Their policies would be unconstitutional if applied in the US itself. These groups influence those in political power who defer to them to withdraw funding from recipient agencies that provide some abortion care or referral to back up family planning methods, all of which have a low but irreducible minimum rate of failure.

Some USAID-funded family planning agencies that adhere to the common medical professional ethic to consider first the well-being of the patient find that they cannot in ethical conscience decline to offer abortion assistance, and have forfeited USAID funding. This has resulted in their reduced ability to provide contraceptive services, a consequent increase in unwanted pregnancies, and a return to higher national levels of abortion and maternal mortality (Marston, 2003), in some cases related to women's desperate recourse to unskilled abortion, including by self-induction. The ideological anti-abortion motivation of conservative US administrations perverts the original ethical goal of USAID, and exploits the opportunity to impose a domestic policy on populations outside the country vulnerable to the imposition because of their poverty and dependency on US funding for healthcare. This is both dysfunctional by utilitarian criteria, and shows the ethical bankruptcy of policies disrespectful of women's health and self-determination that adherents of such policies promote to defend their value system. It also feeds an emerging perception that globalization may become only "Americanization," and may fuel resistance outside the US to acceptance or imposition of the globalization concept.

REFERENCES

Bartlett, K.T. (1990). Feminist legal methods. *Harvard Law Rev, 103,* 829–888.
Beauchamp, T. & Childress, J. (2001). *Principles of biomedical ethics (5th ed.).* New York: Oxford University Press.
Cook, R. Dickens, B., & Fathalla, M. (2003). *Reproductive health and human rights: Integrating medicine, ethics and law.* Oxford: Oxford University Press.
Flood, C. (2000). *International health care reform: A legal, economic and political analysis.* London: Routledge.
Global Forum for Health Research. (2000). *The 10/90 report on health research.* Geneva: Global Forum/World Health Organization.
Gostin, L. (2000). *Public health law: Power, duty, restraint.* Berkeley: University of California Press.
Lane, S.D., Rubinstein, R.A., Cibula, D., & Webster, N. (2000). Towards a public health approach to bioethics. In A. Cantwell, E. Friedlander, & M. Tramm, (Eds.), *Ethics and anthropology: Facing future issues in human biology, globalism and cultural property (Vol. 925, pp. 25–36).* New York: New York Academy of Sciences; Annals.
Mann, J., Tarantola, D., & Netter, T. (1902). *AIDS in the world: A global report.* Cambridge, MA: Harvard University Press.
Mann, J.M. (1997). Medicine and public health, ethics and human rights. *Hastings Center Report, 27(3),* 6–13.
Marston, C., Cleland, J. (2003). Relationships between contraception and abortion: A review of the evidence. *International Family Planning Perspectives, 29,* 6–13.

O'Reilly, M. (1993). Nazi medicine: The perversion of the noblest profession. *Canadian Medical Association Journal, 148*(5), 819–21.

Pollack, R. (2003). Gaps and inequities in America's health care system. *Health Matrix: Journal of Law–Medicine, 13*, 415–27.

Reich, W.T. (1999). The 'wider view': Andre Helleger's passionate, integrating intellect and the creation of bioethics. *Kennedy Institute of Ethics Journal, 9*, 25–51.

World Health Organization (WHO). (2001). *Maternal mortality in 1995*. Geneva: WHO.

Chapter 5

World Health
A Mobilizing Utopia?

M. MANCIAUX AND T.M. FLIEDNER

In his book, entitled *Utopia* and published in 1516, Sir Thomas More described an imaginary island with a perfect social and political system, where a fair monarch rules over nice, honest, and well-tempered people. This "place of nowhere," from the Greek word sou, (not), and topos, (a place), would be heaven on earth; unfortunately, it does not exist. However, throughout history, some heretofore only imagined utopias have become realities: Who, at the beginning of the 20th century, would have believed in smallpox eradication? A goal of a utopia can be mobilizing, especially for visionaries, and the founding fathers of the World Health Organization (WHO), in 1946, were realistic yet visionary, scientific yet humanistic, people.

In spite of some tremendous achievements in the field of health since the end of the second World War, so much remains to be done that new visions, new utopias, must mobilize new thoughts and energies and take up new challenges. Although almost all chapters in this book address this idea, this chapter aims to present a snapshot of the global outlook of world health in space and time. After a promising start, where do we stand now? What are the critical health problems confronting us individually and collectively? What are the existing resources and how are we to mobilize them? Which values and ethical issues are at stake? Is it possible to combine, in order to improve health globally, an evidence-based approach with a utopian vision? These points will be critically reviewed.

A few years ago, the WHO Advisory Committee on Health Research (ACHR) published *A Research Policy Agenda for Science and Technology to support Global Health Development* (WHO, 1997). Because it is still valid and valuable, we, the authors of this chapter, who were also involved in preparing that book, will sometimes refer to it.

HISTORICAL BACKGROUND

It is not by chance that WHO was founded after the second World War. Wars, besides being sources of tremendous human suffering and material damage, also engender important breakthroughs in knowledge, science, and technology, which, in turn, might be beneficial or detrimental to health. Moreover, they highlight the value and benefits of peace for human and world development and of international cooperation for the health and good of human beings.

The terrible individual and collective trauma caused by six years of a war that transformed, because of its worldwide scope and terrific, inhumane forms, the moral conscience of all the world, also created a propitious climate for establishing some international instruments and organizations to promote a better, peaceful future. Quite logically, the pre-existing International Office of Public Hygiene of the League of Nations and the previous model of the International Society of Public Health, created in the late 19th century, paved the way for a new, more comprehensive and welcome institution: the World Health Organization.

Adopted by the International Health Conference (New York City, July, 1946), and brought into force in April, 1948, the WHO Constitution is a remarkable instrument and still valid. It begins by defining health: an ideal to strive toward, maybe a utopia, yet a mobilizing and innovative concept (WHO, 1999). Proposing a bipolar, well-balanced definition of health (what it is, what it is not), associating its three components—physical, mental, and social—and assimilating health to welfare, represented, at that time, a visionary and stimulating advance, whatever criticism might be made of this definition. Emphasizing the importance of infirmity as a crucial threat to health was also pioneering: Accidental injuries, as well as invalidity resulting from the aging population, now represent a huge burden for individual and public health.

Moreover, the Constitution states: "The enjoyment of the highest attainable standard of health is one of the fundamental rights of every human being without distinction of race, religion, political belief, economic, or social condition".

The text goes to enumerate a series of principles on peace and safety, cooperation and interdependency, health inequalities, child and human development, the benefits of progress in scientific, medical, and psychological knowledge, and the need for public cooperation and governmental commitment in order to improve the health status of populations. These principles, enacted more than half a century ago, should again inspire and stimulate global and national health policies. Let us quote this basic text further:

> The health of all peoples is fundamental to the attainment of peace and security and is dependent upon the fullest co-operation of individuals and States.
>
> The achievement of any State in the promotion and protection of health is of value to all.

Unequal development in different countries in the promotion of health and control of disease, especially communicable disease, is a common danger.

Healthy development of the child is of basic importance; the ability to live harmoniously in a changing total environment is essential to such development.

The extension to all peoples of the benefits of medical, psychological, and related knowledge is essential to the fullest attainment of health.

Informed opinion and active co-operation on the part of the public are of the utmost importance in the improvement of the health of the people.

Governments have a responsibility for the health of their peoples, which can be fulfilled only by the provision of adequate health and social measures.

A new impetus was provided in 1978 by the WHO–UNICEF Conference on Primary Health Care held in Alma-Ata. Prepared after several experiments with the so-called basic health services, the Conference made this statement: "The existing inequalities in health between and within countries are politically, socially, and economically unacceptable." By the end of the meeting, both organizations issued the now famous slogan: "Health for All by the Year 2000." Even translated into: "primary health services for all," it stood as a utopian objective. However, the emphasis put on primary health care proved useful, especially in developing countries, particularly through formulating a list of specific priorities. For instance, for children, breast feeding, growth monitoring, immunizations, and so forth.

Is global health improvement economically unacceptable? The 1993 report of the World Bank entitled *Investing in health* clearly demonstrated with a lot of data, references, and tables, that "Good health is a goal in itself (World development report, 1993)." Unfortunately, as far as developing countries and, by extension, the poor everywhere are concerned, the investment in and the fight against health inequalities proved insufficient! Should one put this into terms more constraining for the human conscience since health inequalities are also ethically unacceptable? In a concrete and realistic statement, the great French demographer Alfred Sauvy said, thirty years ago: "L'égoïsme, aujourd'hui, c'est la solidarité" (selfishness, today, is solidarity), meaning: If the rich West wants to keep its advantages of all kinds, it has to share with the poor. One more utopia!

We have enough knowledge to improve world health. We have enough money to start, for the benefit of all people, with the principle of equity: more for the most needy. We have the health personnel, indeed, more or less well-trained. Why do we not succeed, despite brilliant breakthroughs such as smallpox eradication? There are many reasons that we shall address later on. Let us quote but a few: lack of political will at all levels; insufficient mobilization of other sectors; under-controlled population growth; and incessant conflicts and wars throughout the world. So many lost opportunities and new challenges: HIV/AIDS is the major new challenge, but not the only one. Health protection and promotion are, more than ever, urgently needed.

In this respect, the Ottawa Charter, promulgated in 1986 by WHO, Health and Welfare Canada, and the Canadian Public Health Association, offers an operational tool to be used for promoting health in various contexts (WHO, 1986). Its five points, all of equal importance, constitute together a comprehensive program for action: develop personal skills, create supportive environments, strengthen community action, reorientate health services, and build a public health policy. These appealing guidelines should be implemented in constant and vivid cooperation between all concerned. However, the narrow and vertical specificity of organizations and services make this difficult. In the last part of this chapter, we shall propose some measures to help revisit and implement this worthwhile instrument.

WHERE DO WE STAND TODAY?

For a long time, through several development decades, the improvement of the world's health has been seen, in theory, as a phenomenon of catching up: The less developed countries should progressively get nearer to the industrialized ones through a double transition—demographic, with a reduction of their birth rate, and epidemiologic, by a decrease of the major killers, mainly communicable diseases, infectious or parasitic. Malaria eradication was on the WHO agenda at the beginning of the second half of the 20th century. Medical and scientific breakthroughs (antibiotics, immunizations against various diseases, progress of surgery, prevention, etc.) led to an illusion of the omnipotence of medicine. The following quote evokes both the naïve hope that the transfer of medical technology alone could solve many health problems and the disillusion of failure:

> "If I were asked to compose an epitaph on the twentieth century, it would read "Brilliant in its scientific discoveries, superb in its technical breakthroughs, but woefully inept in its application of knowledge to those most in need . . . " We are now experienced; and all that remains is the problem of translating what is current common knowledge and routine medical and health practice to the other two thirds of the world: the implementation gap must be closed." (Fendall, 1972)

Mothers and children are often considered among the most vulnerable groups of the population, especially in developing countries. In 1990, the World Summit for Children had aroused the hope of the world for children. The leaders of various countries had promised to reach ambitious objectives by the year 2000, such as the reduction of infant and maternal mortalities and progress in the rates of immunization. An evaluation realized in 2001 showed the gap between hope and reality.

- The first objective aimed at reducing by a third the infant and the under five-year-old children mortality rates between 1990 and 2000. The reduction achieved was of 14%. But some tremendous disparities still remain from a country to another. What is more, the post-infant mortality rates have soared in several countries mainly because of the HIV/AIDS epidemic whose prevalence makes it the most dramatic indicator of socio-economic inequalities.

- The objective of reducing mortality from diarrhoeal diseases has been almost achieved, particularly thanks to the increasing use of oral rehydration.
- As far as immunization is concerned, in SubSaharian Africa only 47% of children are vaccinated against diphtheria, whooping cough, and tetanus.
- In the field of nutrition, the objective was to reduce by half the rates of malnutrition in children. The rate has been reduced by an average of 17% in developing countries, but has increased in SubSaharian Africa.
- As for women's health, no real progress is noticed. The objective was to reduce by half maternal mortality but no real improvement has been made. The risk of death during pregnancy or delivery is still very high in all developing countries, especially in SubSaharian Africa, where it is higher than anywhere else in the world, with 1/13 against 1/4,000 in industrialized countries. Still in Africa, only 37% of deliveries take place with the help of a qualified person.

Malaria, which remains a very deadly infection, especially in children, must also be mentioned. So must be tuberculosis, back in force as a consequence of the HIV/AIDS epidemic. Moreover, a new social morbidity has emerged along with street children, AIDS, war orphans, the consequences of children's exploitation in labor, sexual abuse of children, and the development of numerous addictions and child trafficking networks.

However, it would be wrong to compare point-by-point the health problems prevailing in developing countries to those well-known in the developed nations. What makes the difference is accessibility to care. Nowadays, most of the important health problems are global, and must be dealt with on a global basis.

Here, again, a specific and critical situation exists. Emerging countries have now simultaneously to face the "traditional" pattern of communicable diseases of the third world and the chronic pathology of the industrialized countries.

HIV/AIDS deserves special mention. This modern plague illustrates at once the bridge between nations and the gap which separates them, as far as therapeutic resources are concerned. According to the 2003 World Health Report, of the estimated 6 million persons needing treatment for HIV/AIDS, only about 400,000 received it. Coverage is lowest in the African region: 2%. Indeed, accessibility to care is a major problem; however, a global strategy (global both geographically and in the quality of care received, including prevention) is badly needed to control this world threat, and the promises made at the end of each major international meeting should be kept.

It is difficult to measure with reasonable precision the burden of disease currently affecting world health. It is even harder to anticipate the near future. Besides the ancient diseases that we believed to be definitely conquered and that now are re-emerging, new plagues are arising. The fight for health must be a permanent engagement.

PROBLEMS OF CRITICAL SIGNIFICANCE TO INDIVIDUAL AND GLOBAL HEALTH

Health policies and services are used to identify priority problems. They are, indeed, logical tools for planning and acting. However, health problems are evolving rapidly, and the prioritization should be periodically revised; it varies according to places, and national priorities must be adapted to local conditions. Finally, defining priorities leads to accepting "posteriorities," in other words, health problems judged to be less urgent and less important, and too often neglected— orphan diseases are an illustration of this trend. Another approach, one that is in our opinion more operational, is that of critical significance and globality of health problems.

A **health problem** will be considered **significant** if it:

- contributes substantially to the burden of illness in a population, in terms of prevalence and/or severity;
- has the potential of becoming a significant risk to community health status and general welfare;
- represents a major and identifiable financial cost to the community and/or the health care system;
- is amenable to improvement, thus increasing political and public pressure for corrective action.

A **significant health problem** will be considered **global** if it:

- affects people in many regions;
- affects people in only one or a few regions, but has the potential and probability of affecting people in many regions;
- cannot be solved by one region alone;
- is limited to a certain region, although research results can prove useful for other regions;
- calls for international and interdisciplinary response, research, and development.

Another aspect of this approach is the ability to think in terms of causality. Critically significant evolving problems are complex. Many causal and contributing factors influence human health; however, many of these factors are not yet fully understood or, perhaps, even identified. Population dynamics, mobility and migration, urbanization, industrialization, employment, energy, environment, food supply and nutrition, and social behavior all impinge on the health of individuals, families, communities, societies, and the environment—in short on the health of all. For instance, rapid aging of the population and changes in lifestyles and the environment account for the increasing prevalence of cancer, cardiovascular diseases, diabetes, accidents, suicide, dementia, and other chronic conditions. As already mentioned, the double burden of communicable disease and diseases of affluence in developing countries is being aggravated by the spread of the AIDS pandemic and the resurgence of such ancient scourges as malaria, tuberculosis, and cholera. Many of these health problems transcend national boundaries, calling for global solutions through international coordination and cooperation.

The traditional medical approach—symptom(s), diagnosis, treatment—does not fully apply to public health. We now know that all conditions of ill health are multi-factorial in their origin, and thus require a plurisectoral management. Let us elaborate in few words on the main determining factors that, in fact, interact with one another in a complex process.

Population Dynamics

The exponential growth of the world population, although moderate, is still increasing, especially in the less developed countries. From 6 billion people at the end of the 20th century it would reach a possible 12 billion by the end of this century. More significant still is the inequitable distribution of population density in relation to resources. Pressures from migration and refugees are evident. The effect of an older age structure in populations, already felt in developed countries, will soon affect the developing ones. Reproductive health and healthy aging constitute priorities for health services.

Industrialization, Urbanization

For all the benefits that industrialization and urbanization have brought, there has been a price to pay in overcrowding, exhaustion of energy and other non-renewable resources, habitat destruction, pollution, and an adverse impact on human health. This is especially the case in megacities or in the slums, where the overpopulation, the loss of privacy, and the worsening of living conditions pave the way to violence.

Environmental Health

The current destruction of the natural ecosystem will lead inexorably to the future destruction of the human habitat on this finite planet Earth unless drastic changes take place quickly. Climate change and ozone depletion are frequently cited, yet far more imminent are the effects on safety and quality of food, water, air, land, and the living and working environment. In the second half of the 19th century, the concept of public health started with development of private and public hygiene. It is now time to promote environmental health as a top priority and the involvement of modern public health.

Food, Nutrition, Water Supply

Many areas of the world already face insufficient or absolute lack of nutritious food and a safe water supply. Not surprisingly, foodborne or waterborne diseases constitute a big load in the burden of diseases. The potential of science to protect existing sources, and to provide new sources, of food and water is enormous. It must be mobilized.

Behavioural and Social Problems

In all countries, individual and social behavior is a major determinant of human health. Indeed, modern industrial life is creating new problems of affluence and lifestyle, including stress, substance abuse, violence, and a loss of sense of responsibility to self and others. Modern human growth has been described as "restless, ruthless, jobless, voiceless, and futureless." Mental conditions are increasingly recognized as major contributors to morbidity and loss of quality of life, but there is still much unknown that requires multidisciplinary research. The positive side is that collective healthy behaviour can be the best assurance for the attainment of health for all.

Poverty

Poverty ranks first among the social problems (Spencer, 1996). "The relationships between poverty and health are amongst the most constant and strong ever found in public health." (Haan et al., 1989) This statement by Haan et al. is reinforced by the common observations made in all countries, whatever their stage of development: Economic growth and improvement of health go together, up to a certain level. Unfortunately, the reverse is also true: The current financial difficulties and the bad health status of many people in many countries confirm the accuracy of this statement. Policies of structural adjustment have been detrimental to health, education, and social services almost everywhere that they were implemented. And, in contrast to the WHO definition of health, ill-health of underprivileged persons and groups is a state of physical, mental, and social disadvantage (*mal-être*).

Scientific and Medical Resources

In addition to the highly visible advances of modern molecular biology, practice and achievements in disease control and delivery of health care owe much to a range of other sciences. Other biomedical sciences—physical sciences and engineering, environmental sciences, social and behavioral sciences, educational sciences, economic sciences, information and communication technologies and public health sciences—all contribute to the effectiveness, acceptability, and sustainability of the effort to attain better health for all.

Biomedical sciences

After the enthusiastic hopes that arose following the discovery of penicillin, the chief disappointment in the accelerating race against the pathological microorganisms has been the rapid failure of our repertory of anti-bacterial antibiotics and the risk of a virtual desert of chemotherapeutics for viral infections. The second disappointment has been the emergence, or re-emergence, of infectious diseases, including AIDS, haemorrhagic fevers, and drug resistant iatrogenic infections.

The endless race against these organisms must be complemented by the fight against constitutional diseases, including cancer, cardiovascular and other non-communicable diseases, and hereditary and/or chronic diseases. The solutions are not simple; nevertheless, there has been a revolution in molecular biology and genetics, including the inter-species transfer of genomes, the elucidation of DNA and the mapping of the human genome. All raise important practical and ethical issues, but also open the doors to major applications in public health.

Physical Sciences and Engineering

A scientific and technological scene that contributes to human health is developing rapidly. In addition to molecular genetics and biotechnology, many other new diagnostic and therapeutic possibilities are emerging. These include laser technology, "designer" drugs, and surgical and prosthetic materials as well as imaging and visualization technologies. Information and communication technologies allow the effective gathering and utilization of public health information. Modern computing technology and the use of computational logic provide new opportunities for system modeling and for the use of advanced decision support at all levels of the health system.

Environment and the Hygiene Revolutions

The industrial revolution in the 18th and 19th centuries brought home the realization of the capacity of mankind to despoil and upset the balance of his natural environment. The response was first a hygiene revolution, drawing on physical, social, and biomedical disciplines and sciences, to find ways to ensure clean air, water, and living conditions, and to develop antimicrobial agents. Progress, however, was slow and inequitably distributed.

Today, in the face of rapid change, including nuclear energy and the dawn of a new age of information communication, nothing less than a second hygiene revolution is called for. This must begin with the worldwide assessment of human health in the environment, including monitoring of exposure, studies of environmental effects on life balance, assessment of human health in a changing environment, and assessment of interactions, using new bio-indicators, diagnostic tools, and sensing technologies. Global environmental epidemiology must attain a new dimension through risk assessment methodologies, appropriate indicators of exposure and effects, and the study of combined effects of mixed exposures. This should include integrated chemical and biological monitoring, supported by modeling of complex systems including food chain, energy flows, population change, and industrialization in relation to eco-systems. These ideas offer the beginnings of a second hygiene revolution, using all available and relevant scientific tools and intellectual resources, which may provide new repair and coping mechanisms to ensure the health of all mankind and of our planet.

Public Health

Public health is not a discipline in itself, it is a broad domain where various disciplines meet. The main characteristic that distinguishes public health from clinical medicine is its focus on the population at large, at various levels, from nations to groups of people linked by some common features. From its very beginning, public health has been concerned with classical hygiene designed to prevent the dissemination of diseases, including the notion of containment by the "cordon sanitaire." Engineering sciences, particularly those concerned with safe water and sanitation, continue to make a tremendous impact on health and human development.

As it applies throughout the life cycle at the individual, family, and community levels, public health embraces action and research on human reproduction, maternal and child health, adolescent health, occupational health, and health of the elderly. This is the field of social medicine, which is the meeting point where medicine, science and public health must merge for the common good. Research on behavior either conducive or destructive to health, including diet and lifestyles, is central to the public health approach. Poverty, as a fundamental determinant of ill health, is itself an important field for social research, drawing on sociology, economics, and other human sciences.

Mobilizing Science, Technology, and Medicine

Progress in some other scientific domains and technological breakthroughs may help medicine in its fight to contribute to world health, for instance in the social, behavioral, and educational sciences, health economics—crucial for the equitable optimization of shrinking resources—information and communication technologies, new materials, and products and instruments.

However, there is a basic requirement: One must bring the above sciences, the entire scientific community, and other relevant partners together to address the main issues, assume priority tasks, and develop the needed products, leading to the best scientific advice, technological development, and interventions—at the service of the greatest number of humankind.

Equally important is the mobilization of communities at all levels—including the world community—with a view to putting Health for All high on the local, national, and world agenda.

This mobilization of existing scientific resources and their use in improving population health is indeed a valuable objective. However, there is a need for an adequate methodology in planning, research, and development. The Research Policy Agenda referred to at the beginning of this chapter offers interesting openings.

First, starting from the existing data and from the various scientific resources previously mentioned, it is possible to prepare, for a country, a region, or a group of people, a visual health information profile (VHIP) under five headings: disease conditions and health impairments; food and nutrition; health care system(s); socio-cultural characteristics; and environmental determinants. If displayed along the radius of a circle in five sectors corresponding to the above-mentioned headings, the existing data provide a visual representation of health and health related problems in a given situation and time. This display makes the comparisons easier in space and time. Such a graphic indicates, also, the shortcomings in health information and the needed research.

The modern information and communication technologies can be used for further developments detailed in the Research Agenda: construction and functioning of a planning network for health research (Planet HERES) and the building of intelligent research networks (IRENEs) in order to facilitate intra- and international cooperation for health and health research and development. Such an approach allows the scientific community to become a partner in promoting global health.

Value Systems and Ethical Issues

Another chapter in this book is devoted to value systems and health care ethics; therefore, we shall only deal with some specific points.

We envisaged earlier the current perspectives on concepts of health and disease, health, nutrition and demographic trends, man-made environments, and health development. All, indeed, have ethical implications, and the ethical dimensions of these issues must be considered carefully, taking into full account their benefits as well as potential adverse effects.

While providing ways and means of solving major health challenges, science must help define the right balance between the protection of individual rights and public rights, both at various political levels and worldwide. Another ethical issue deals with human behavior vis à vis health. Many health problems, especially but not exclusively in the industrialized countries, are associated with behavior detrimental to health, at individual (risk taking) and collective (pollution, man-made disaster) levels. Other problems—permanent or universal, such as gender discrimination, mass population displacements, the AIDS pandemic—call for ethical approaches based on redefined societal value systems.

The new technological methods of collecting, retrieving and exploiting information facilitate its use, but may also increase the risks of misuse. Therefore, safeguards should be introduced to protect the privacy of people involved—with their informed consent—in any type of activity or research involving human beings. Steps need to be taken to ensure the confidentiality of personal data and the intimacy of private life. Health for all cannot develop without confidence and trust among the professionals themselves and between them, the users, and decision makers of health care.

Is ethics able to help, according to a well-known saying, "reconcile science with conscience" in the field of health? Probably so, if, not confining itself to medical bioethics, it becomes truly an ethics of life and health sciences. Indeed, medical ethics has experienced, in half a century, a tremendous change, evolving from the Hippocratic tradition to the development of bioethics linked to dramatic progress in science and technology, and then to the concept of equity in health access and care. However, as health is more and more seen as a human right, new ethical questions arise—a critical one is how to balance efficiency and ethics in the delivery of health care in a context of limited resources. This question is central to the renewal of the Health for All strategy. Increasingly, ethics stands at the crossroads of science, technology, health, and human development. And in the new field of evidence-based medicine, doctors and their co-workers must indeed conform to well-known principles that constitute the common denominator, or, better still, the humanistic core of classical ethics. However, some other principles are worth considering, namely: The principle of reality, including realistic appraisal of facts, constraints, limits, and opportunities, and of the results of medical activities; and the principles of responsibility, vis à vis the persons and groups needing health care. The German ethicist Hans Jonas has enlarged this responsibility into two directions. First, mastering the progress of technology and its application to health care, in order to prevent, or at least to control, its possible side effects. Second, to feel responsible—and act consequently—for the fate of the next generations. This second point calls for applying the principle of precaution in the control of the potential risks linked to the dissemination of new sources of energy, especially nuclear power. When one thinks of the strong links between environment and health, this responsibility for the future of the human species constitutes an essential principle of what is often called macro- or mega-ethics.

Another crucial concern already emphasized is the link between poverty and individual and public health. The principle of equity, advocated by WHO, calls for a fight against these unacceptable inequities—iniquities—between the rich and the poor in terms of health status, life expectancy, burden of disease, and handicapping conditions. Such a combat must address the cause, the roots of poverty.

As in Aesop's language, globalization may be either the best or the worst thing. It is the best when it develops international unselfish cooperation based on the feeling of our common belonging and acts in humanism and solidarity. It is the worst when it spreads a toxic culture, when it increases inequities, and when it encourages the confrontation between the right to health and the marketing of health care. The ethical choice is quite obvious.

Finally, ethics may be summed up as the respect of the dignity of every human being, whatever his/her race, religion, political belief, economic and social condition, age, gender, or health status. This is a burning and urgent obligation!

WORLD HEALTH TOMORROW: A VISION FOR THE WORLD COMMUNITY

If we are to implement the WHO slogan by the end of the current century and to make a utopia become a reality, a general mobilization is needed. The last three World Health Reports: 2002, *Reducing risks, promoting healthy life*; 2003, *Shaping the future*; and 2004, *Changing history*, pave the way for action.

First, a balance must be found between knowledge and action. On the one hand, research is essential to our understanding of health, disease, process of aging, behavior, and society. On the other hand, the amount of knowledge available today is largely sufficient to orientate much of our action for individual and public health. Evidence-based medicine, as valuable as it is, must not ignore the observation-based approach. We have a lot to learn from both.

Second, as already mentioned, cooperation between all health and health- related disciplines is vital, and the latter, health-related disciplines, are many. Health is too serious a problem to be entrusted to doctors alone. The reorientation of health services advocated by the Ottawa Charter must put more emphasis on prevention. Although suggested by the Charter, the mobilization of these sectors is not rated at the same level as the others. Nevertheless, it deserves to be highlighted as a specific goal, since intersectorality is crucial for achieving health. Sectors that need to be involved include finance, local government, education, information and media, agriculture, social welfare, defense, water and sanitation, private sector, religious sector, non-governmental organizations, and so forth. However, the number and variety of partners involved—varying according to the nature of the joint activities—increases the risk of people being lost between so many tasks and participants. One key role of the health sector is to act as a bridge between the community and other sectors, and another is to train and empower community members for complex joint venture. This is not wishful thinking, and some successful experiments clearly demonstrate the feasibility of such an approach.

Third, the empowerment of individuals and communities—two key recommendations of the Ottawa Charter—are crucial for health for all. However, it would be counter-productive and cynical to make people responsible for their health without providing them with the ways and means needed to exercise such responsibility. Ethics represents a safeguard against such practices.

Fourth, political will is crucial. It has prevailed throughout the process that led to the birth of the United Nations, including WHO. Such an impetus and engagement, both at national and international levels, is necessary if one wants the utopia—health for all—to become a reality.

Finally, to revert to the opening of this chapter, it is not necessary to reinvent what was so wisely codified almost sixty years ago. The vision needed is entirely explicit in the seven statements on the first page of the WHO Constitution. It is urgent to implement the guidelines that its founding fathers handed on to mankind. The necessary mobilization must be global: **All together for Health for All!**

REFERENCES

World Health Organisation. (1997). *A Research Policy Agenda for Science and Technology to support Global Health Development* (vol. 3, p.164). Report on the 35th session of the Global Advisory Committee on Health Research (ACHR), Geneva.

World Health Organization. (1999). *Constitution of the World Health Organization. Basic documents* (42th ed). Geneva.

World Bank. (1993). *Investing in health*. World development report. New York: Oxford University Press.

World Health Organization. (1986). Health and Welfare Canada Public Health Association. Ottawa.

Fendall, N.R. (1972). Auxiliaries and primary healthcare. *Bulletin of the New York Academy of Medicine.* 43, 1291–1303.

Spencer, N. (1996). Poverty and child health. Oxford, NY: Radclife Medical Press.

Haan, M.N, Kaplan, G.A, Syme, S.L. (1989). Socioeconomic status and health : old observations and new thoughts. J.P. Bunker, D.S. Gomby, & B.H. Kehrer (Eds.), *Pathways to health. The role of social factors* (pp. 76–138). Mento Park, Californie: The Henry J. Kaiser Family Foundation.

Section II

Systems

Chapter **6**

Health Policies versus Public Policies

ANDRZEJ WOJTCZAK

INTRODUCTION

Around the globe, health care systems are in a state of continuous reform and, in some countries, even in crisis. The media are full of concern about the unsatisfying health status of the people, health care quality, and about accessibility and the ineffective efforts to improve it. In spite of fast growing medical knowledge, advanced health technologies, and management techniques, the same old problems persist: rising costs, unsatisfactory quality and access to health care, and lack of secure health care benefits. We talk about an urgent need of substantial improvement, but we seem to have run out of good ideas and are becoming increasingly vulnerable to politically welcome, but technically bad, ideas. Even more disturbing is the fact that there is no clear vision for the future of health care. Although it is often said that the current problems emerged due to present economic difficulties, in fact they are a result of accumulated policy decisions made over the years. Health care definitely needs innovative policies, but not necessarily brilliant ideas from out of the blue, proposed without honest analysis of former failures and mistakes within the socio-economic situation of a specific country. It needs also a strong leadership able to enlist the support of politicians, policymakers, professionals, and consumers. Although leaders cannot change the course of the economy nor the basic values of respective societies, they can innovate, build consensus, develop institutions, propose mechanisms, and motivate the implementors. Leadership in the development of health policies has to start with a good understanding of the vision and values prevailing in a given society.

HEALTH CARE VISION AND VALUES

Health care systems are the products of broad public policies, and reflect fundamental societal values and cultures that differ from country to country. The vision of a health care system should be consistent with a country's existing values, and not with values we would like it hold or that exist and seem to function well in other countries. Therefore, we are very unlikely to be able to build an effective health care system without meaningful dialogue with policymakers, professional experts, and relevant organizations about societal values in the framework of political and economic conditions. Unfortunately, many recent reforms have been made with very little or no meaningful discussion with all pertinent partners. The requirement for building a coherent and sustainable health care system is to link vision and values with leadership.

In spite of deep economic and societal differences, almost all developed countries in Europe as well as in Canada, Australia, Japan, and countries with rapidly developing economies in Asia, possess relatively similar values and visions of health care policies. In these countries, access to some form of health care services is regarded to be a *human right,* and such values as *universality, equity* or *public administration* of the health care system are not an equivocal, even if the method of achieving them may vary. Although the health care systems may not always deliver the same services to all citizens and residents, equity—a principle that means everyone gets the same benefits, the same access, and the same quality of services—is in this group of countries, and, in particular in Scandinavia and Canada, is a prevailing value.

Universality of access to some form of health care services is achieved by such indirect means as mandatory coverage imposed by a government, but provided by individuals (e.g., Singapore) or by employers and labor groups (e.g., Germany) or in more direct form where the national health system owns, delivers, and pays for health services available to all citizens and residents (e.g., the United Kingdom). In Canada, the Health Act of 1984 has reinforced universality, equity, and public administration, observed even by the private sector.

Although many countries still are skeptical about *markets* and *competition* in health care, this attitude is changing. Some countries have started to promote privatization and market mechanisms to energize their health care (e.g., Central and Eastern Europe). Yet, too often the markets fail in health care and in health insurance, and there is a rather widespread view about the necessity and importance of the regulating role for *governments* or government-like organizations.

On the other hand, in the United States a different and in many cases even diametrically opposed view to the above set of health care values prevails. There is a lack of political consensus on such values as *right to health care*, guaranteeing availability to all citizens, and *equity*, guaranteeing everyone the same benefits, access to, and quality of services. The concept of equity is more appealing to

Americans as a goal for justice than for health care. Being against any kind of monopoly they highly value *pluralism, choice,* and *individual responsibility* in health care. If people choose to be uninsured, that's their choice and their problem. The scope of individual responsibility is extended to covering one's own health insurance. *Competition* is a value in itself, and very unique for that country are *volunteerism and community service.* Although the U.S. public shows *ambivalence towards the government's* role in public life, it nevertheless believes that government should play an important role, especially in helping the elderly and the poor to get access to health services. Generally, the public wants a mixed public and private model of health care and there seems to be a consensus that people should have the possibility to trade up for "better" health care services with their own money. It is ironic that the two most popular programs—Medicare and Social Security—are the fruit of governmental initiatives.

HEALTH VERSUS MEDICAL CARE

Usually, health services are understood to be a synonym of medical care, provided by doctors and hospitals. However, more and more physicians and others are realizing that lifestyles, occupation, education, housing, and socioeconomic status have at least as much impact on people's health as genetics or medical interventions. It is realized that many chronic conditions, such as high blood pressure, diabetes, and heart disease, can be controlled by exercise, proper diet, and avoiding alcohol and other harmful substances, and that healthy aging is more heavily influenced by lifestyle than by genetics. It is estimated that only 10–25% of the improvement in health status can be attributed to medical interventions. The rest is the legacy of improved nutrition, improved public safety, and more important, improvements in income, education, and wealth distribution in society. The most salient gains in the health status of the population can be achieved through broader social and economic interventions. Also the policymakers, government, and people are being increasingly aware that what creates health depends to a great extent on broad societal and economic factors and not on even the most advanced medical care. Although data show that the single most important variable in improvement in life expectancy and health status of a population is universal access to health care services, in the United States this is still not considered politically acceptable value.

Therefore, if we really want to improve the health of communities and not only secure better medical care, it is necessary to broaden our vision of health care services and include health promotion as a goal of universally accessible health care. Such an approach should be an integral part of our health policy systems and should be an important challenge that every society must face. Unfortunately, the public likes wellness and health promotion as general concepts, but when it comes to practical realization, surgery or medical interventions take precedence over prevention, for instance, in resource allocation. Here rests the irony in the health care versus medical care debate.

THE GLOBAL CONTEXT OF HEALTH POLICIES

With the leadership of the World Health Organization (WHO), the concept of *health care as a human right* has been re-shaping international health policy and influencing the formulation of policies at national levels. From its inception the organization has been playing the role of coordinator, initiator, and supporter of various campaigns and programs focused on fighting diseases of social relevance, such as tuberculosis and malaria.

The realization that many health risks are associated with modern, prosperous lifestyles and with the physical and socioeconomic environment in which we live, resulted in the adoption, by the Thirtieth World Health Assembly, in 1977, of a resolution widely known as "Health for All" (HFA). The follow up event, the International Conference on Primary Health Care, organized in 1978 in Alma-Ata, unanimously adopted a declaration stating "primary health care is the key to attaining the goals of the 'Health for All' policy." The HFA resolution and the Alma Ata declaration, both emphasized *equity* in health and *universal access* to health-oriented services, with special emphasis on primary health care and intersectoral cooperation. They both emphasized the development of national "Health for All" policies and strategies that promoted essential healthcare, accessible to all individuals and families in a way that they could afford, and with their full involvement. It also stressed the importance of "promoting health and preventing diseases" as a requirement for improving the health of the people. These policies, accepted by most countries around the world, have been dominating health care philosophy until quite recently. In some countries, the health of the people has improved, in others it has worsened, and new obstacles have arisen to challenge health progress.

The renewed HFA policy strongly promotes equity in access to health care and accepts primary health care as a valid basis for the development of comprehensive health service systems. It promotes improvement of life expectancy and quality of life through reducing the burden of diseases and disabilities and by forward-looking health promotion and disease prevention. It is now widely realized that health is an outcome of the actions of many socioeconomic sectors such as agriculture, education, transport, and employment, and not only the health sector per se; it needs the participation of private and public capital and institutions and also of the people themselves who must take a measure of responsibility for their own health.

In 1996, the European health policy based on such values as human dignity, equity, solidarity, and professional ethics was reiterated by the representatives from

Ministries of Health of 46 countries who met in Ljubljana, Slovenia. They adopted unanimously the declaration, which states that financing of health care systems should enable universal coverage and equitable access to necessary health care for all people as the road to improvement in the health status of the population. It also states that the reforms of health care systems should adopt the primary health care philosophy to ensure protection and promotion of health, prevention and treatment of diseases, rehabilitation, and care for the terminally ill. (The "Ljubljana Charter on European Health Policy"—EURO 1996).

Although in many countries governmental policies formally guarantee universal access, most health systems are unable to afford all the services needed by their populations and satisfy the insatiable health demands of an expanding rapidly aging population and changing epidemiological patterns. Therefore, in spite of that declaration, most health care reforms have focused on attempts to incorporate various market-derived mechanisms to achieve cost cutting, with less emphasis on improvement of the health of the population.

The observed successes of marketplace competition in controlling health care costs have started to slowly shift health security from the once unquestioned governmental responsibility to the private sector. In many countries, the private health option was welcome not only because it might help control health care costs or rationalize existing health resources, but also because the private sector health plans, in contrast to mandated single risk-pool public systems, might increase choices. For this reason, the public and private health sector leaders are gradually examining how to combine the innovations of the competitive marketplace with the larger social values of solidarity and health justice. The question is how to secure universal access to health care and attract private sector investment, and how the public sector can be successful in competition with the private sector in the open marketplace. The extent to which a private sector finances health care for a segment of the population that then no longer requires public subsidies will decide how much of governmental resources might be available to pay for population-based, community-wide health measures. All these provide both private and public health sector leaders an opportunity unprecedented in health care history, to establish the legitimacy and operational effectiveness of private health care systems and to forge public-private partnerships that serve the public interest.

However, the private sector must accept that in most societies, public opinion and policies consider health care to be a public good, distributed according to need, accessible to all, and financed on the basis of one's ability to pay. It must also be made clear that government is not the bureaucratic enemy of the private sector, and that without strong social safety nets and political and civil stability the private sector cannot flourish.

It must be noted that virtually all modern civilizations reject reliance on the marketplace for basic public health measures. On the other hand, in the midst of heated discussions and the daily power struggle to determine who will control health resources—doctors, drug companies, health plans, hospitals, government—the common and noble purpose of health care, important for all major stakeholders, is often neglected.

HEALTHCARE SYSTEMS

Although in most countries health care systems rank within the top largest economic sectors, health care is still too often considered to be a very expensive social expenditure based on high moral imperatives. The economic value of the creation of permanent and socially useful jobs by a robust health sector is too often forgotten; for instance, in the United States spending on health care is four times greater than spending on the military.

Among the various factors influencing health systems one of the most important is the sources of financing. To a great extent these sources determine the policies that influence the nature of a health system, with great implications for equity and accessibility of health care. The tax finance system imposes a larger share of the burden on people with higher incomes and user charges, and private insurance imposes a greater burden on those who use health care more. As resources for health care are always limited, it is not possible to do everything for everybody. Therefore, difficult choices that must be made all the time raise ethical questions regarding equity and access to health care.

In the majority of developed countries health care is a public responsibility. It is well recognized that every health system has flaws and that there are no ideal solutions for all existing problems, because every health system is a compromise between various factors such as accessibility, cost, quality, and service responsiveness that reflect the values of a particular country. Moreover, health care systems are frequently marked by fragmented care, inequitable access and uneven clinical quality, and rationing by under-funded systems. On the other hand, government interventions have increased almost everywhere and the ways and details of their application vary greatly.

Based on a recent international comparative survey published by Harvard University School of Public Health, the British public in 1998 felt more positively about health care services than it did ten years earlier, which can be linked to recent governmental financial support to the National Health Service System. In contrast, in 1998, Canada's system was less popular than it was in 1988, perhaps as a result of the austerity programs put in place in the early 1990s which led to longer waiting lists for services. The very low rating of the United States health care system in 1998 may be related on one hand to too-high expectations from the people, and on the other hand to the existence of 44 million people with no health insurance and, additionally, perhaps also to the fact that another 60 million are uninsured in any two-year period because they change jobs or lose work. There is also widespread uncertainty and insecurity about health care among a large number of the U.S. population under 65 years of age.

HEALTHCARE REFORMS

In general, the health policy objectives of reforms undertaken by governments in many developed countries during the 1990s have stressed equity in access to health care, macro- and microeconomic efficiency, consumer choice, appropriate autonomy for providers, and decentralization of health systems management.

A number of countries started to introduce elements of market-style incentives with continued public-sector ownership and operation of facilities. This hybrid approach has been given a number of different names: internal market, public competition, and quasi-market. The design and implementation of this type of planned market has been important in health care reform in Sweden, the United Kingdom, Finland, Italy, and Spain, as well as in various Central and Eastern European countries and the Commonwealth of Independent States (former USSR).

In countries with publicly operated command-and-control health systems, most of the reforms were market oriented—aimed at improving the performance of health-care institutions, quality of care, patient choice, decentralization, and administrative flexibility. By introducing the market-derived competitive incentives into the operation of their health systems, they hoped to achieve more with fewer resources. However, if the objective of the reform is an improvement of health care services and health status of the population, introduction of cost-containing mechanisms and improvements in financial and administrative effectiveness are not enough.

Therefore, the countries of the Central and Eastern Europe that were introducing profound political and economic changes substantially diminished peoples' access to health care services. Here, much blame can be directed to the international donor agencies and their experts for uncritical promotion of market mechanisms or exporting models from particular countries instead of taking a more country-specific view, because external assistance is not a major source of financing of health services in any country. On the other hand, in Northern Europe, where reform began, there has been a substantial retreat from the market-oriented incentives toward the original publicly planned coordination and cooperation.

There is no single concept of a market that can be adopted for use within a health care system, but, rather, market-style mechanisms. These include a number of different specific instruments, such as consumer choice, negotiated contracts, and open bidding that can be introduced on the funding of various parts of the system. On the other hand, all markets are regulated, and even in the absence of government intervention, a private sector regulates the market. Bureaucratic market regulation by public and private agents is unavoidable if there is to be competition in healthcare.

In the opinion of two world authorities in health economics—Professors Robert Evans (Canada) and Uve Reinhardt (U.S.A)—after several decades of experience in the developed world, it is fair to say that efficient and competitive markets for health care cannot exist. A truly private marketplace would require that the poorest and sickest in the population be excluded from access because they cannot afford the care they need.

If the philosophy that favors market forces dominates, the role of increasingly competitive for-profit organizations in the health care arena will grow into an enormous influence on the way in which limited health care resources are allocated, who is cared for, and what kind of care they receive. This situation is not acceptable to the majority of societies. It is not possible to finance a modern health care system wholly or even primarily through private markets. In all systems, the bulk of funding comes from the government, which is alone able to make the trade-off between public expenditure on health and other sectors. Therefore, the real choice is between an explicitly public, universal system of financing, and a mix of public and private mechanisms. This latter option yields a system heavily based on public funding but without a corresponding system of public regulation and control.

In Europe, governments reforming their economies are retaining their welfare states. The Europeans have decided to pay a price in some inefficiency of health systems for their political values, even though this might seem strange and irrational on the opposite side of the Atlantic. They are reinforcing the role of government, as there is no such thing as voluntary universal coverage for all citizens without a government mandate that obliges the individuals or their employers to purchase health insurance.

Cost-containment Measures

The common problems around the world have to do with cost and the inability to pay for health care on the one hand, and quality and accountability on the other. It is fair to say that all developed countries in the world have similar concerns about costs of health care and responsiveness to an increasingly demanding public.

Cost containment is a persuasive theme in all health policy, whether the debate is taking place with health care expenditures at 7% of gross national product, as in Japan and the United Kingdom, 9%, as in Canada and Germany, or 14%, as in the United States. According to the OECD in 1997 the highest health care expenditures per capita (adjusted for cost of living differences) were in the United States ($4,090), then in Germany ($2,339), Canada ($2,093), and France ($2,051), and in Japan and the UK, only $1,741 and $1,347, respectively. The OECD median was $1,747 USD per capita.

In Europe the history of health care cost control began with the cost-conscious voluntary insurers using a variety of devices to keep costs under control, so to keep premiums low and thus to attract a larger membership. Then came the government, which controlled costs by introducing regulations restricting the health insurers or vetoing any increases in compulsory health insurance premiums levied on patients. In countries which had inherited multiple insurers, their number was reduced, thus rationalizing administrative costs. Increasingly, hospitals planned to prevent wasteful duplication and expensive equipment and drug prices were regulated; the positive or negative lists of drugs which health insurers were prepared to cover were introduced, and the costs of sales promotion were limited.

At present in the European Union, the most commonly used methods that have successfully contained costs have been *global budgets* introduced from the top down, imposing for all or large part of expenditure a budget ceiling on individual hospitals, irrespective of ownership. This has led to reduced lengths of stay and the development of alternative health services to in-hospital care. The consequence of global budgets is *rationing* with apparently no negative consequence to the overall health status. Other methods have been *technology assessment* and *management of innovation*, methods that have been especially valued by the policy-making elites in such countries as Sweden, Canada, and the United Kingdom, where technology assessment is a much more central part of policymaking, controlling new technology and its diffusion. In this model relatively unproven technologies are either not approved or not reimbursed because they fail to pass hurdles of both efficacy and cost-effectiveness.

In the United States, health care has never been fully accessible and affordable for all citizens; yet, in spite of this, expenditures on medical care are among the highest internationally. However, the doctors, medical facilities, and health care delivery for the insured and those who can afford are considered the world's best.

In the United States, the public gives the highest priority to innovation; new technologies and cutting-edge medical care systems, which have led to an extravagant health system that uses technology with little or no difference in health outcomes. Innovation results from the strong pressures from interest groups on legislators and new regulatory mechanisms that too often turn out to be so many paper tigers. This is why the United States has been less successful than most developed countries in providing a sensible balance in cost containment, quality of care, and outcomes in terms of health status. Professional standards review organizations, certificates of need, and comprehensive health planning, to name but a few, have been relatively unsuccessful.

The lesson is that the countries that have applied methods containing costs from the top down have had much greater success than the United States' competitive models. Countries that started off cost-containment policies in the 1970s have maintained around the same share of GNP on health care spending, showing that macro-management of health care costs work. On the other hand, the slow down in the rate of health care costs in the U.S. in the mid-1990s attributed to "managed care" was relatively small and short-lived. Nevertheless, many still subscribe to the illusion that regulation is the enemy of competition, although elsewhere it has been shown to be one of the necessary conditions. However, it is necessary to stress that there is still no known mechanism that can contain costs indefinitely.

Managed Competition

Until the early 1980s, managed care providers supplied services at a cost much lower than the fee-for-service sector while imposing little or no rationing. According to the theory of managed competition, its sponsors, such as large employers, assist consumers in selecting among competing health plans on the basis of cost and quality. The idea was that consumers would make much more cost-conscious decisions about their choice of health plan because they were making decisions with their own money. Among different forms of managed care organizations, the most common in the U.S. is the *health maintenance organization* (HMO), which combines delivery and financing of health care services in a single system, providing an extensive package of services for a fixed annual fee, in an expected to be more efficient and high-quality way. Perhaps most important was the fact that health plans and integrated systems would be caring for a defined population and would support health promotion to keep people healthy, as well as keeping medical care costs down. It was really the very promising and stimulating framework of health care services hiding behind the rise of managed care in both the public and private sector.

Managed competition in the United States was a default policy for a quarter of century, consistent with American values such as competition, pluralism, individual accountability, and a limited role for government. It certainly has altered the landscape of U.S. health care, in spite of the fact that still over 80 percent of health care is provided by the nonprofit hospital sector. However, the managed care industry has managed mainly costs, but not care, with as yet unproved effect on quality and outcomes. It was also reluctant to include health behavior interventions in the coverage because preventive efforts incur costs up-front, while future, far down-the-line payoffs are uncertain. More recently managed care has been shifting away from a defined-benefit model to a defined-contribution model in which consumers are being asked to pay a higher share of their health care costs out of pocket for a higher level of coverage, superior benefits, or perceived improvements in quality of services. This shift from defined benefit to defined contribution is pervasive and applies to both the public and private sectors.

By 1998 it became increasingly evident that managed competition could neither permanently reduce health care cost inflation nor eliminate the costs associated with the rise of medical technology, increased utilization and pricing of new pharmaceuticals, or the rise in medical utilization for visits, tests, and procedures, and health care costs, as well as insurance premiums for employers, were on a rise again. The managed care plans instead of turning profits, turned losses. At present, even insured citizens are increasingly unhappy with access to and the quality of received medical care, and doctors are frustrated with different limitations put on their medical decisions. From the viewpoint of physicians, managed care is "maddeningly complex." Alain Enthoven, a professor at Stanford University and a "father" of managed care concluded: "Physicians are angry over their loss of authority, autonomy, and income. They want more money and freedom to practice." John Cochrane (1999), a former editor of Integrated Healthcare Report, expressed a similar opinion.

It now seems clear that employers and governments must give up their fantasy that managed care and, in particular, HMOs, have some magic ability that can provide a painless path to keep medical costs down. Managed competition is certainly in some disarray and can be questioned as the basis for health care policy. You cannot have a health care system in which benefit managers and health plan executives are happy, and patients and their doctors angry and disappointed. This growing dissatisfaction with managed care, coupled with the failure of some of the significant players in pure-market health care, led to questions about whether the traditional HMO approach is a viable answer for the future.

Certainly managed care won't go away, and, because there is still no alternative, one can expect that the most objectionable elements will be removed. Whatever course is taken by the health insurance industry, some of its potential for quality improvement and cost control, which are desirable to prevent another explosion of health care costs and for the elimination of inefficiencies, will remain. However, the problem is that competition cannot control the pressure on costs imposed by the expanding arsenal of new technology. Once increased competition squeezes out any remaining inefficiency in the system, it can produce further savings only when competing providers begin to impose serious restrictions on the availability and quality of care offered. This will bring back the present problems that it intended to solve.

Managed Care in the World

For the past few years managed care has been seen as a model and has become the mantra of health care. In various forms and to differing extent it was introduced in many countries with the great hope of making the health system cost-effective, improving quality of care, and of better financial status for the health personnel. In spite of significant interest in this very attractive concept, no one really wanted to replicate the U.S. model into their country's health system except for some elements such as privatization and competition that might stimulate government-run health care services to be more responsive to an affluent and sophisticated public. Moreover, managed care offers some potential in the areas of medical management (medical utilization and medical costs), demand management (identifying ways of intervening in the demand for health care), systems of accountability for cost and quality, and concepts of empowering consumers with education and providing new information, thereby preventing unnecessary and excess utilization of health services.

Alain Enthoven said in 1989: "It would be, quite frankly, ridiculous to suggest that we have achieved a satisfactory system that our European friends would be wise to emulate." Therefore, only some of the tools and concepts of managed care could have value globally if they were selectively applied and properly executed to fit a country's cultural and societal values, circumstances, and the political and economic environment.

DRIVING FORCES FOR HEALTH POLICY
IN THE NEW MILLENNIUM

Among the various driving forces that play an important role in the transformation of a healthcare system, a few seem to be front-runners.

Rising Public Discontent

One of the most important factors to contribute to the process of health system transformation in developed countries is a rising public dissatisfaction with health care, because health benefits have been eroding and consumers have to pay more for health insurance and health care services. This results in an increasing number of people who cannot afford to be insured, and in a rising number of uninsured or marginally insured groups.

In Europe's austere postwar environment, people were satisfied with the high marginal tax rates in exchange for a reasonable level of security through the social safety net, which made social services, like health care, available on a socially equitable basis. However, at present, because the economy has expanded, and because the marginal tax rates have risen to levels approaching 60 percent (or even more in the Scandinavian countries), European states are starting to run out of people to tax. On the other hand, there is increased sophistication and demand among the emerging middle classes that are no longer simply willing to accept the social welfare bargain of the postwar period. So there are growing calls from certain quarters, such as physicians and private health insurers, for privatization of the system. These pressures exist also in the United Kingdom and Canada, although the majority of citizens of these countries still remain committed to preserving a single-tier health system.

Consumerism in Health Care

A new phenomenon in health care is a growing consumerism that is responsible, at least in part, for a shift in health care values. This is due to the rising education levels of consumers, growing incomes in the top tiers of society, and the revolution in communication technology. Although consumerism in health care is presently most visible in the United States, it is spreading fast as a global phenomenon. Consumers are becoming more active due to better education, relentless coverage of advertising and healthcare issues in the media, and the Internet. The Internet, unlike broadcast media, knows no boundaries and opens up the possibility of both health care information exchange and electronic commerce across national boundaries. It leads to the creation of a more informed, skeptical, and demanding public. New consumers are also hungry for current, accurate, and understandable information about their health and available services. However, they need reliable and truthful information about technology, about what works and what doesn't, and what really contributes to health and what doesn't. They want to be involved in all choices related to their health care, including choice of plans, providers, and medical decision-making; they also reach out to alternative therapies as part of their medical care. Moreover, consumers are often ahead of the health professions in adopting electronic means of getting information, handling transactions, and communicating.

This increased emphasis on informed and empowered consumers leads to important questions: Will there be a slowdown in the rate of increase in health care spending, or will spending go off the charts? To date, increasing consumer involvement has driven up health care spending, because patients often demand more costly treatment even against the doctor's better judgment. However, there is a hope that by giving consumers information and treatment alternatives, patients, when presented with various treatment options, will choose a more conservative, less invasive, and less costly treatment. However, consumers with limited knowledge based on what they believe is best may demand inappropriate treatment for themselves or for their families.

There is a hope among health care administrators that consumers will trade up to more expensive forms of care with their own money. However, such an assumption seems to be premature, especially outside the United States, as traditionally health care has not been a market good for most consumers, and a third party has paid for rising health care costs. The question still remains, to what extent will consumers be willing to pay for the health care services they want, or will they continue to demand that third party payers share the cost?

The growing role of consumer in healthcare decision making points to a far-reaching trend and this will change the way health care services are accessed, financed, and delivered in the future. Consumer expectations will fuel demand for more and better services. Actually, the movement toward consumerism is not adequately reflected in the thinking of health care policymakers and legislative leaders.

Important drivers of consumerism in health care are *patient advocacy groups* and a wide range of *disease-related advocacy groups*. They have increasing power in the health system and have demonstrated an ability to significantly change the course of public policy. Advocacy groups are likely to grow more important in the future, and the Internet has provided a platform and vehicle for creating and sustaining them. Also an important contributor to the rise of consumerism in health care is aggressive marketing from pharmaceutical companies. Once prevented by regulation, this industry now sees *direct-to-consumer (DTC) advertising* as a major force in building brand and product awareness in the minds of consumers, and encourage users to visit their doctors and ask for the product by name.

Alternative Medicine and Self-care

The Internet is already revolutionizing the way people get their healthcare information and on how they should manage their diseases or family ailments; they act on new information and make decisions. It is part of a broader trend that consumers are taking charge of their own health due to growing skepticism in conventional medical care and in unbiased and honest professional services. As the Internet continues to grow, the way people access medical care will change, resulting in an increase in *self-diagnosis* and *sell-care*. The rise of alternative medicine not only reflects consumer preferences for natural products but also in some way shows discontent with the response of allopathic medicine to their health needs. In an atmosphere of recession and privately paid health care, self-care and less costly alternative medicine will tend to expand as individuals adjust to their new economic circumstances. Also the rapid growth in the number of people with chronic medical conditions is giving rise to increased interest in self-care.

Growing Role of Community in Health Services

An important challenge for improving health care services is to find ways to make community-based integrated health care systems work more effectively, providing also a greater continuity of care. Even though much of health care financing and policy direction comes from the national level, the local communities must be encouraged to create solutions that will improve the care and health of the people. The best examples are the World Health Organization programs—"Healthier Communities" and "Healthy Cities"—that have been adopted by a number of organizations that aim at stimulating people's interest in understanding the role communities play in fostering health.

The concept of an integrated community health system is an important scenario with a future impact on rationalization of health care delivery and meaningful change in financing health care. It will require the will of all local community stakeholders to work together to create solutions for themselves.

FUTURE TRENDS IN HEALTH CARE

At the beginning of the new millennium, health care systems seem to be ready for change. On the one hand were the fast growing global market and dazzling new medical technologies and, on the other, critical situations of health care systems in many countries are stimulating thinking about where the health care systems are heading. Unfortunately, there is lack of a clear vision for health care systems and what is more astonishing, a lack of meaningful dialogue and discussion among the various players as to how to solve problems and have compassionate, effective, and sustainable health care systems. Although all predictions for the future remain elusive, there is a need for possible scenarios as road maps for the future to provide clues about what may lie ahead. Their real value is to highlight the key opportunities and threats that demand planned responses.

First, we need to decide how far we are going to pursue the principles of universality and equity of publicly financed health care, and when we are going to admit that health care concerns also the private sector, calls for private resources, and needs people to co-pay for some of the services?

Second, we have to decide how long we are going to tolerate the present practices of managed care with giant health plans, incentives for frustrated doctors, and unsatisfied consumers who scramble to get what they need (and want) from an unresponsive health care system?

Third, we have to be clear about whether we are going to accept the principle that only the people themselves are responsible for their health, and for their choice between paying growing health insurance premiums for the necessities of daily life, without health being a government obligation?

These dilemmas indicate clearly that health care desperately needs *a new vision*. One of the main causes of the current difficulties about its future is that we have never, or only rarely, tried to connect all the elements of the health system together in an effort to find solutions. Therefore, we urgently need a societal debate on a broader vision of health, with greater understanding of its determinants, health behaviors and administrative and economic policies, all of which influence the health status of individuals and communities. This should provide a clearer view of the necessary elements and the requirements of a comprehensive health care system.

It is not possible to conceive a health care system run by market forces exclusively, nor a system in which the market doesn't participate. The notion that the health care field can be left to the consumers and providers is not only naïve but clearly an ideological nirvana. In a case of domination-of-a market scenario, in which health care will be available only to those who are able to pay, the disparities between the choice and quality of care available will grow. At one end of the spectrum there will be the wealthy, able to purchase the high-cost and marginal-benefit services; at the other end will be those unable to pay, for whom care comes primarily from charitable and public facilities, at a level far below that offered by the private sector. Consequently, a growing inequity in health care access and quality will evolve. It remains to be seen what degree of disparity in levels of medical care will be tolerated before the public demands the government's intervention to guarantee basic health rights and preserve the social order.

Therefore, governments—at federal, state, and local levels—are likely to maintain an important role as mediating organization in almost any scenario—as payer, provider, regulator, or enabler. In most countries, governments are already playing this role. There has to be some form of subsidy for both the poor and the elderly to ensure their access to some form of health care. However, we must also recognize the legitimacy of the roles played by the market, the independent sector and private organizations, because the future of health care seems to depend on mixed public–private forms, mediating between patients and providers. Both government and the independent sector have an important and increasing role to play, and none of these sectors is likely to disappear in the health care system. Public-private exchange is essential to resolve many of the challenges facing the health care system and health in general. Nevertheless, we need to look more closely at how government finances can be used more effectively, and ensure that technology, pharmaceutical and medical product companies are in a dialogue with the payers, and not just with the providers, as is the case now.

Progress toward a better health of the population cannot be made without universal access to health care services. However, it must be broadly recognized that there is no such thing as voluntary universal coverage. Progress toward universality will require an explicit recognition of floors and ceilings; a floor below which no citizen can fall, and the right to trade up with one's own money for the desired better health care services. We need honest consumer public debates about various conflicting health care values and about what is an acceptable level of service as a basic floor, and how much variation and difference between rich and poor we are prepared to tolerate.

The above-mentioned policy drivers—public discontent, growing consumerism, managed care, technological innovation, a broad use of the Internet, and the re-invention of the importance of community-based health care—will certainly affect health system development in the future. The movement toward consumerism in health care, fuelling demands for more and better services, will heavily influence how health care services are accessed, financed, and delivered. Consumerism is compatible with a growing focus on building healthy communities and strengthening the continuum of care in each community. The concept of an integrated community health system is an important scenario for the future impact on rationalization of health care delivery and meaningful changes in financing health care.

The role of leaders in health strategy development will be one of the most important factors in successful implementation of a needed new vision. The leaders have to develop a long-term strategy of health care and they have to create a supportive environment and build consensus through debate and dialogue around social values. On the other hand, to reform it it is necessary to seek the active support, participation, and leadership of the doctors who are the caregivers and decisionmakers in the delivery system. It is high time that physicians are brought back into the mainstream of development of a new vision for the future of health care. They must also decide about the future of specialty care that is becoming continuously narrower. Another area seeking doctors' contributions is the huge variation in medical practice standards. The reduction of these variations is unlikely to occur only through federal government regulations without the active involvement of physicians. Information technology and the Internet certainly will play an important role here.

Finally, there is an urgent need for new research and pilot experiments in health policies and in the marketplace. Different foundations, academics, and the media can play an important role in educating the public and the providers about factors improving people's health, the role and responsibilities of governments, and about the crucial contribution of health to the social and economic development of countries.

SELECTED BIBLIOGRAPHY

Abel-Smith B. (1996). The escalation of health care costs: How did we get there? Health care reform: The will to change. *Health policy studies* (Vol. 8, pp. 17–30). Paris: OECD.

Abel-Smith B., Figueras J., Holland W., McKee M., & Mossialos, E. (1995). *Choices in health policy: An agenda for the European union* (Office for Official Publications of the European Communities). Luxembourg: Dartmouth.

Dekker E., & Van der Werff, A., (Eds.). (1990). *Policies for health in European countries with pluralistic systems.* Copenhagen: WHO Regional Office for Europe.

Dekker E. (1994). Health care reforms and public health. *European Journal of Public Health, 4* (2), 281–286.

Enthoven, A. (1989, December). What can Europeans learn from Americans about financing and organization of medical care? *Health Care Financing Review,* Annual Supplement, 49–63.

Evans R.G. (1996). Marketing markets, regulating regulators: Who gains? Who loses? What hopes? What scope? *Health policy studies* (Vol. 8, pp. 95–110). Paris: OECD.

Jonsson B. (1996). Making sense of health care reform. *Health policy studies* (Vol. 8, pp 31–46). Paris: OECD.

Maynard A. (1991) Developing the health care market. *Economic Journal, 101,* 177–186.

Reinhardt U. (1987). Health care spending and American competitiveness. *Health Affairs, 8* (4), 5–21.

Saltman R.B., & Figueras, J. (1997). *European health care reform; analysis of current strategies* (WHO Regional Publications, European Series No. 72). Copenhagen. WHO Regional Office for Europe.

Saltman, R.B., Figueras J., & Sakellarides, C. (Eds.). (1998). *Critical challenges for health care reform in Europe (p. 424)*. Buckingham, Philadelphia: Open University Press.

Wojtczak, A. (1998). Health, disease and society in view of WHO health policy. *Japan Journal of Clinical Pathology, 46*(3), 203–210.

Wojtczak, A. (1998). *WHO health philosophy: A half-century of development (pp. 19–29)*. Opus Honorarium to B. Paccagnella, Studies of University of Padua.

Wojtczak, A. (2000). The concept, evolution and present problems of managed care in the United States. *E-Journal of Public Health Education, 2*, 70–81. Retrieved from http://www. aspher.org/D_services/I-JPHE/I_JPHE_Journal.htm

Wojtczak, A. (2002). *Health Care Systems*. In encyclopedia of life support systems (EOLSS). Global Perspective in Health, Oxford, UK. Retrieved form (http://www.eolss.net)

World Health Organization. (1978). *Declaration of Alma Ata; Report of the International Conference on Primary Health Care in Alma Ata* (Conference held September 6–12, 1978 Alma-Ata, USRR; Health for All Series No.1). Geneva, WHO.

World Health Organization. (1981). *Global strategy for Health for All by the year 2000* (WHO Health for All Series No. 3). Geneva: WHO.

Chapter 7

A Medicine Based on Evidence

J. Szczerbań

From its earliest beginnings, medicine—the discipline devoted to heal human beings—naturally began collecting evidence of good practice and of failures, and to learn from experience. These early databases of causal relationships and information about results developed, through the centuries, into a considerable repository of knowledge, tradition, and critique. In attempting to update this repository, contemporary medicine is facing an on-going dilemma in deciding what *new* is to be included and what *old* is to be removed. But the pool of accepted and questioned facts contained in the medical heritage is only one source of the difficulties now being encountered in identifying reliable evidence to be used in medical practice. Medicine *per se* is a combination of science (using strict methodologies), practice (utilizing accumulated and acquired expertise), and art (involving competence and skill), in its understanding and performance. All these components are necessary to practice medicine effectively. Thus, each one of them, although inherently incompatible, has to be reflected in the process of converting information into evidence, to generate guidance for preferred medical practice.

Evidence based medicine (EBM), a coherent basis for the practice of medicine, has been formulated in the face of the undeniably widening gap between available information and adequate absorption. The profusion of information flooding in is, for many reasons, not matched by a general ability to appreciate, evaluate, and utilise what could valuably be accepted. In particular, the dynamic multidimensional development of new health technologies, has itself created a hiatus between opportunity and utilisation. These are the circumstances in which evidence based medicine took responsibility for the rational adoption of scientific advances into effective and efficient everyday clinical practice. A crucial essay, "Effectiveness and Efficiency: Random Reflections on Health Services," by Archie Cochrane, (published in 1972 by the Nuffield Provincial Hospitals Trust), gave birth to the EBM idea.

Evidence based medicine, as a specific concept, was subsequently pioneered in the 1980s by a group from MacMaster University, Canada (Guyatt, 1991), and the self-explanatory term "evidence based medicine" accurately reflected their intention. The group conducted several studies into conceptual views of teaching, and functional aspects of clinical medicine, in the new scientific environment (the paradigm shift). The EBM idea, as it is now understood, has thus emerged in response to an unprecedented development of new medical technologies and methods adopted into clinical use.

DEFINITIONS

It is natural that the idea of EBM, now widespread and affecting a variety of medical specialties, would be differently interpreted according to specific applications. Thus, there are several descriptions of the nature of EBM. Some sources describe EBM as a *medical movement*, suggesting by this that the development is stimulated by natural needs, is self-promoting, and engages the whole medical profession, both direct users and supervisors. It asserts further that the movement is " ... based upon the application of the scientific method to medical practice, including long-established existing medical traditions not yet subjected to adequate scientific scrutiny" (www.nationmaster.com/encyclopedia). This definition also places attention on an important part of EBM—tradition, which is not necessarily recognized in standardized algorithms of treatment.

A concise characterization of the EBM core is given by Sackett et al. in their classical definition: "EBM is the conscientious, explicit, and judicious use of current best evidence in making decisions about the care of individual patients (Sackett, Rosenberg, et al., 1996). This formulation may be considered a prototype, and is quoted as such in the literature. It became a standard description of EBM and the concept itself has achieved great impact. Scientists, practitioners, scholars, and, last but not least, patients have consciously accepted the notion as pertinent to their needs and perception. EBM, directed to a wide range of users, has been developing into an auxiliary branch of health care, placed between theory and practice.

A comprehensive, explanatory account is given by W. Rosenberg et al., who interpret EBM as "the process of systematically finding, appraising, and using contemporaneous research findings as the basis for clinical decisions. Evidence-based medicine asks questions, finds and appraises the relevant data, and harnesses that information for everyday clinical practice" (Rosenberg & Donald, 1995).

MEDICINE IN FLUX

It seems that decisionmakers have not always fully realized that health care in the near future will undergo a substantial further transformation. The current common model of health care is oriented to disease and requires a basis of hospital medicine but, due to infiltration of the new information technologies into every sphere of human activity, this model is going through alterations that will require new steering instruments, refreshed intellectual preparedness, updated know-how, and additional resources. This infiltration, not infrequently spontaneous and, hence, unintended, is triggering new options for resolving clinical problems. Such new tendencies in medicine can be illustrated by the now commonly adopted, highly effective, and economically sound procedures of noninvasive surgery and video surgery, which restrict the extent of classical surgical interventions. There are new, efficient imaging diagnostic methods (computer image modeling techniques, CT, NMR, etc.). Ultrasound has become a routine reference diagnostic tool. There is also a wide range of other methods with functional diagnostic capacity. These examples illustrate a shift that was not at all perceived only one or two decades ago. Several surgical procedures, once classical, have disappeared from the operating lists. A noteworthy example is gastric resection for peptic ulcers. The surgery that was performed routinely for that condition for many years has lost its ground-ings after evidence came to light of the infectious etiology of the disease, which is caused by *helicobacter pylori*, and could consequently be successfully treated by antibiotics. The changing milieu of medicine needs rational, methodical, scientifi-cally justified evaluation and verification of the accumulated resources now at the disposal of medical practice. An abundance of options calls for solutions that are optimal, approved and scientifically justified.

The fundamental nature of these transformations needs clarification. Is it just the advancement inherent in any active domain, affected by adding new experience and new findings? Or is it a radical shift that affects the entire concept, role, prospect, and place of medicine within the global socio-economic system? The fact that decisive changes were not a consequence of "internal conversions," but resulted from influences from other domains of science and technology, such as informatics, creates a new situation. The change is not solely the result of an advance in traditional medical disciplines. On the contrary, the added value to medicine has been a result of an adoption of the new technologies driven by the needs of medical practice. This kind of merger effect supports the view that progress occurs on the borderline of two disciplines. In these circumstances, evidence based medicine should be the subject of continuous adjustment; regularly revisiting the status of health research and practice is therefore a prerequisite for the effectiveness of EBM.

Specifically, the immense inflow of new diagnostic and therapeutic applica-tions requires systematic assessment of their validity and applicability. The profu-sion of available optional proposals provided in the literature, which are sometimes misleading or confusing, calls for systematization and verification of the informa-tion to confirm its scientific rigour, prior to use in an individual patient. In short, practitioners have to be provided with credible evidence on which to rely in their day-to-day decisions. The process of converting research findings into practical recommendation is the essence of EBM.

Another EBM incentive is theoretical. The new environment in which modern medicine has to operate urges an innovative approach to research and medical practice. Applied research, practically oriented, has been brought to the forefront of attention. Comprehensive understanding of the cause-and-effect chain is needed. The concept of traditional academic medical education thus requires reconsideration: to shift, for example, from focusing on pathophysiology and basic sciences to better understanding of clinical manifestations of disease (Haynes, 2002).

THE ESSENCE OF EBM

The theoretical foundation of the EBM programme renewed attention to Thomas Kuhn's concept of the scientific paradigm, described in 1962 in his important book, *The Structure of Scientific Revolution* (Kuhn, 1970), and defined as ways of looking at the world that express both problems that can legitimately be addressed and the range of admissible evidence that may bear on their solution (www.cche.net). Notwithstanding Thomas Kuhn's concept of revolutionary shifts in science development (once enthusiastically received as admissibly interpreting discernible scientific facts, a view now not commonly shared (Franklin, 2000)), the paradigm concept is a convenient approach by which to explain the entirety of the transformation process. The shift of paradigm in medicine, mentioned above, conveniently reflects the meaning and mission of EBM.

Kuhn identifies evidence as a necessary component of the paradigm structure: It is a basic prerequisite of any scientifically sound solution. This logic was adopted in EBM theory and explicitly expressed in its name. Resolving medical dilemmas, one of the highest responsibilities of human action upon another individual (interfering with his/her biological integrity), is the essence of medical practice. Thus EBM, by addressing this priority, has recalled medicine's primarily pragmatic character and, in doing so, has expressed the need to bring closer together two components of contemporary medicine that had been drifting apart: biosciences and curative medicine.

The general idea of EBM is thus duly encapsulated in its definitions. Complementary comments concern EBM in action. Obtaining physicians' support and partnership in employing the evidence-based medicine appears to be an urgent issue. But there are other issues that need exploration. The original design of the EBM function probably did not strive to expand the already far-reaching extent of health development. Sackett et al., in focusing on practical aspects of EBM, concisely outlined its role as "integrating clinical expertise and the best external evidence" (Sackett et al., 1996). But the consequences of such a systemic integration have further implications and involve other parallel issues, such as the chain of problems linked to EBM. These are, for example: orientation of research, medical education priorities, relationship of official and traditional medicine, quality of care, patient safety, economic aspects of health services, and the like. Furthermore, a worrying increase in expenditure invested in research having a disproportionate return to public health prompts questions about priorities of investment.

Naturally, the wide range of problems logically but unintentionally linked to evidence based medicine can cause some confusion in perceptions of EBM, diverting it from its prime task and perhaps diluting its focus. By definition, it is a method designed to use the best evidence to assist optimal clinical judgment (Lloyd, Werk, et al., 1999). The promoters of EBM, interested in preserving the original meaning of EBM as a practical tool helping practitioners to trace and apply scientific advances, had at the outset warned against abusing the promulgated concept with unrealistic expectations; the appropriate place for EBM is solely in any situation where there is doubt about an aspect of clinical diagnosis, prognosis, or management.

The entire process of care is a result of several specific, interacting steps and components. These are, *inter alia:* recognition of the health problem (diagnosis), planning of therapeutic and diagnostic procedures (prescribing), application of treatment (therapy), monitoring of the process, servicing and nursing the patient, documenting the process (evaluation), evaluating intermittent and immediate sequelae and, eventually, the long-term final outcome (outcome). The EBM concept aims to treat the clinical routine as a *process*, with emphasis placed on the process of clinical judgment and decisionmaking as a logical and objectively justified sequence of events. Thus, the traditionally significant role of personal experience in "good practice," which is the result of empirical individual conviction, is strengthened and converted into a transparent process led and controlled by generally recognized evidence.

EBM thus encourages the habit of asking the questions *why? how?* and *when?* and of answering them all according to scientific requirements. This is particularly valid in surgery, where several methodological and technical options for the intervention may be available and where crucial questions about indications for surgery, timing, and tactics for surgical procedure have to be answered. A variety of competing methods may need to be considered, on the basis of rational reasoning backed by the evidence. So EBM is not only a *sine qua non* for unraveling the complexities of contemporary medicine, it is also a guide for navigating through the potential labyrinth of medical options.

CONTROVERSIES AROUND EBM

Critics may argue that EBM is nothing but *existing* health research (with special reference to clinical medicine). Medicine is a branch of science; all its clinical interventions are the results of research. Medicine does not accept methods that are not grounded in science. The pertinence of research evidence to clinical usage is a matter of competence; using research in support of clinical decisions is a matter of individual behaviour. All these remarks are valid, and do not conflict with EBM. EBM builds on the same principles with the aim, however, to streamline the process of applying research to practice and to make scientific advances directly usable wherever feasible. Concern has also been expressed that EBM is "chasing" after practicalities; in the process of translating science into practice it may subvert its original sense of seeking information, or perhaps, under the influence of lobbying bodies, it may derive premature or inappropriate conclusions. These are possible inconveniences, but they are of an "operational" nature; they do not contravene the method of EBM. Actually, EBM has triggered a general interest in research and reinforced the perceived standing of medicine in public opinion. It has enhanced the scientific background of medicine.

Clarity of the concept on the one hand and vagueness associated with its applicability on the other, have raised awareness of the possible misinterpretation of the EBM mission (Lloyd, et al., 1999). A crucial question appeared along with the promotion of evidence based medicine: How does the concept relate to established medicine? Is it a new science, a new trend in medicine, or just a new application of a conventional discipline? (Bauchner, 1999)

Such controversies and doubts, natural when an old, well-established concept is revisited anew, do not discredit EBM as a tool for careful usage. Discussions around EBM have revealed once more that medicine is too complex a domain to be treated in a simplified manner. And, it is interesting and encouraging to note that prominent clinicians, with undoubted scientific backgrounds, are defending the autonomy of medicine. Nevertheless, it is important to appreciate that EBM does not disregard medicine's integrity. It is using medicine "as it is" or as it should be.

But discrepancies among professionals do exist about the way in which EBM is to be conducted. Justified concerns exist about the credibility of evidence and the methods by which it is identified. The concerns warn against credulous acceptance of the method that would put EBM in danger of "becoming a new and unchallenge-able orthodoxy following its own political agenda" (Goodman, 1999). Some critics of EBM, in defending the role of the human factor in problem-solving, argue about hazards resulting from the employment of automatic "prompters" as a substitute for personal competence. This point particularly concerns the clinical professional expertise accumulated collectively at an individual health centre, especially in clinical "schools." Similarly, reservation has also been expressed about whether a resourceful health system, in the light of its entire multidimensional diversity, dynamically drawing from research, is able to accept a strict regimen of proce-dures; restrictive health care policies may happen to be counterproductive or even harmful. This concern may be especially valid for academic institutions inclined to contest the innovations in the course of exercising their academic autonomy.

THE ROLE OF RESEARCH

The role of research in modern society is not contested; nor is its relevance to EBM. The issue of research utilization is critical. What kind and quality of research is to be applied for EBM purposes? To what extent can research outcomes be translated into evidence to support practical applications in clinical medicine? What still remains research hypothesis and what is established fact? Who is to decide on this, and how? Questions such as these could be multiplied, but health research results can be ambiguous and their verification in clinical outcomes can be uncertain, so answers to these questions are not obvious, but are needed. Ethical constraints on clinical experimentation, the interactions of unknown or concomitant factors modifying a clinical picture, inadequate response to standard treatment by the individual patient—all these (to mention but a few) are responsible for difficulties in practising medicine. The current inclination to standardize medical actions by merging collective experience and knowledge into consensus statements, although alluring, is not always feasible. Nevertheless, there are some relevant procedures that can help—for instance, meta-analysis. This is a quantitative method of combining the results of independent studies (usually drawn from the published literature) and then synthesizing conclusions, which may then be used to evaluate therapeutic effectiveness, to plan new studies, and so forth; its applications are chiefly in the area of medical research (L'Abbe, Detsky, & O'Rourke, 1987). However, the psychological tendency to report positive results and to hide the negative ones is a bias to meta-analytical data and may undermine confidence in clinical trials; that risk needs to be carefully avoided.

In passing, it should be stressed that any political embargo on research is against the nature of the EBM concept[1]. Knowledge *per se* is neither ethical nor anti-ethical. But the way it is applied, and for what purpose, carries an ethical connotation. Scientific evidence in morally controversial areas could be biased, as happens, for instance, with research into therapeutic cloning and the use of embryos as a source of stem cells (Sandel, 2004). Therefore, science and scientific research, with their function to search for new knowledge, should not be restricted by decree. So, what is controversial? Some of the applications of knowledge—such as the splitting of the atom resulting in A-bomb development. Subsequently, an embargo on proliferation of nuclear weapons was imposed by international treaties, so it is therefore possible to control the use of research products (even conceding some breaches in the control), without imposing an embargo on research itself.

---

[1] "When prominent scientists must fear that descriptions of their research will be misinterpreted and misused by their government to advance political ends, something is deeply wrong." E. Blackburn: Manipulation of Science for Political Ends. Bioethics and the Political Distortion of biomedical Science. *NEJM 150; 14. 1379–80. April 1.2004.*

Behind the issue of standard performance there is another point in question: Is a practitioner obliged to implement standard approaches and advances in practice, or is this a matter of his choice? The answer depends on the system within which the practitioner operates and by which his activity is supervised. Some systems (such as managed care in the U.S., for example), due to their constitutional philosophy, are rather strict in applying the advocated norms of demeanour. It is rather unusual nowadays that an individual practitioner operates entirely outside any organization (corporation) or supervisory scheme, even if his/her institution formally does not belong to any corporation. The health care infrastructure and function, with all its legal foundation and tradition, varies widely from country to country and this determines intrinsically the status of EBM in given circumstances and attitudes towards it. Although academic schools and hospitals, medical professional associations, and quality assurance organizations, by definition, represent and implement evidence-based principles within their sphere of interest and influence, EBM is still regarded to a large extent rather as a desirable option than as a requirement.

In periods of resurgence of paramedical practices, there is a special need to reinforce the standing and comprehension of scientific medicine. EBM, with all its components, is perfectly designed to accomplish this task. The side-by-side existence of two health care alternatives: the official, academic medicine of so-called western type and another, "natural" or "popular" medicine, with its variants and different orientations, is not only confusing for the lay public but also can divert the patient from effective treatment. The EBM viewpoint on paramedicine still needs consideration; the problem is complex and multidimensional. Several branches of popular or traditional medicine, for example, traditional Chinese medicine, have through the accumulated experience of many years gained a favorable reputation and deserve attention, especially when supported by research studies. Several national research centres have been set for research on the validity of traditional procedures; the need for scientific certification of such procedures is acknowledged by the research authorities of traditional medicine who promote its place within the western health care system (Critchley, Zhang, et al., 2000; www.cochrane.org/colloquia/abstracts/capetown).

Whatever their nature, associations for research and educational organizations have a special role in promoting the concept of EBM. Under their influence there is a growing tendency to follow EBM policy as the only rational set of guidelines for health care services. In a modern world dominated by science and technology, evidence based medicine is an obvious component of modern culture. It is a product of progress and civilization. Ignoring the achievements of modern sciences in a deeply scientific branch of knowledge such as medicine would divert medical practice from rational thinking and professionalism. If this happened, the resulting impact on a most sensitive and responsible aspect of human activity—decisions and practices concerning human beings—would be inadmissible in an orderly society, and contra-indicated in any legal system.

VERIFICATION OF RESEARCH FINDINGS

Perhaps the most debatable aspect of EBM theory and practice is the methodology of converting research outcomes into "evidence," in other words, verifying the interpretation and conclusions from research findings. In order to serve efficiently in extracting valid evidence at the right time to assist in real problems, EBM recognises that an abundance of information is a real obstacle. The difficulty of browsing through immense lists of references, along with the accumulating stock of research, will be ever-growing. Ambiguity of data, if not critically assessed, can provide "evidence" of any pre-assumed concept. The situation well illustrates a paraphrased saying by Sir William H. Ogilvie "Whatever you want to believe, you can prove your theory in literature."[2]

Some difficulty in evaluating evidence in medicine lies in its very nature. The biological response of individuals to whom a standard procedure is applied may differ considerably due to many unknown factors. Medical evidence cannot be constructed on the basis of "mathematical" or black-and-white principles. It commonly contains a certain degree of approximation emerging from statistical calculations and averaging. Furthermore, in areas where the outcome of health care strongly depends on performance (as in surgery, for example), the approximation is even greater.

Due to their complexity and because of ethical constraints, scientific and technological advances in medicine require rigorous trials and practical verification before being recognized for clinical application. On the basis of consensual expertise the practically validated procedure for a specific problem is then validated and becomes the "gold standard".

A quantitative, numerical way of ranking data in human sciences (as also in medicine) for such validation could be questioned as being too "hard" for what is in fact rather "soft" material. Nevertheless, the principle of using measurable criteria in clinical research is rational. Numerically expressed data are computable, and hence are readily able to be compared, evaluated and generalized. Such treatment of data is a key to converting seemingly independent observations into evidence. By systematizing complex components of the clinical picture, the grading system allows the reporting of results in a relatively uniform and understandable manner. (The objection mentioned is actually a caution that statements in clinical medicine require critical appraisal.)

It is natural that introduction of any methodology for evidencing data, that is, applying scientific rigor to voluntary choices, will raise criticism about its validity. However, measurable and comparable data analyses obtained from prospective

---

[2] Sir William Heneage Ogilvie, British surgeon. (1887–1971). The original saying refers to experimental work.

randomized clinical trials are universally accepted as the standard for clinical research. If, in 1965, there were 100 randomized controlled studies in the United States, then today, more than 10,000 are published yearly (Ellrodt & Keckley, 2001). Statistical analysis to calculate the significance of the results obtained in the studies thus became indispensable.

To be converted into clinically useable evidence, any research should undergo a methodical process of scrutiny and further clinical monitoring. A rigorous scheme for evidencing research findings practised in scientific circles consists of several steps. Research results are submitted to thorough clinical trials. After being verified in the clinical setting and proved to be acceptable, diagnostic or therapeutic usage of such results is permitted. For novel procedures that modify the conventional approach to treatment, the evidence is subjected to further trials to prove its effectiveness against other methods before being recommended as the method of preference. This rigorous and costly process of translating research into practice is to ensure the patient's safety and to make sure that optimal care is offered according to the standards available at the current stage of knowledge. Immense research projects spontaneously carried out in innumerable laboratories and clinical settings are in fact inspired by just this process of validating evidence and optimising effectiveness.

E-HEALTH AND EBM

Perhaps the most significant recent advances leading to new developments in medicine are those of the ever-novel electronic communication technologies. In fact, unlimited and instant individual access to relevant information contained in innumerable databases and on-line publications, with the opportunity to retrieve original research resources, is the key to the success of evidence based medicine. Informational technology has allowed medicine to enter cyberspace with the development of new domains such as e-Health, a new sphere of knowledge currently under development with a number of practical outcomes. Utilising expansive communication capabilities, e-Health will increasingly play a crucial role in providing updated and accurate health information. Specifically, health informatics, a tool for professional intercommunication and interaction, enables the practitioner to enrich his/her experience and knowledge to optimise the quality of their clinical performance.

Governments and inter-governmental organizations, having recognized the potential of emerging communication technologies and their significance for health ecosystems, began adjusting their national health systems to utilise the new opportunities for health care development. In many instances, e-Health creates a new line of communication between consumer and provider, bypassing a once indispensable link—the doctor. Direct on-line dialogue is widely used in "direct-to patient" advertisements of pharmaceutical products. Any information is useful if the message transmitted is honest, reliable, and sufficiently complete. This condition is particularly valid for health. It is not uncommon, however, that commercial competition generates information that is misleading, if not harmful. For instance, direct-to-patient advertisement of drugs may suggest that avoidance of medical advice is possible. It may also imply that a recommended drug is free of side effects. Warnings that accompany the product's commercial announcement (on the attached information note, advising the patient to consult a physician) could easily be overlooked or neglected by the consumer in the face of persuasive arguments about the drug's benefit. On the other hand, the Internet does contain pages specially developed to communicate to a wide public on the advances in and potential of modern medicine, which are intended to help them overcome barriers of ignorance or concern when confronting medical realities. However, complex professional information addressed to the lay public, although or specially because of transmission in a simplified language, may be confusing or misleading. Yet an EBM "open dialogue" between practitioner and patient makes the mysterious process of the medical prescription both transparent and comprehensible. Transparency of medical procedures thereby ensures quality and, at the same time, provides the practitioner with a mechanism for patient's self-control of medical actions.

The above remarks simply underline the point that information technology, like any potent instrument, is to be used with prudence and purpose. The easiness of entry of information onto a web page indicates potential misuse of the Internet. Concern about validity of the retrieved information is naturally crucial. Setting up a mechanism to ensure credibility of information is an indispensable prerequisite of EBM efficiency. To preserve the ethical standard of disseminated messages, mechanisms for monitoring ethical aspects of health-related communication are needed and have been initiated.[3]

MULTIDISCIPLINARY SCOPE OF EBM

When first launched, the EBM idea evoked reactions from both practitioners and scientists. Questions and critical comments were raised, necessitating further clarifications.

Discussions concentrated around definition, methodology, practicality, conversion of research into evidence, reliability, and usefulness of evidence; these discussions have contributed appreciably to both theory and practice of evidence based medicine. The large quantity of published material on all aspects of EBM (theoretical and methodological reviews, analytical and critical essays, manuals,

---

[3] The International Code of Ethics for Health Care Sites and Services on the Internet.

research papers, correspondence, editorials, etc.) underscores the importance and timeliness of the concept. The distinct clinical specialties supported by specific areas of research, as well as different public health agencies and programmes, have come to define their own scope and orientation within EBM. These subdivisions of the EBM framework are dedicated either to different clinical specialties (surgery, medicine, obstetrics, ENT, anesthesiology, etc.) or to specific public health subjects (nursing, health promotion, primary health care, family medicine, ageing, epidemiology etc.). Accordingly, several descriptive explanations of the relevant idea to evidencing procedures in different areas of public health can now be found in the literature. (A glossary would contain such terms as evidence based nursing, evidence based pediatrics, evidence based health care, evidence based mental health, evidence based social services, etc.) In fact, any specific area of human activity, where decisionmaking could be guided by credible evidence, may adopt the EBM concept, appropriately adjusted. The common denominator for this is the methodology of identifying credible evidence.

THE MEDICAL CURRICULUM AND EBM

As a new trend in medicine, EBM demands an updated strategy of teaching curricula, in respect to both medicine and its practical component. Discussion of theoretical and methodological aspects of teaching medicine is naturally an on-going activity, and a number of leading academic authorities, together with relevant organizations, are engaged in the process of optimization of medical education. From a conceptual point of view there are two competing general options: "academic" and "professional." However, if treated as an intrinsic part of medicine, EBM offers an expanded model of teaching. In these circumstances, it is hardly surprising that discussions on how best to incorporate EBM into medical curricula are actively under way.

The argument for treating the medical profession as a technical service is that, nowadays, the practice of medicine requires from the performer several technical skills and expanded, sophisticated knowledge, and that teamwork (one of important characteristics of present-day medicine) characterises the model of healthcare. Accordingly, performance is the decisive factor of quality service; perfection is the ultimate goal. The entire progress of medicine is linked to scientific and technological achievements and the current concept of EBM is based on this reasoning.

There is justified concern that the teaching of contemporary medicine risks being overloaded with information of remote relevance or with simplified mechanical formulas. To avoid this risk it is necessary, regardless of trends or temptations, to give precedence to the brain over artificial intelligence (while not neglecting the latter).

In pursuance of the task of presenting data to the medical practitioner in utilizable forms, oversimplification could easily occur. The risk that evidence, when provided with too general an interpretation, might not sustain scientific rigour is not exaggerated—especially when the practitioner employs information in a mechanical way, without conscientious assessment. To avoid incompatibility of the evidence with the clinical problem, the practitioner needs to be taught science: its horizons, methodologies, and its research process. This will help him to comprehend the consistency of the evidence extracted from research. Thus, in order to meet actual EBM requirements, the medical teaching model should suitably integrate its dual domains: science and practice. A concern about overvalued "practicalities" in educational curricula, which could possibly lead to the conversion of an academic school into a professional one, is to be balanced by care for intellectual values. Contemporary medicine, notwithstanding its pragmatic shifts, is deeply anchored in science; thus it requires a well-balanced approach. Teaching EBM techniques, that is, dealing with evidence, is a specific syllabus item that is being developed by several medical schools and EBM centres. For example, a sequence of components as follows has been identified: (a) the clinical question (defining the clinical problem); (b) the best evidence (finding); (c) critique the evidence (evaluating); (d) apply the evidence; (e) and evaluate the performance (http://library.umassmed.edu/EBM/about.html).

By its very nature, EBM does stimulate the practitioner towards learning. Reference to the literature in support of a physician's decision means that the educational role of EBM is perhaps one of the strongest elements of its mission. The well-recognized problem that arises following the adoption of an EBM programme—the need for teaching EBM—has, to some extent, overshadowed the process of self-learning so far.

Continuous education—a prerequisite of modern quality healthcare practice—requires regular reference to the literature, updated research, experience, and shared expertise. Continuous education is also a tool for tracing research findings and for gaining shared clinical experience. In other words, continuous education (and self-education) in this sense is a means for keeping track of relevant advances in science and technology.

QUALITY ASSURANCE

Inherent within the EBM system is inscribed the quality assurance model. Quality is an inseparable component of EBM. In fact, the *raison d'etre* of EBM is to ensure quality for health care, to guarantee the optimal outcome of curative efforts—the prime aspect of treating human patients. Maintaining the quality of standards in health care, without referring to EBM, is simply impossible, because the indicators of quality to which to refer for purposes of comparison do not exist.

What principles would then be available to guarantee quality? One might argue that a value system other than EBM could contain the quality patterns. In theoretical terms, this might be true—providing however, that behind this hypothetical system there is an unquestionable validation. The grounds on which such a system would be based are obscure. On the contrary, the entire base of knowledge that is being used to practice contemporary medicine and which has proved historically to be efficient comes from science (combined with experience originating from science as well).

Quality assurance programmes are designed to investigate effectiveness, efficiency, safety, and standards of the health services and strategies and to identify measures for their achievable improvements. Because the primary goal of EBM was to enforce sustainable quality assurance of medical services, all efforts undertaken in pursuance of optimizing the entire health delivery system meet, in EBM, an efficient guardian of quality.

Sizeable investments in health care are not necessarily paying off in terms of the outcome of medical efforts. The main means to cover this gap is through the establishment of workable systems of quality assurance. This, with reference to EBM, is to ensure the rational exploitation of all available best resources (knowledge, technology, skill, experience) compatible with established actual quality/efficiency standards. Indeed, the success of the health care system depends on coherent interaction of these elements. Quality assurance is a means to generate, measure, and regulate those interactions. It is worth noting that sophisticated health care technology is prone to increasing the likelihood of human errors or of technical failures, both of which are important origins of departures from established quality criteria (http://www.eolss.net). EBM is able to play important roles here, both in referring clinical problems and dilemmas to research sources and in supporting the operation of quality assurance systems.

CONCLUDING REMARKS

To apply evidence based medicine correctly, with optimal benefit to the patient, no functions other than what EBM is designed for ought to be expected. EBM is, as an extensive discussion in the literature has clarified, neither new medicine nor a fad, but a new approach to the practice of medicine in the changing scientific and technological environment. It is an orientation towards the best possible exploitation of options offered by modern medical sciences and applied technologies for health care. Indeed, EBM restores the basic function of medicine by equipping the medical practitioner with knowledge of the most rational health care applications, while preserving, even strengthening, the cognitive role of the biomedical sciences. A balanced relationship between science and the practice of modern medicine is an important target of EBM: by referring to scientifically grounded evidence, EBM highlights the role of science; by asking questions from medical practice, health research is stimulated to find the answers. From the outset, medical practice was supported by rules of physics and chemistry—where scientific rigour is a methodological principle. Thus medicine, as a multidisciplinary domain, is a good example of how advances of different sciences can be absorbed; the multidisciplinary platform of medicine strengthens its scientific background.

Among other controversial points about EBM, the role of the individual practitioner's experience and skill in good medical practice should not be overlooked. Disregarding this would mean rejection of acquired competence as an important factor of good medical practice; and pressing for the exchange of an individual practitioner's expertise for some external expert systems is not necessarily preferable. On the other hand however, linking two incompatible elements—measurable, objectively verified research data belonging to medical science with the non-measurable elements of medical art—can create a methodological inconsistency.

Identification of proper, scientifically valid evidence is a crucial task and key to the rationality of EBM. EBM is valid only when the research from which the evidence is derived is credible.

Meta-analysis—an achievement in finding reliable evidence from clinical trials—may be subject to biased conclusions, because of the psychological tendency to exaggerate positive results and hide negative ones. Additionally, a biased stance by expert groups could affect the credibility of evidence. Furthermore, at the level of clinical decision-making, distinguishing real from estimated evidence is a matter of individual intellectual and professional aptitude.

In short, the perfect method for evidencing research data does not exist. Safeguarding the scientific purity of medical approaches is the common denominator of EBM, but in selecting evidence to fittingly resolve a specific clinical problem, it is sometimes unavoidable to rely upon the discretion of the decisionmaker. Here scientific rigour and personal experience meet.

Despite the presumed rationality of EBM principles and its manifest presence in clinical decisionmaking, clinical reality is often ruled by customary tradition, local habits and experiences nurtured in the past. Medical decisionmaking and practice can also be dominated by arbitrary decisions dictated by the hierarchical structure of the workplace. Critical observers of clinical realities think that sometimes persons in charge elaborate their own standard for evidence; these largely depend on personal preferences. A jocose description of such a stance refers to alternatives to Evidence Based Medicine as: vehemence based medicine; eloquence based medicine; providence based medicine; diffidence based medicine; nervousness based medicine; confidence based medicine, and so forth (Isaacs & Fitzgerald, 1999).

Difficulties in clinical reasoning may arise from insufficient, inconclusive, and misleading data. In situations when the clinical picture does not provide a consistent basis for diagnosis, the only solution is to expand diagnostic procedures and tests. But prudence in striving to betterment must be observed. Additional investigations, apart from consuming time (often precious) and resources (often inadequate) can lead to over-investigation, exhausting critically ill patients and aggravating the underlying illness. Over-investigation is as equally undesirable as over-treatment. In medicine, abundance can be as detrimental as indigence. Both can perhaps divert the course of disease and affect the prognosis. Indeed, there are reported cases where frequent and endless diagnostic investigations led to secondary distress and health impairment of the patient.

In the increasing globalization of competition, competitiveness of hospitals and outpatient clinics operating in a free-market economic environment forces them to observe standards, because these lead to their ranking according to efficiency. Certain health systems are checking such institutions with appropriate benchmarks of performance prior to contracting their services Transparency of operating health systems is thus an important argument for utilising EBM in everyday medical practice. EBM applied appropriately strengthens a physician's sense of security by maintaining his/her actions within accepted limits.

A critical insight into the reality of operating health care systems leads to the question of whether EBM needs active implementation or whether its obvious logic will make it self-promoting? Heterogeneity of the health care infrastructure and inequalities of rendered services urge active promotion of EBM principles at all levels of relevance: at hospitals, health centres, outpatient departments, individual practices, professional associations, and medical schools. Although widespread appreciation of EBM idea does exist, a holistic approach to EBM with the support of influential authorities is still needed in order to enhance the system and strengthen its performance.

Everything mentioned above points to EBM as a potent scientific tool to be applied with due recognition of its complexity. Manipulation of apparently readily available knowledge is contrary to the scientific method that must be scrupulously observed when dealing with humans.

REFERENCES

A paradigm shift. The Centre for Healthcare Evidence (University of Alberta, Edmonton, Canada) (http://www.cche.net)

Bauchner, H. (1999). Evidence-based medicine: A new science or an epidemiologic fad? *Pediatrics, 103*, 1029.

Critchley, J.A., Zhang, Y., Suthisisang, C.C., Chan, T.Y., & Tomlinson, B. (2000, May). Alternative therapies and medical science: Designing clinical trials of alternative/complementary medicines—is evidence-based traditional Chinese medicine attainable? *Journal of Clinical Pharmacology, 40*(5), 462–7.

Ellrodt, G., Keckley, P.H. (2001, August). Where medicine and technology meet. Health management technology web site http://healthmgttech.com/archives/h0801medicine.htm

Franklin, J. (2000). Thomas Kuhn's irrationalism. (from The New Criterion Vol. 18, No.10, June. www.newcriterion.com

Goodman, N.W. (1999). Who will challenge evidence-based medicine? J R Coll Physicians London May–Jun; 33(3):249–51. comment in Clin Med. 2001 Mar–Apr;1(2):154.

Guyatt, G.H. Evidence-based medicine [editorial]. (1991). *American College of Physics Journal Club, 1991, 114,* A-16.

Haynes, B.R. (2002). What kind of evidence is it that evidence-based medicine advocates want health care providers and consumers to pay attention to? *BMC Health Services Research, 2,* 3.

Isaacs, D., & Fitzgerald, D. (1999). Seven alternatives to evidence based medicine. *BMJ, 319,* 1618.

Kuhn, T.S. (1970). *The structure of scientific revolution.* Chicago: University of Chicago Press.

Liu, J., Li, T., Lin, H., & Wang, S. (2000). The need for systematic research in traditional Chinese medicine: Department of Epidemiology. Third Military Medical University, Chongqing, China web site www.cochrane.org/colloquia/abstracts/capetown)

L' Abbe, K.A., Detsky, A.S., & O'Rourke, K. (1987, August). Meta-analysis in clinical research. *Annals of Internal Medicine (Review), 107*(2), 224–33.

Lloyd, N., Werk, L.N., Bauchner, H., & Chessare, J.B. (1999, December 1). Medicine for the millennium: Demystifying evidence based medicine. *Contemporary Pediatrics, 12,* 87.

Rosenberg, W., & Donald, A. (1995, April). Evidence based medicine: An approach to clinical problem-solving. *BMJ, 310,* 1122–1126.

Sandel, M.J. (2004, July). Embryo ethics—The moral logic of stem-cell research. *New England Journal of Medicine, 351,* 207–09.

Sackett. D.L., Rosenberg, W.M., Gray, J.A., Haynes, R.B., & Richardson, W.S. (1996, January). *Evidence based medicine: What it is and what it isn't BMJ, 312*(7023), 71–2.

Szczerban, J. Quality Assurance. Encyclopedia of Life Support Systems (EOLSS) web site (http://www.eolss.net)

The University of Massachusetts Medical School (UMMS) web site http://library.umassmed.edu/EBM/about.html

www.nationmaster.com/encyclopedia

Chapter **8**

The Promise of Technology

PIERRE B. MANSOURIAN

INTRODUCTION

The last 150 years have been marked by unparalleled advances in science, technology, and industry. The health sector has been one of the main beneficiaries of such progress.

It is often argued that health technologies are responsible for excessive health care costs, and are not affordable by, and somewhat irrelevant to, the poor, being at best marginally efficacious.

While the criticisms are often justified, it is also true, as this chapter tries to show, that tremendous progress has been achieved in the prevention and control of disease; technology, in general, holds the promise for further gains.

The general theme of Science and Technology (S&T) is introduced first, together with a description of global inequalities within S&T and within the health sector.

The issue of cost is also discussed, followed by an overview of major, promising trends and prospects in technological development.

As in other aspects of Technology, health technologies become cheaper over time, thus improving their global accessibility and affordability.

SCIENCE AND TECHNOLOGY FOR THE WORLD

General Principles

The triumphs of scientific discovery and technological innovation have greatly increased society's comprehension of the ambient world and the benefits that can be derived from it. However, these benefits have been unevenly distributed across nations and within them. The process of rapid accumulation of knowledge and skills has not yet reached more than a billion people worldwide who are still living in absolute poverty.

One of the central issues of the new millennium is the need to build capacity in developing countries so that they can adapt to the challenges of continuous change. Achieving this objective will require universal access to information and to financial and technical resources, as well as the ability to use them constructively. Thus, it is necessary to formulate national policies and establish international arrangements that promote and protect the interests of all.

Historical Trends

Twenty-five years ago, at a Conference organized by the United Nations, (Davies & Mansourian, 1992) the Vienna Programme of Action on Science and Technology for Development was adopted. The global context was then very different, characterized by the North–South debate, lingering East–West conflict, and Governments' preoccupation with fostering technological capabilities. There was, at the time, little participation by the private sector, particularly in developing countries. In this environment, direct foreign investment was viewed by many developing countries and Central and Eastern European countries as a mechanism for control over their economies by firms based in developed countries, particularly multinational corporations. The international context changed considerably in the early 1990s. The end of the Cold War was followed by increased cooperation between countries of the former Eastern and Western blocs, and privatization, liberalization, and globalization began to span all continents. International agreements governing trade in goods and services, and investment and intellectual property rights were discussed and signed. Consequently, many developing countries adjusted their policies to nurture the development of enterprises, particularly small and medium-sized ones. This adjustment was accompanied by the transfer and diffusion of foreign technology and managerial know-how, various collaborative arrangements, partnerships, and networking within and between countries. Despite the obvious tensions created by such global changes, the process witnessed an increased diffusion of information and communication technology and a major restructuring of the system of production and work organization thereby affecting employment and international flows of money, people, goods, and services.

Future Needs

Can society afford not to get involved in the assessment of new technologies? The consequences of any technological innovation in the next century can no longer be viewed solely in terms of its benefits to specific groups or organizations, but should be assessed in terms of its full economic, social, and environmental impact on society at large. The assessment needs to be carried out with the full participation of all those concerned; of particular importance to the public are questions related to biotechnology and information and communication technology.

Furthermore, the ability of economic and social actors to generate and absorb new knowledge is fundamental to the dynamic functioning of innovatory systems. So, in the area of education, for example, priority should be given to (a) the elimination of illiteracy; (b) increased investment in higher education, especially in the physical and biological sciences; and (c) the promotion of vocational training.

Partnerships between private and public sectors are desirable, provided they are congruent with overall human development needs.

SCIENCE AND TECHNOLOGY DISPARITIES

Except for China and India, and possibly a few other countries, the gap (Mansourian, 2002-04) between high-income (a proxy for the rich North) and low-income countries (a class used as proxy for the poor South, notwithstanding big variations between, say, Southeast Asia and SubSaharan Africa) is large and growing. An example of calculations is given by the following approximate ratios (per capita, rich versus poor, OECD, World Bank, and UNESCO data, ca. 2002)

GNP/cap. (PPP, USD)	30 : 1
Telephones (fixed and mobiles) per 1,000	150 : 1
PCs/1,000	500 : 1
Patents	500 : 1
Publications	50 : 1
Energy use (Kg of oil equiv./cap.)	10 : 1

(PPP = purchasing power parity, adjusted dollars).

A basic difference between the "haves" and the "have-nots" lies in the extent of their scientific and technological development. Data derived from UNESCO and other sources point to a differential in R & D funding of the order of 100 : 1 per capita. Such disparity is reflected in output measures, such as publications and patents.

These figures emphasize the need for strong pro-development policies, with appropriate economic and financial support. It may be worth recalling that the total amount of official donor assistance (ODA) is a little more than 50 billion dollars per year (of which 12–15% is for health), that is, of the same order as the annual R&D expenditure of the pharmaceutics transnational corporations.

HEALTH DISPARITIES

Gaps can be assessed also by simple measures of health, such as mortality (World Health Reports, 2002-03). For example, the World Health Organization (WHO) has proposed a compartmentalization of the world into five mortality regions:

Group A countries have low levels of mortality—both child and adult (male and female)—and include OECD countries and Central Europe.

Group B countries have intermediate levels of both child and adult mortality and include most of Latin America, the Eastern Mediterranean, Southeast Asia, and China.

Group C countries have the same levels of child mortality as group B, but much higher levels of adult male mortality. All are located in Eastern Europe and Central Asia.

Group D countries, in Asia and SubSaharan Africa, have high levels of both child and adult mortality.

Group E countries are all located in SubSaharan Africa and have extremely high levels of adult male mortality and—in most of them—extremely high levels of female mortality (attributable in large part to AIDS).

WHO has also embarked on measuring health gaps in terms of "Disability Adjusted Life Years" (DALYs). DALY is a metric which combines information about mortality and disability into a single figure, expressed in the time domain. In other words, there are X DALYs lost due to a particular disease or risk factor.

At the turn of the century, about 20% of global DALYs lost were due to lower respiratory infections, perinatal conditions, diarrhoeal diseases, and HIV/AIDS. Projections for 2020 describe a different picture, with the principal causes of disease burden being ischaemic heart disease (5.9%) unipolar major depression (5.7%), motor vehicle accidents (5.1%) and cerebrovascular disease (4.4%).

In terms of risk factors, malnutrition has been shown to account for about 16% of the global disease burden, and poor water supply and sanitation for about 7%.

All these calculations have been used, obviously, to portray differentials among countries, within countries, and across regions.

GLOBAL COSTS OF HEALTH TECHNOLOGY

The World Bank and WHO have defined a minimum package to improve health in poor countries (World Development Report, 1993). It consists of two components: (a) Essential Public Health Interventions (EPHI) and (b) Essential Clinical Packages (ECP).

EPHI includes an expanded program of immunization; school health including deworming, micronutrient supplementation, and health education;

information on health, nutrition and family planning; tobacco and alcohol control programs; monitoring and surveillance, vector control, and programs for prevention of AIDS.

The second includes short-course chemotherapy for tuberculosis, management of the sick child, prenatal and delivery care, family planning, treatment of sexually transmitted diseases, and emergency care (such as pain control and management of minor trauma).

It was calculated at the time (1993) that these measures could avert more than 15% of the disease burden in low-income countries and more than 30% in middle income countries.

However, it has been reported (Sachs, 2001) that in some of the world's poorest countries, "the average of many basic interventions is falling, not rising. In many of these countries, the percentage of mothers whose childbirths were attended by trained mid wives or doctors is falling. Despite the importance of vaccination for child survival, levels of childhood vaccination stagnated or dropped in many poor countries in the 1990s" ... In his report of the Commission on Macroeconomics and Health (CMH), Sachs calculates that the annual net financing gap (in 2002 U.S. dollars) for all recipient countries would be 22.1 billion USD in 2007 and 30.7 billion USD in 2015 (Sachs, 2001).

One of the major estimated benefits would be that, by 2010, around 8 million lives per year, in principle, could be saved by the essential interventions against infectious diseases and nutritional diseases recommended in the CMH report.

Looked at on a per capita basis, these costs are not excessive, because they translate into 34 USD per person, per year (considering the average of 2,000 USD in high-income countries), of which nearly half could be covered by the least developed countries themselves. On balance, these calculations assume that low-income countries could devote 5% of their GNP to health (vs. approximately 10% in high-income countries).

The proposals of the CMH have been partly implemented, for example, by the creation of a Global Fund to fight AIDS, tuberculosis, and Malaria. The Global Fund has already in its 2-year existence committed USD 3 billion for 310 grants in 129 countries (www.theglobalfund.org). These three diseases combined kill more than 6 million people each year.

There is another way to look at the technological cost equation. It may be observed (World Development Reports, 2002-03) that high-income countries, on average, are spending in excess of 10% of their GNP on health (i.e., more than USD 2.5 billion per year, meaning some 2,500 per cap.). The differential per capita, therefore, is roughly 40:1. Most of this is due to technology, in the sense of products, services, and infrastructure.

The double burden of disease (communicable and non-communicable) needs no more emphasizing—people in low-income countries will be in need of, and expecting, modern health care. Hence the importance of affordable, up to date, "appropriate" technologies. One of the end products of scientific and technological progress, by essence, is a decrease in cost (e.g., computer memory) and there is no reason why, if looked at on a longer time-horizon, the reasoning could not apply to health.

TECHNOLOGICAL ADVANCES, TRENDS AND PROSPECTS

It has been argued that if the South were to spend as much as the North on health (by no means an insurance for good results), the expenditure would be 40 times greater per capita, that is, in excess of 12 trillion USD (Mansourian, 1995). This is more than twice the total GNP of all low-income countries combined. Because no one could ever envisage expenditures of this magnitude, it is understandable that all expert advice would focus on essential, preventive care, and cost-effective interventions.

In the long run, all these "appropriate" technologies are also dependent on the state of progress of science, which eventually translates into technologies, which in turn feed back into scientific knowledge.

It is therefore impossible to dichotomize technology into one for the poor and one for the rich.

Critical Issues: a Brief Overview

In relation to methodological issues for health development: (a) identifying, utilizing, and improving existing knowledge; (b) health measurement and monitoring; (c) "knowledge-based" assessment of health; (d) health data interpretation; (e) modeling and simulation; and (f) priority setting methodology; all of these are of top relevance to promote the R&D efforts required to improve health status and health care, particularly in underprivileged populations.

Contemporary technological advances have had important social consequences, for example (a) increased reliance on brain work rather than physical work and (b) growing mobility of labor. Major industries have developed, which are bound to impact health globally. Of particular significance are those related to biotechnology and to informatics.

Health technologies can be categorized as (a) preventive, (b) diagnostic, (c) therapeutic, (d) rehabilitative, and (e) auxiliary. Key technology drivers for the next ten years are thought to be: genetic engineering, nanotechnology, robotics, and artificial intelligence (AI).

Examples of genetic engineering can be found in drug design. The present cost of developing a new drug is of the order of 500 Mio. USD, and the time from conception to marketing spans about ten years. The goal is to reduce cost and time by 50–60%. To assist in this task, industry uses huge databases for millions of individual DNA sequences that are robotically tested, ultimately leading to the selection of a small number of active substances.

The second area, nanotechnology, is promised a brilliant future, with biochips reaching sizes smaller than one tenth of a micron. Computer chips already are as small as a quarter of a micron.

In the robotics area, surgical and minimally invasive techniques are currently in use and are amenable to wider application. Catheterizable robots are also susceptible to be used extensively.

The relevance of AI to public health is to assist the decision-making process. As has been the case in other sectors, "Knowledge Engineering" and "Computational Logic" techniques can prove useful. The task here is to measure health levels in a population, to have the capacity to analyze data, to distill information out of such data, then to synthesize the information to augment the knowledge base. The whole process should be able to improve the objectivity and rationality of decision making.

Major Developments

In an article entitled "Medicine gets cheaper," Peter Huber (a Manhattan Institute Senior Fellow) argues that the cost of health care in the U.S. has been declining steadily for the last 50 years (www.forbes.com/huber). This, of course, is not a widely held view. A characteristic statement is that "whatever it cost to develop the whooping cough vaccine or to distribute it free, the cost must merely have been dwarfed by the economic gains that came from freeing up mothers to engage in other pursuits." The same reflection could apply to other major health problems of the last century, which are now either preventable or curable, for instance, poliomyelitis and tuberculosis.

While vaccines and antibiotics have reduced the large amount of personal care that was required before their advent, thus freeing up manpower to augment economic productivity, spending on hospitals and physicians has gone up sharply.

Most of these dollars are spent buying time: in the U.S., 31% on hospital care and 22% on physician and clinical services. Prescription drugs account only for 11% of the "on-budget" health spending.

Vaccines and antibiotics have already demonstrated that they can change the economics of health care fundamentally. Initially, R&D costs are very high, but manufacturing is relatively cheap. Early on in a pharmacological assault, health technology is more expensive (more for the products, the skills, and the facilities). The argument is made, however, that as the results improve over time, the technology is able to displace and reduce the costs of manpower and infrastructure.

As Peter Huber concludes: "Yes, very difficult and expensive problems, as engineering problems go. But when well-engineered molecular machines displace manual labour, costs don't rise, they fall" . . .

PHARMACEUTICALS AND HEALTH CARE

The following sections highlight some strategic developments in the technology of pharmaceuticals (Financial Times, 2003):

Pharmaceuticals and biotechnology: A striking feature of the early 2000s has been a rapid rise in the number and value of biotechnology companies, followed by a rapid fall. Yet, since the beginning of 2003, the global biotechnology index has risen again, as a number of major clinical trials have been making progress, especially in the area of cancer therapy.

Pharmacogenomics and pharmacoproteomics: Since the human genome was mapped in 2000, life sciences companies have competed to put the identification of the human body's 30,000 genes to useful medical effect. One of the most challenging development concepts is the process of tailoring pharmaceuticals to a genetic profile. The principle is to use knowledge about genes—and the disease-causing proteins that genes express—to shape drug design. Hence, the term pharmacogenomics and, next in line, pharmacoproteomics.

Gene therapy: During the 1990s, several hundred trials of gene therapy were carried out, mainly on a small scale, for a wide range of disorders. Unfortunately none produced a clear-cut cure and, by the end of the decade, disillusion had set in. The dawn of the millennium brought better news: Researchers reported success with gene therapy for a form of haemophilia and for severe combined immunodeficiency (Scid), a life-threatening failure of the immune system to develop. Despite all its problems, gene therapy remains a very active field of biotechnology. According to a recent report (by Technical Insights), more than 300 companies are involved in gene therapy development and 500 clinical trials are in progress.

The original concept of gene therapy was to introduce correctly functioning genes to replace or augment ones that are not working properly because of an inherited disease such as Scid or haemophilia. But applications run far wider than that, because a gene could, in principle, be introduced to produce any therapeutic protein in human cells, for instance, dopamine for Parkinson's disease.

Cancer has a big potential for application of gene therapy. It is possible, for example, to introduce genes that make toxins to eliminate tumour cells, or to introduce genes that will stimulate the patient's immune system to fight cancer more effectively.

Aside from deciding which therapeutic gene to use, the biggest technical issue has been delivering the gene safely and efficiently to the target cells. Most gene therapy "vectors" are viruses that have been disabled genetically so that they lose their capacity to cause viral illness while retaining infectivity. Several types of viruses are in use, including adeno-associated viruses, lentiviruses, retroviruses, and herpes.

Drug delivery: Since the modern pharmaceutical industry evolved out of the chemicals industry at the beginning of the 20th century, pills that dissolve in the gut have been sufficient to deliver the majority of medicines. But the complex biological molecules such as antibodies, enzymes, and genes now being developed by the biotechnology industry are broken down in the gut before they can be absorbed. This has created a growing market for delivery technologies and devices to get them intact to their site of action.

New inhalation delivery techniques could revolutionize the use of established biotechnology products. Several companies are developing inhalers to deliver insulin via the lungs. These are still in development, but, if successful, could end the need for diabetics to constantly inject.

Patents: At the 2001 summit arranged with the World Trade Organization (WTO) at Doha in Qatar, trade ministers issued a statement that patent protection should not impair access to essential drugs; they gave a green light for poor countries to take advantage of exemptions in the trade rules that allow them to override patents. One issue was not resolved at the talks, however. Only countries with a domestic drugs industry could take advantage of these loopholes. The question of whether poor countries could import cheap copies of patented drugs from a third country was left open.

Since then, there has been deadlock. Developing countries have pushed for the right to "parallel import" essential drugs and many see the issue as a test of the good faith of the developed countries for negotiations on other charged subjects such as agriculture. Meanwhile the U.S. government, strongly backed by the pharmaceuticals industry, has argued that the right to import generics should be limited to AIDS, tuberculosis and malaria, three of the biggest epidemics facing the developing world. Paradoxically, this conflictual situation might create technological opportunities for developing countries, for example in the production of generics.

ADVANCES IN BIOMEDICAL ENGINEERING

The 20th century has witnessed considerable achievements in engineering, particularly chemical engineering, electrical engineering, electronics, and computing. The last two are creations of the 20th century and have contributed in major ways to biology and medicine.

GENERAL TRENDS

In a historical review article, F. Nebeker (2002) makes the following statement:

> The individual achievements of biomedical engineering have been astounding.

Exploratory surgery is almost a thing of the past, having been replaced by medical imaging. Tissue engineering has made great advances, including the creation of synthetic structures that the body recognizes as its own and the growth of a patient's own tissue in vitro for later transplantation back into his body. Microelectronics has been used to restore some control over paralyzed limbs. Cochlear implants allow the profoundly deaf to hear well enough to carry on a conversation. Artificial silicon retinas have been implanted in the eyes of blind patients. Computer-based simulators are beginning to be used in surgical training. And many other important achievements might be named.

Controversy, too, has increased the prominence of medical technology. It has been blamed for the huge increases in health-care costs. It has been criticized for dehumanizing medical care, as patients confront machines in the hospitals and receive computerized bills and health records. Some people have objected to the use of animals in research. And new technologies have raised new ethical issues, such as what measures should be taken to prolong life.

In prospect are advances that will increase still further the role of biomedical engineering. Natural organs may be regrown after injury or disease. Molecular nanotechnology may provide microscopic means for targeted delivery of medications. An all-inclusive lifelong health record (text, images, instrumental readings, and so on), under control of the patient, may be readily accessible. Precise understanding of genetic defects may permit more effective treatment by conventional means, and gene transfer may alleviate or correct problems resulting from genetic defects. Treatment at a distance, especially treatment in the home, may become common.

The following technologies appear to hold a potential for revolutionary impact in the first decade of the 21st century: advanced computer modelling and simulation of physiological systems; high-performance computing and distributed systems; Web-based means for interacting and for disseminating information; advanced medical imaging modalities; biomedical informatics; computer hardware, smart biosensors, implantable devices, and novel instrumentation; human performance engineering; high-throughput methods for genetic engineering; artificial organs and assist devices; rehabilitation engineering; and health-care evaluation systems (Nebeker, 2002).

The most visible achievements for the public have been the impressive variety of medical devices, particularly in the diagnostic domain: imaging technologies (CT, MRI, echography, etc.), but also electrophysiological methods (ECG, EEG, EMG, etc.). There have been advances, too, in the therapeutic and rehabilitation or assistive technologies. Examples of therapeutic technologies, apart from drugs and automated infusion systems, are cardiac pacemakers, defibrillators, auditory and visual prostheses ionizing radiation devices, and lasers. Assistive or rehabilitative devices (such as eyeglasses, canes, braces, hearing aids, respirators, etc.) aim at improving the quality of life and can be life supporting in many instances.

A less well known—and recently developed—area of biomedical engineering is "tissue engineering." Nebeker defines it as "the use of engineering principles, facilities, and theory to design and create tissues and devices to replace structures that have impaired function or have lost their function." As such, this new specialty brings together engineers, cell biologists, histologists, and surgeons in a team to improve the quality of life and to lengthen it. The activities range from the creation of new biocompatible devices, ranging from those made from non-biological materials (typically polymers, ceramics, and metal, all treated to be accepted by the host), to materials on which specially selected cells are grown on a scaffold matrix, some types of which are biodegradable. The cell types are selected to provide a function that is impaired or missing in the host.

The obvious desired characteristics of a tissue-engineered material are: (a) it should provide the impaired or missing function, (b) it should be biocompatible without treating the host to accept it, (c) it should not do more than is needed (i.e., it should not continue to promote unchecked growth, like cancer cells), (d) it should not have any immune or toxic side effects, and (e) it should remodel to become host tissue, indistinguishable histologically from native adjacent host tissue.

A significant body of research has been conducted during the past decade showing that tissue repair scaffolds, derived from native extra cellular matrix (ECM), can induce constructive remodeling of missing or severely damaged tissues. Use of these scaffold materials is associated with tissue healing that includes differentiated cell and tissue types such as functional arteries and veins, innervated smooth muscle and skeletal muscle, ligament, cartilage, and specialized epithelial structures. These differentiated cells are highly organized and the remodeled tissue resembles native tissue by the end of the repair process. The source of cells that contribute to this remodeling process has been the subject of considerable investigation, which is ongoing.

"One of these ECMs, derived from porcine small intestine sub-mucosa (SIS), has remodeled to become smooth, cardiac, and skeletal muscle, and tendon, ligament, and bone. It has remodeled to become a vein, an artery, the cusp of a heart valve, and even a vocal cord. It is an excellent wound dressing from pressure and diabetic ulcers. The active factors in SIS are under investigation and the FDA has given approval for orthopedic use and soft-tissue repair" (Nebeker, 2002).

FOOD TECHNOLOGIES

Another area of technology which is often overlooked, is that of food technologies (WHO, 1995).

They are used to ameliorate the nutritional quality and safety of food, to control contaminants, and prevent recontamination during or after processing. Some examples are heat treatment (including pasteurization and sterilization), freezing, irradiation, and disinfection with chemical agents and high pressure technologies (to kill microorganisms). In other cases, for example, for the control of contaminants, acidification, fermentation, drying, or freezing can be used.

Most foodborne diseases are preventable through the utilization of appropriate food technologies.

CONCLUSION

Biomedical technology promises great improvements in disease control and patient care. However, it is probable that cutting edge technology will continue to be viewed as an expensive luxury by many public budget managers.

They will plead for simpler "appropriate" technologies. Such views are understandable and legitimate.

At the same time, it is imperative to try to reduce the health inequalities within and between countries and regions.

This requires technological innovation which, like in any other sector, will be expensive initially, but can recover its development costs by and large, over the long term.

Considering the massive resources involved, the private sector is in a position to contribute as a major player. It has been demonstrated however that to leap forward, private-funded R&D often relies on public-funded R&D, which does seem to be more cost-effective.

REFERENCES

Davies, A.M.,& Mansourian, B., (Eds.). (1992). *Research strategies for health.* Published on behalf of the
    World Health Organization, Hogrefe and Huber Publishers.
Financial Times, November 2003.
Mansourian, B. (1995). ACHR news, *bulletin of the World Health Organization,* 73(2), 259–264.
Mansourian, B. (2002-04). Health science and technology: Gaps and opportunities. *Bull. Seanc.
    Acad. r. Sci. Outre-Mer,* 48, 475–486.
Nebeker, F. (2002). Golden accomplishments in biomedical engineering. Special issue of EMB, (entitled
    'Charting the Milestones of Biomedical Engineering).
    Note: special thanks are due to the Executive Office of IEEE and to their IPR team for permission
    to reproduce sections from Dr. Nebeker's chapter.
Sachs, J.D. (Ed.). (2001). Macroeconomics and health: Investing in health for economic development
    (Report of the Commission on Macroeconomics and Health).
World Health Reports. (2002-2003).
World Development Report. (1993). *Investing in health.* World Bank.
World Development Reports. (2002-2003).
WHO/FNU/FOS/ 95.12, World Health Organization, 1995.
www.theglobalfund.org
www.forbes.com/huber

Chapter 9

Critical Inquiries on Technology Utilization

ARMINÉE KAZANJIAN

INTRODUCTION

The emergence and diffusion of various types of health care technologies over the last two decades has been characterized by unprecedented vigor in development and proliferation. The degree to which such interventions have been embraced in the 'rational' health care environment of developed countries is hardly less than astonishing, given that the great majority have received little or no examination to scientific standards, which might demonstrate benefits or risks to health.

It is clear that the momentum of the overall process can be understood only by examining issues that go decisively beyond the clinical effectiveness of any given technology, or its latest application. With a broad cross-disciplinary analysis of the relevant processes, calling into consideration the social, economic, and political contexts within which these technologies have materialized, a more consistent picture emerges.

Under such analysis, benefit for the health of the population is not revealed to be the principal, or necessarily as even a subsidiary, impetus. We can, however, identify marketing strategies which have created the 'need' for product, test or intervention and which have been able to operate forcefully, without necessarily serving the health interests of the population groups they target.

Critical examination of specific technologies applied in public health can de-lineate some of these forces, and bring to light previously tacit assumptions that have driven technology use. Critical health technology assessment starts from a premise that clinical care does not simply reflect scientifically proven diagnos-tic and treatment protocols, but is embedded in, and shaped by, specific social, economic, and political contexts. Medicine and science take their place among other beliefs and practices that reflect and support the cultural values of society. Clinical medicine may therefore be viewed, not as a simple description of pre-existing biological realities, but as a reflection and perpetuation of complex societal power relationships.

From this perspective, it can be seen that a process of medicalization has, in the developed world, led natural life-cycle phenomena to become labelled as "disease." The general public is inundated with media coverage about "discovered" disease (Gifford, 1986; Skrabanek 1985), and the ensuing anxieties provide fertile ground for commercial exploitation. Social studies of medicine have repeatedly demonstrated how market forces may create and capitalize on a climate of risk and reassurance, which then drives the use of health technologies, regardless of whether they lead to an improved health outcome. This has been shown for pre-natal ultrasound (Rapp, 1995), electronic fetal monitors (Bassett, 1996; Kunisch, 1989), predictive genetic and other screening (Marshall, 1996; Nelkin, 1996), hormone therapy (Haraway, 1990), and mammography (Gifford, 1986; Lock 1996), among others (Koenig, 1988; Strother-Ratcliffe, 1989).

This chapter seeks to demonstrate that forces beyond sustainable claims of health benefit are operating to support the use of some mainstream health care technologies. A brief survey of four such cases follows: bone-mineral density (BMD) testing, cholesterol testing, prostate-specific antigen (PSA) testing, and laser treatment for benign prostatic hyperplasia (BPH). These modalities range in unit cost from inexpensive to very expensive, with some gender-specificity.

BONE-MINERAL DENSITY TESTING

In an internationalized marketing effort, many aspects of women's life-transition have been repositioned so as to conform to a bio-medical model. One of the most conspicuous recent examples is the targeting of women's bone density as a focus of concern. Early (and hence of necessity, repeated) use of technology to measure bone-mass has been presented as the only hope for preventing bone fractures.

Mainstream media advertising in the developed regions of Europe, North America, and elsewhere has promoted a range of technologies and pharmaceuticals aimed at women, presented in the context of managing an apparent epidemic of the disease identified as osteoporosis. The diagnosis of this condition is widely believed to be reliant on the technology that measures bone-mineral density (BMD).

In the early 1980s, most women had never heard of osteoporosis. Beginning in 1982, sponsored by a pharmaceutical company, an 'education' campaign was launched to create public awareness of osteoporosis as an important women's health issue. The company clearly stood to benefit from increased public awareness of osteoporosis, and women who sought advice from physicians about prevention might easily end up with a prescription for hormone therapy (Mintzes, 1998).

The campaign included radio, television, and magazine coverage, such as various articles in *Vogue*, *McCall's*, and *Reader's Digest*. As Whatley and Worcester explain, by the mid-1980s, women had not only heard of osteoporosis, they had become frightened of what seemed to be the inevitability of postmenopausal hip fractures and of a life of disability and dependency (Whatley, 1989).

In 1993, an industry-sponsored conference convened by the World Health Organization (WHO) redefined osteoporosis strictly in terms of BMD thresholds (WHO, 1994). The WHO definition establishes four thresholds based on reference populations of healthy young women—these are used for diagnosing osteoporosis and determining intervention. Using the WHO standards, 22% of all women over age 50 are defined as having osteoporosis and 52% as having osteopenia. (Ringertz, 1997).

It is important to appreciate, however, that there is no epidemiological basis to support the cut-offs used by the WHO study group. The "epidemic" observed to have swept the globe in recent years is consequently more apparent than real (Green, 1997).

Whole population screening of women using densitometry has, in fact, been widely discredited (Barlow, 1996; Coupland, 1996; Green, 1997), yet BMD testing of all women at or near menopause presumably to prevent fragility fractures 25–40 years later is still being advocated. And, moreover, on the basis of the strength of the WHO conference definitions, unless women maintain bone mass at peak levels throughout their life span they will be labeled as "at risk," or "diseased." As a result, despite mounting evidence that BMD measures have a very low positive predictive value, entire cohorts of middle-aged and older women are labelled with their BMD measures.

The reasons why BMD testing retains an appeal for women and their health care providers do not emerge from the debates on clinical effectiveness, which have centred on estimating when to screen and how many fractures need to be prevented before the intervention can be deemed cost-effective (Hailey, 1996; Marshall 1997). We have, therefore, to ask why women seem placidly to accept commercially motivated interventions and associated technologies that have no relationship to their health needs.

A cross-disciplinary perspective, and in particular a range of critical social studies tools, can explore the social environment in which life processes such as menopause are being medicalized. Critical analysis shows that BMD testing has been effectively diffused because it is marketed and promoted in ways that draw on, and perpetuate, two trends in western popular culture: (a) the medical model of the aging female body; and (b) the fear of aging and its association with disability, dependency and immobility.

The Medical Model

It may be surprising to the western peri-menopausal "patient" that in many cultures, as shown by cross-cultural research, the onset of menopause may bring increased social status to women. In the technologically driven societies however, the feedback loop between popular and scientific knowledge has created and perpetuated the notion that the aging female body is a diseased body.

Since the mid-nineteenth century, female life cycle transitions in Western societies have been increasingly medicalized, that is, interpreted by physicians as a series of events that should be subject to medical management (Lock, 1993; Kaufert, 1988; Kaufert, 1986). Biological changes associated with aging are spoken about in a language of decay and abnormality. The biochemistry of women of reproductive age is taken as the standard measure for what is normal and healthy; and aging women's bodies are understood in terms of "endocrine deficiency disorder," a hormone deficiency disease that is to be treated with estrogen supplements (*Kaufert, 1988; 1986; 1982*). Although passage through the life cycle is both a social and biological process, the focus of attention in medicine has been increasingly confined to biological processes, such as "failing ovaries."

Popular magazine articles and books on menopause contain essentially the same message: The subject matter focuses on biological changes associated with menopause, and rarely puts menopause into a larger context or discusses the subjective experience of individuals (Lock, 1993).

It is, unsurprisingly, a short journey from the well-entrenched medicalized model of menopause to the medicalization of bone-mineral loss. BMD testing "works" in Euro-American societies because it has emerged out of, and in response to, culturally accepted norms about women's bodies and women's roles in society as legitimate concerns of the medical sphere.

The Fear of Aging

Aging is associated with a cluster of meanings involving emotional and physical losses, including declining social status and degradation of self image as the western cultural ideal of youthful femininity can no longer be met. The social meanings associated with aging also include deeper fears of disability leading to loss of independence (Whatley, 1989).

Featherstone and Hepworth (1991) have commented on the fear held of the aging body in contemporary Euro-American societies. They refer to the "mask of aging," the physical signs of "decay" such as wrinkles and grey hair, from which women dissociate themselves. As they note, such a conception of aging "sets great store on the belief that aging is a potentially curable **disease**" (emphasis in original) (Featherstone, 1991).

Once the fear of becoming diseased has been created, women are made to feel personally accountable for managing their risk of disease and for future illness, and are encouraged to take appropriate measures to prevent such disease (Hubbard, 1990; Gifford, 1986; Nelkin, 1996; Koenig, 1988; Posner, 1991). Given that menopause has been defined in terms of hormone deficiency (and osteoporosis is increasingly defined in relation to that deficiency), any woman who wishes to avoid the "diseases" of aging will have to be tested for BMD and, if deficient, will have to take homone therapy.

Psychological side-effects of BMD testing, which result from being labeled as "at risk" will only add to the anxiety caused by popular media coverage about a new disease. The negative impact of labeling is well-described (Goffman, 1963). The identities and life experiences of women labeled as being at risk will be altered significantly—in the absence, let be it noted, of physical symptoms or disease.

But when concepts of risk, that is, probabilities of epidemiology, are transposed into everyday clinical practice, it is inevitable that an identified risk will be interpreted as something from which the patient suffers. Being at risk has come to mean being diseased, and disease must be treated.

In short, on-going medical intervention has come to be seen as necessary to prevent the body from aging.

In this susceptible market, medical technologies aplenty are developed and promoted to meet the need. No matter that the social determinants of health are important risk factors for individuals and populations alike. Adverse social conditions are hardly fertile ground for commercial exploitation. Social determinants are therefore ignored, in favor of ever more intent targeting of groups 'at risk'.

The implications of the 1993 redefinition of osteoporosis for the lives of women remain largely unexamined by scientific research. At the very least, testing and labeling large cohorts of pre- and peri-menopausal women as abnormal in BMD is leading to increased dependency on BMD testing and associated interventions. Repeat testing becomes necessary and hormone therapy would be administered over many years in order to ensure that women retain normal levels of bone density.

But what could be a more powerful inducement to embrace technologies than the marketing of fear? In the time leading up to the WHO redefinition of osteoporosis, drug companies, aware of a massive potential target population of baby-boomers, readied themselves to capitalize on a fearful generation. The economic implications of repeatedly testing and treating female baby boomers from age 50 until they turn 85 are truly staggering.

CHOLESTEROL TESTING

Another new "disease," the condition of "high cholesterol," has become an especial focus of a veritable new pharmaceutical industry in itself. This condition is easily detected by the testing technologies that have become a commonplace of general practice care; a large armory of drugs has been made available to treat it. As these drugs are very widely prescribed to a broad demographic of middle-aged men, women, and the elderly, it is not surprising that they have proved hugely commercially profitable. Yet what benefit is to be derived by use of cholesterol testing and treatment technologies?

Cholesterol has long been identified as a cornerstone of both clinical and public health strategies aimed at reducing the burden of heart disease. A number of clinical practice guidelines, which generally recommend cholesterol testing in men and women with risk factors for coronary heart disease (CHD), and in men and women with previous myocardial infarction (MI) or angina (Savoie, 1997), have been developed throughout the world. Guideline developers justify the use of cholesterol testing by considering it an important element in the overall assessment of an individual's risk for heart disease (Working Group, 1997).

Whether recommended as a stand-alone test or as part of a heart disease risk assessment, the question remains: What is the contribution of cholesterol testing? In other words, what more do we know about an individual's risk of heart disease after cholesterol testing that we didn't know before? Does adding cholesterol testing to the overall assessment of an individual's risk of heart disease provide useful information likely to alter individual patient management and achieve better health outcomes?

The utility of cholesterol tests has been examined to show, in typical scenarios, the contribution made by a cholesterol test in the overall assessment of an individual's risk profile for CHD. Even in individuals with higher cholesterol levels, a sensitivity analysis (Savoie, 1999) has shown that the net contribution of cholesterol testing remains well below 10%. In other words, while elevated cholesterol is a statistically significant risk factor for CHD, its clinical utility is very limited.

When examined together with other risk factors for CHD such as hypertension, diabetes, smoking, and left ventricular hypertrophy, cholesterol testing provides very little additional information and does not significantly help identify individuals at increased risk of CHD. Even in individuals with multiple risk factors for CHD, an elevated cholesterol test provides little additional information to help identify those individuals at risk of developing CHD. Analysis (Savoie, 1999) shows that, based on the evidence, the net contribution of cholesterol testing is unlikely to change patient management.

The reasons why cholesterol testing is of such limited utility are linked first to the low prevalence of heart disease in the individuals tested and, second, to the significant overlap between the cholesterol levels of individuals who develop and who do not develop heart disease. In a key study, Wald et al. reported on the range of cholesterol values of middle-aged men with and without heart disease (Wald, 1994). These authors found a very important overlap between the cholesterol levels of men who developed and those who did not develop coronary heart disease. This overlap implies that for any cholesterol level, the tests will more often than not lead clinicians to draw inappropriate conclusions, by suggesting that individuals are at risk of heart disease when in fact they are not, or that they are not at risk of heart disease when in fact they are. The effect of prevalence on post-test risk of disease has been well described.

Existing cholesterol testing guidelines provide little information on the utility of cholesterol testing and no discussion of the clinical implication of pre- and post-test risk of heart disease. The limited data they provide is compatible with the test utility as estimated by the Framingham risk equations (Anderson, 1990). The Canadian Working Group, for example, report post-test risk of heart disease ranging from 0.7% to 12.4% in individuals without heart disease but with risk factors (Working Group, 1997).

A further issue to consider when examining the utility of cholesterol tests is that a growing body of literature has concluded that the benefits derived from lipid-lowering interventions, mainly statins, were independent of the baseline cholesterol levels (Rosengren, 1998; Grundy, 1998; Cullen, 1997). This implies that something else beside cholesterol levels should determine eligibility for treatment, factors such as age, sex, and the presence or absence of heart disease.

Although most current guidelines support the use of cholesterol testing either as a stand-alone test or as part of an individual's risk assessment for heart disease, the analysis has shown that the utility of cholesterol testing is very limited. It tells us little more about an individual's risk of heart disease than can be determined by examining other risk factors (such as hypertension, diabetes, smoking, and left ventricular hypertrophy). In addition, the contribution of cholesterol testing is such that based on the evidence patient management is not likely to be affected by its addition.

Two Further Examples

Prostate-related technologies applied to men. The first is a screening procedure, prostate specific antigen (PSA) testing. The second is a device used in a hospital setting, laser treatment for benign prostatic hyperplasia (BPH).

PSA Testing

The rise in the incidence of prostate cancer has been another "fear and anxiety" topic of considerable media interest. The marketing of fear in relation to aging is again at play, because if the recorded increases were shown to be "real," this would naturally be of great concern to men. Yet, when the utilization rates of testing for prostate specific antigen (PSA) are related to variation in the rates of prostate cancer incidence and mortality in a geographically defined population, the results support the hypothesis that trends in prostate cancer incidence and mortality are due, at least in part, to fluctuations in prostate cancer screening/case finding intensity (Green, 1993; 1999).

On the face of things, it might be assumed that earlier detection of cancer in individuals would lead to earlier treatment, and therefore to better outcomes. But there are at present important knowledge deficiencies in this field, and a number of authors accordingly argue that earlier detection of prostate cancers with any strategy is contra-indicated.

There are several reasons for caution. A key factor is that the majority of cancers are not likely to progress so as to result in premature death and/or serious illness. At present, it is not possible to predict which prostate cancers will progress dangerously. A recent study concluded that the rate of the rise in the PSA level— PSA velocity—during the year before the diagnosis enhances the ability to identify men who may not require immediate treatment (D'Amico, 2004). Nevertheless, most men with localized prostate cancer are symptom-free; yet side effects from treatment by either surgery or radiation treatment may be severe and life-long. There is also the risk of treatment-related death.

Consequently, the benefits of early treatment for localized cancer are uncertain. There is a real danger that a large number of men who would otherwise live out their normal life-span with asymptomatic prostate cancer will instead be burdened with the emotional impact of a cancer diagnosis, and health problems (impotence, incontinence, urinary strictures, and death) subsequent to treatment.

Currently available evidence does not support the conclusion that screening asymptomatic men with PSA leads to fewer deaths or an improvement in the quality of life for those with prostate cancer. It is quite possible that many men in whom prostate cancer is detected through screening intervention will not in fact benefit from treatment, but will actually be less well off, due to the consequences of aggressive strategies of diagnosis and treatment.

PSA screening is, in itself, an inexpensive technology. But this cannot be used as an argument for its widespread use in a population of asymptomatic men. Routine PSA screening would almost certainly result in significant net harm to the screened population, because many more non-progressive cancers would be detected than progressive. The inevitable result would be removal or irradiation of many more prostates that would not progress to clinical cancer. These treatments, besides being unnecessary, carry the risks noted, together with the heavy costs of initial treatment, and managing the subsequent effects.

PSA screening therefore is not a cost-effective intervention. An effective screening test must lead to more good than harm for the people to whom it is offered. Early detection screening strategies differ from diagnosis in that the physician is looking for disease in people without symptoms; therefore it is particularly important to observe the injunction of Hippocrates, "above all, do no harm."

Yet in the currently inadequate knowledge of the natural history of prostate cancer, it is not possible to predict reliably the natural course of a given tumor. But many, if not most, asymptomatic men, when faced with abnormal PSA results, might naturally fear the worst, and be prepared to undergo aggressive treatment and experience serious complications in large numbers. As we have noted, labeling, in this case as having cancer, can itself be emotionally and socially devastating.

Any move to introduce wide-scale screening in asymptomatic men would inevitably initiate a chain of ever more invasive and risky procedures in this population, perhaps culminating in radical prostatectomies in those with essentially normal prostates. This must be a clear violation of the precept 'first, do no harm.'

Laser Treatment for BPH

In general, the device industry is the least regulated in the health sector—with sometimes deleterious effects on patient populations. The development of lasers has been (in common with many technologies) pursued by industries unrelated to health. Uncertainties in laser use in health care have discouraged most companies from investing in these applications. But laser treatment of benign prostatic hyperplasia (BPH) has emerged as a potentially huge market for the laser industry, and consequently an attractive technology for development and application.

Laser technology for BPH is expensive and necessarily hospital-based. For present purposes, it is enough to note that diffusion rates and patterns are dependent on its use by academic physicians and specialists who are eager to develop programs of research. Again, it may be thought that efforts to establish evidence on the use of a given technology might serve to clarify the benefits of its use.

In Canada and the United States, lasers have been approved as safe to treat a general category of soft tissue, skin, glandular, and connective tissue problems. In the United States, however, which has more rigorous control of medical devices than in many other countries, the Food and Drug Administration specifically notified laser manufacturers in 1992 that they could not market lasers for treatment of BPH.

Elsewhere there is much less clarity. A study in a Canadian hospital setting (Bassett, 1996), sought to examine the basis for introducing laser technology for BPH, and for establishing a clinical program for its use. It found that the process set up to consider this question did not bring about consensus between representatives of the participating professional groups: urologists, the device industry, the hospital authority, and evidence-based methodology researchers.

The local urologists primarily saw the new BPH technology as an addition to their therapeutic armory, which they were entitled to build up within the hospital and deploy in patient care. They regarded the technology assessment process, not as a means to improve patient care, but as primarily bureaucratic, designed to prioritize competing budget requests.

The laser industry representatives were determined to stay ahead in the technology market, which meant maintaining a high profile for their products among urologists. Consequently, they targeted the clinicians (the urologists) themselves, rather than the representatives of the hospital that would purchase the technology.

The hospital technology-assessment representatives considered the technology in terms of individual patient care, in wider terms of population health and community needs, and also with regard to hospital resources within the entire health region hospital group.

The evidence-based methodology researchers focused on the strengths and weaknesses of effectiveness evidence and its relevance to the hospital. Their concerns were with the weaknesses of both efficacy evidence and relative efficacy evidence. This perspective argued that without sufficient evidence there could be no basis on which to select between varieties of laser technology and other competing technologies.

What emerged clearly from this study was that various groups had divergent rather than convergent priorities and agendas. It illustrates that in the diffusion of technologies, hidden and often self-serving dimensions may exist in hospital technology acquisition processes. Without adequate scrutiny, it is clear that the acquisition of technologies (here, for the treatment of BPH) may reflect the predominance of marketing efforts by the device industry. Companies approach clinicians directly, urging them to use their powerful influence on purchasing decisions, regardless of the evidence on effectiveness that can be related to public-health benefits for the population.

CONCLUSION

It can be established that the recently heightened profile of women's health issues, such as osteoporosis, and men's health issues, such as prostate cancer, are based more on economic premises than on sound evidence from technology assessment. The marketing of fear over impotence, infertility, and the "diseases" of aging is manifestly capable of supporting whole industries of health care products, suddenly found necessary to combat the discovered epidemics of our age.

Clearly, the sensibiliies of the target populations are part of the social sphere in which marketing forces can operate successfully. In the west, the cultivated "vanity" of women, or "sexuality" of men are susceptible to fears of inadequacy in a competitive cultural atmosphere promoting these values.

While the developed Euro-American societies have been the cradle for nurturing the commercially advantageous phenomenon of creating demand by identifying potential epidemics, it can hardly be overlooked that large populations in the developing world represent a hugely attractive target for applying the same concept. Certain regions are now producing much wealth for select groups, and consequently offer an almost perfect market for technologies that can be easily promoted as attractive commodities.

But what is the health-need? If a society has been not merely content that its members accumulate the wrinkles, graying hair, and other manifestations of the advancing life-cycle, but has honored them, why should it seek to embrace the medicalization of their status? Costs to society are enormous and extend beyond inefficient ways of financing health systems. There are serious implications regarding opportunity costs: funding is diverted from more effective, basic public health interventions, such as nutrition, which yield more certain and widespread benefits for population groups.

In addition, negative results on screening tests usually lead to large numbers of further testing for follow-up and one or more therapeutic interventions including invasive surgery or use of pharmaceutical products with high harm-to-benefit ratios. The human cost to unnecessary treatment, including emotional and psychological harm, is rarely quantified when economic analysis is undertaken.

To resist this globalizing phenomenon, it is important that health-care professionals and decisionmakers have a clear sense of the variety of forces seeking to propel it forward; and of how important is the need for scientific standards of assessment of health-care technologies. When the evidence on effectiveness clearly does not support the pattern of diffusion, a critical approach should be applied so as to provide a broader perspective within which power relations and private interests can better be understood. Appropriate mechanisms that bring together technology assessors, healthcare providers, policy makers, and non-governmental organizations, are required for taking results of scientifically rigorous comprehensive assessments and translating these into public policy, and more importantly, for identifying cases where regulation and controls are needed to constrain the use of unproven technologies.

The ultimate goal of critical inquiry is to produce evaluative frameworks that will make transparent disparities among population groups that are created through inappropriate use of health technology, and to produce decision support tools that promote equity in health and healthcare.

REFERENCES

Anderson, K.M., Odell, P.M., Wilson, P.W.F., & Kannel, W.B. (1990). Cardiovascular disease risk profiles. *American Heart Journal, 121*, 293–8.
Barlow, D., Cooper, C., Reeve, J.,& Reid, D. (1996, February). Department of health is fair to patients with osteoporosis. *British Medical Journal, 312*, 297–8.

Bassett, K. (1996). Anthropology, clinical pathology and the electronic fetal monitor: Lessons from the heart. *Social Science and Medicine, 42*(2), 281–92.

Bassett, K., & Kazanjian, A. (1996). Incorporating clinical effectiveness debates into hospital technology assessment: The case of laser treatment of benign prostatic hyperplasia. Vancouver, BC: British Columbia Office of Health Technology Assessment.

British Columbia Council on Clinical Practice Guidelines (1996). Cholesterol testing. Vancouver (BC): The Council.

Brown, J., & Kerns, V. (1985). *In her prime: A new view of middle-aged women.* Massachusetts: Bergin and Garvey.

Coupland, D., Lentle, B., Aldrich, J., Connell, D., & Janzen, D. (1996). Recommendations for the measurement and quantification of bone mineral density. *British Columbia Medical Journal, 38*(5), 265–8.

Cullen P, & Assmann, G. (1997). Treatment goals for low-density lipoprotein cholesterol in the secondary prevention of coronary heart disease: Absolute levels or extent of lowering? *The American Journal of Cardiology, 80*, 1287–94.

D'Amico, A.V., Chen, M.H., Roehl, K.A., & Catalona, W. (2004). Preoperative PSA velocity and the risk of death from prostate cancer after radical prostatectomy. *New England Journal of Medicine, 351*(2), 125–35.

Featherstone, M., & Hepworth, M. (1991). The mask of ageing and the postmodern life course. In M. Featherstone, M. Hepworth, & B.S Turner (Eds.), *The body: Social process and cultural theory* (pp. 371–389). London: Sage.

Gifford, S. (1986). The meaning of lumps: A case study of the ambiguities of risk. In C.R. Janes, R. Stall, & S.M. Gifford (Eds.), *Anthropology and epidemiology: Interdisciplinary approaches to the study of health and disease* (pp. 213–246). Dordrecht: Reidel.

Goffman, E. (1963). *Stigma: Notes on the management of spoiled identity.* Englewood Cliffs, NJ: Prentice-Hall.

Green, C.J., Hadorn, D., Bassett, K., & Kazanjian, A. (1992, September). *Prostate specific antigen in the early detection of prostate cancer.* Vancouver, BC: British Columbia Office of Health Technology Assessment.

Green, C.J., Bassett, K., Foerster, V., & Kazanjian, A. (1997). *Bone mineral density testing: Does the evidence support its selective use in well women?* Vancouver, BC: British Columbia Office of Health Technology Assessment.

Green, C.J., Gallagher, R.P., & Kazanjian, A. (1999). *A population-based study of the relationship between prostate specific antigen testing utilization rates and patterns of prostate cancer incidence and mortality.* Vancouver, BC: British Columbia Office of Health Technology Assessment.

Grundy, S.M. (1998). Statin trails and goals for cholesterol lowering therapy. *Circulation, 97*, 1436–9.

Hailey, D., Sampietro-Colom, L., Marshall, D., Rico, P, Granados, A., Asua, J., et al. (1996). *Statement of findings. INAHATA project on the effectiveness of bone density measurement and associated treatments for prevention of fractures.* Edmonton, AB: Alberta Heritage Foundation for Medical Research.

Haraway, D. (1990). A manifesto for cyborgs: Science, technology, and socialist feminism in the 1980s. In L.J. Nicholson (Ed.), *Feminism/Postmodernism* (pp. 65–107). London: Routledge.

Health Services Utilization and Research Commission. (1995). *Cholesterol testing and treatment guidelines.* Saskatoon, SK: The Commission.

Hubbard, R. (1990). *The politics of women's biology.* New Brunswick: Rutgers University Press.

Kaufert, P. (1998). Menopause as process or event: The creation of definitions in biomedicine. In M. Lock & D. Gordon (Eds.), *Biomedicine examined* (pp. 341–49). Dordrecht/Boston/London: Kluwer.

Kaufert, P. (1982). Myth and the menopause. *Sociology of Health and Illness, 4*, 141–66.

Kaufert, P., & Gilbert, P. (1986). Women, menopause, and medicalization. *Culture, Medicine and Psychiatry, 10*, 7–21.

Kazanjian, A., Cardiff, K., & Pagliccia, N. (1995). Design and development of a conceptual and quantitative framework for health technology decisions: A multi-project compendium of research underway. British Columbia Office of Health Technology Assessment.

Koenig, B. (1998). The technological imperative in medical practice: The social creation of a "routine" treatment. In M. Lock & D. Gordon (Eds.), *Biomedicine examined (pp. 465–496)*. Dordrecht/ Boston/London: Kluwer.

Kunisch, J.R. (1989). Electronic fetal monitors: Marketing forces and the resulting controversy. In K. S. Ratcliffe (Ed.), *Healing technology: Feminist perspectives (pp. 41–60)*. Ann Arbor: University of Michigan Press.

Lock, M. (1993). *Encounters with aging: Mythologies of menopause in Japan and North America.* Berkeley and Los Angeles: University of California Press.

Lock, M. (1996, November). Social and cultural issues in connection with breast cancer testing and screening. *Genetic testing for breast cancer susceptibility: The science, the ethics, the future.* Paper presented at International Bioethics Conference, San Francisco.

Logan, A.G. (1994). Lowering the blood total cholesterol level to prevent coronary heart disease. *Canadian Task Force on Periodic Health Examination. Canadian guide to preventive health.* Ottawa, ON. Canada Communication Group.

Marshall D., Sheldon T.A., & Jonsson, E. (1997). Recommendations for the application of bone density measurement: What can you believe? *International Journal of Technology Assessment in Health Care,* 13(3), 411–19.

Marshall, K. (1996). Prevention. How much harm? How much benefit? Physical, psychological and social harm. *Canadian Medical Association Journal,* 155(2), 169–176.

Martin, E. (1991). The egg and the sperm: How science has constructed a romance based on male and female roles. *Signs,* 16(3), 485–501.

McKinlay, S., Brambilla, D., & Posner, J. (1992). The normal menopausal transition. *Human Biology, 4,* 37–46.

Mintzes, B. (1998). Blurring the boundaries: New trends in drug promotion. *Health Action International-Europe.*

Nelkin, D. (1996). The social dynamics of genetic testing: The case of Fragile-X. *Medical Anthropology Quarterly,* 10(4), 537–550.

Parsons, T. (1967). *The structure of social action: a study in social theory with special reference to a group of recent European writers* (2nd ed.). New York: Free Press; London: Collier-Macmillan.

Posner, T. (1991). What's in a smear? Cervical screening, medical signs and metaphors. *Science as Culture,* 2(2), 167–87.

Rapp, R. (1995). Real time fetus: The role of the sonogram in the age of mechanical reproduction. In G.L. Downey, J. Dumit & S. Traweek (Eds.), *Cyborgs and citadels: Anthropological interventions in the borderlands of technoscience (pp. 32–64).* Seattle: University of Washington Press.

Ringertz, H., Marshall D., Johansson C., Johnell O., Kullenberg R.J., Ljunghall S. & et al. (1997). Bone density measurement: A systematic review. A report from SBU, The Swedish Council on Technology Assessment in Health Care. *Journal of Internal Medicine,* 241(suppl 739):i–iii, 1–60.

Rosengren, A. (1998). Cholesterol: How low is low enough? Reaching target levels may be better than relative reductions. *British Medical Journal,* 317, 426–7.

Savoie I., Bassett K., & Kazanjian, A. (1997, August). Supporting clinical practice guidelines development: An appraisal of existing cholesterol testing guidelines. Vancouver, BC: BC Office of Health Technology Assessment.

Savoie I., Kazanjian, A. (1999). Will it change patient management? What we really get from cholesterol testing. Vancouver, BC: BC Office of Health Technology Assessment.

Shiva, V., & Moser, I. (1995). *Biopolitics: A feminist and ecological reader on biotechnology.* London; Atlantic Highlands.

Skrabanek, P. (1985). False premises and false promises of breast cancer screening. The Lancet, 2, 316–320.

Strother Ratcliffe, K. (1989). Health technologies for women: Whose health? Whose technology? In K. S. Ratcliffe (Ed.), Healing technology: Feminist perspectives (pp. 173–198). Ann Arbor: University of Michigan Press.

Wald N.J., Law, M, Watt H.C., Wu ,T, Bailey, A, Johnson, A.M., & et al. (1994). Apolipoproteins and ischemic heart disease: Implications for screening. The Lancet, 343, 75–79.

Whatley, M.H., & Worcester, N. (1989). The role of technology in the co-optation of the women's health movement: The cases of osteoporosis and breast cancer. In K. S. Ratcliffe (Ed.), Healing technology: Feminist perspectives (pp. 199–220). Ann Arbor: University of Michigan Press.

WHO Study Group. (1994). Assessment of fracture risk and its application to screening for post-menopausal osteoporosis. Geneva, Switzerland: World Health Organization.

Working Group on Hypercholesterolemia and Other Dyslipidemias. (1997, March). Detection and management of hypercholesterolemia (Interim report).

Chapter 10

Therapeutic Patient Education for Chronic Diseases

JEAN-PHILIPPE ASSAL

Because of social progress, improved medication, and increasing life expectancy, chronic diseases—whether among the elderly or the young—are becoming more prevalent, their treatment more demanding, and more important to health care delivery and decisionmaking. The medical profession and society are being forced to develop new strategies and more imaginative approaches to meet the growing needs.

Long-term education of the chronically ill is proving to be one of the most successful key strategies to meeting the challenge, which is for an extended management system that adds pedagogic, psychological, and sociologic dimensions to traditional responses. It should also expand the role of the physician and health care team beyond the established biomedical approach.

The treatment of diabetes mellitus illustrates this remarkably well, representing a model of novel approaches applicable to the management of an ever-increasing mass of chronic diseases. In this context, taking the example of insulin-dependent diabetes, four significant phases in long-term patient therapeutic education can be distinguished (Fig.1).

First Phase: 1921

The discovery of insulin introduced a radical correction of a metabolic problem that was theretofore fatal (Fig.2).

STAGES IN THE TREATMENT OF DIABETES MELLITUS

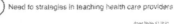

	INSULIN +	ANTIBIOTICS +	EDUCATION +	MANAGEMENT
morbidity	short-term complications		long-term complications	
	Diabetics	hospitalizations (days/year) (5.4) (1.7)		↓ 50% { eyes / kidneys / nerves
	Non Diabetics	(1.2) (1.2)	(+)	(?)

	1921 insulin	1946	(oral agents) Antibiotics	1972 Drugs, diet + patient education	1983 ———— 1993 Stockholm/DCCT
medical approach	**Specific Biomedical**		**Non specific Biomedical**	*Biomedical + teaching + psychosocial*	*Biomedical + teaching + psychosocial + management of follow-up*

research		Biomedical	Bio-psycho-social	Bio-psycho-soc. + Management of follow-up
		Pharmacology +	Human sciences +	Management of follow-up Training health care providers

J.Ph. Assal

(+) Worsening of health care in the absence of "charismatic leader"   (?) Need to strategies in teaching health care providers

Figure 10.1. The four phases in the history of the treatment of diabetes.

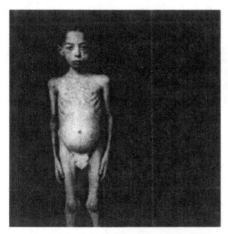
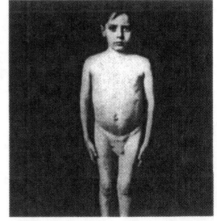

Figure 10.2. One of the earliest children treated with insulin. On the left, the first day of insulin injection; on the right, three months later.

Second Phase

The advent of antibiotics, which made it possible to control many infections that caused severe metabolic failure. Many diabetics had to have limb amputation for osteomyelitis secondary to an infected neuropathic foot!

In these two phases, improvement in the control of diabetes was due to research and treatment in the biomedical field, diabetes-specific for insulin, and non-diabetes-specific for the antibiotics.

Third Phase: 1972

The arrival of pedagogy and patient education in the field of therapeutics, thanks to the work of Leona Miller (Miller & Goldstein, 1972). For instance, among the Mexican-American population of Los Angeles, which has a large underprivileged patient community, this physician introduced a patient education programme that reduced hospital stays from 5.4 days per year, per patient, to 1.7 days. This statistically shortened period was the same as that for non-diabetic hospital patients, at 1.2 days/year/patient. For the first time in the history of medicine it was proven on a large scale that the patient's education played a therapeutic role of prime importance. It was shown that even though the medical profession had the advantage of remarkable technical tools for treatment: highly purified insulin, diabetes auto control techniques, and a choice of antibiotics that covered most of the micro-organisms, the patient's education affected the outcome.

The biomedical dimension of a diabetic's treatment was therefore optimal, but its efficiency could only be manifest through another dimension, that of patient education. The epidemiological proof was thus established: Psychosocial and pedagogical approaches came to the rescue of biological therapy.

It must, however, be mentioned that right from the discovery of insulin, several clinicians had insisted, in their own centres, on the role of the patient's training. Examples include E. Allen in London (Jackson), E.P. Joslin in Boston, E. Roma in Lisbon, G. Constam in Switzerland, M. Derot and H. Lestradet in France, and J. Pirart in Belgium. The list can be extended to include every country. These eminent physicians blazed the path—without, however, quantifying their approaches. They did not describe their techniques of patient education. Their experiences had not succeeded in motivating the medical profession at the international level. These exceptional clinicians, charismatic personalities, bound by their daily activities, did not have the time or see the need to structure and to organize the training of the medical and nursing professions in their therapeutic environment.

Then came Leona Miller. Her study on the effects of training 6,000 patients, published in 1972 in the *New England Journal of Medicine*, provided a proven and official approval to this method of treatment. To reinforce the biomedical approach, the treatment of diabetes thus benefited from the human sciences: a new challenge for the medical profession, a new role for the physician—that of integrating pedagogy and psychology into medical practice. In centres that applied this integrated approach for diabetes the patients were able to diminish by about 80% the cases of failure, of keto-acidotic coma, and of hypoglycemic coma. As for prevention of amputations in high-risk patients,—those with loss of pain sensitivity or with arterial deficiency–the rate of amputations fell by about 75%.

Thanks to technological improvements, auto control of glycemia made it possible for patients to manage their diabetes on a day-to-day basis. Results have shown that in the 1970s and '80s the auto control of blood sugar was perhaps more useful in the control of acute failures (hypo- or hyperglycaemic comas) than in a permanent improvement of metabolic balance. There is a similar auto control possibility in other chronic diseases also, such as asthma, with regular assessment of peak flow, or in Parkinson's disease, with a recorded diary of the frequency and length of kinetic crises that helps the patient to adapt accordingly the timing of his L-dopa therapy.

Fourth Phase: 1993

The organization of patient follow-up as assurance for long-term metabolic quality control.

The American study of Diabetes Complications Control Trial (DCCT) (Research Group, 1993) and six European studies (Reichard, Nilsson, & Rosenquist, 1993; Wang, Lau, & Chalmers, 1993) analysed the effects of diabetes control on the incidence and long-term progress of complications. These investigations have shown similar results: a fall of about 50% in the incidence of long-term progression of complications involving diabetic retinopathy, kidney disease, and neuropathic deterioration. A study of the activities of all these centres shows that, in addition to patient education, the organization of follow-up of the patients was a determinant factor in long-term metabolic quality control. These centres had structured their follow-up in an optimal fashion, with multidisciplinary teams that included physicians, nurses, dietitians, and psychologists. These investigations, especially DCCT, have shown to the profession the importance of organizing in long-term care and the dynamics of interdisciplinarity within the health care team as well as the regular assessment of the patients' performance.

One example among many is worth citing. In the DCCT investigation, every fortnight the patient had to bring to the physician or the nurse the results of his blood sugar readings and metabolic value controls. He also had to show how he had modified the treatment according to his findings. Telephone and fax were used regularly; telephone terminals were provided so that the patient could have constant access to information and advice on the management of his treatment programme. Guidance by psychologists was included in these services to reinforce the patient's motivation for treatment. This fourth phase shows that education alone is not enough and that it must be completed by organizing the medical follow-up. The accent is therefore on the medical "management" of the patient, an aspect that until now depended on the common sense and personal initiative of the health care team, but which had never been fully thought out within the structure and organization of long-term care. Here is a new field in which expertise must be developed to ensure continuous quality of care.

A diabetes clinic, as in any centre for continuing care of chronically ill patients, can no longer be based entirely on biomedical technology or knowledge, however important these may be at the pathophysiological level. Diabetes mellitus, like any other chronic disease, necessitates medical training based on follow-up techniques and integration of the patient in a continuous process of care.

Here biotechnical and psychosocial dimensions are fundamentally complementary and can no more be separated or opposed, as is often the case with medicine. It behooves the physician to unite these two sectors, quite a difficult mission even today, as little has been done to close the gap between these dimensions of medicine. The treatment and continuing care of chronic patients offers a unique opportunity to develop such an integrated approach.

Experience shows that health practitioners are not sufficiently conscious of the peculiarities of the kind of medicine they practice. They little know how much the type of service they provide (e.g. emergency medicine) can complicate and interfere with the transition to another type of care, such as follow-up of chronic illness. Such problems are seen when a hospital-based physician leaves his institutionalized position and goes into private or community practice.

LONG-TERM FOLLOW-UP OF A PATIENT

An important part of out-of-hospital activity is the long-term care of patients suffering from chronic illnesses such as cardiovascular diseases (arterial hypertension, anginal claudication, cardiac insufficiency), metabolic and nutritional diseases (diabetes, hyperlypedemia, high blood urea, overweight), rheumatological conditions (arthritis, backache, rheumatism), neurological diseases (cerebral arteriosclerosis, Alzheimer's disease, epilepsy, Parkinson's disease), pulmonary conditions (chronic bronchitis, obstructive syndromes, bronchial asthma), and gastrointestinal diseases (gastroduodenal ulcer, colonic conditions, cholecystopathies, hepatitis).

Each one of these conditions has probably been seen within the hospital in an acute stage, such as pulmonary oedema, diabetic coma, herniated disc, epileptic attack, acute asthma, gastrointestinal haemorrhage, jaundice, and so on. There the physician will have learned to treat the emergency and to have "cured" it. However, he or she will not have learned to treat these illnesses on a long-term basis, most of which cannot be cured but can well be kept under control. Although these diseases are different, they share certain common characteristics:

- *Chronic illness*
  - is often incurable;
  - is silent outside acute exacerbations;
  - if there is pain, it tends to be persistent;
  - often there is little relationship between the complaints and biological findings;
  - its progress is unpredictable;
  - may be related to the patient's lifestyle.
- *The treatment*
  - is important for survival and/or daily comfort;
  - has variable effects;
  - often necessitates the training of the patient to ensure its management;
  - implies daily discipline;
  - usually takes the patient's time;
  - often interferes with social life.
- *The patient*
  - may not be cured of the illness, but can control it;
  - must manage the treatment according to various factors related to his private life;
  - outside acute episodes, his illness is usually silent;
  - as soon as surveillance weakens the disease relapses;
  - must be trained to act rapidly in case of crisis;
  - must accept a certain degree of loss of his integrity.
- *The physician*
  - prescribes the treatment but only indirectly controls the illness;
  - must train his patient for treatment; must share his medical power;
  - must manage the illness often in its silent phase;
  - must urgently treat the acute episodes;
  - must be vigilant to detect late complications;
  - must ensure psychological and social support;
  - must be prepared to accept a new medical identity;
  - must be prepared to work as a part of a team.

The medical identity associated with the treatment of acute illness often imprisons the physician in a stereotyped functional mode and prevents him from being fully effective in his new role for long-term care. He is bound by biomedical, pharmacological, and status specificities and finds it difficult to adapt himself to the requirements of long follow-up of these chronic patients, young or old.

Several physicians have developed some very effective approaches to these patients, but unfortunately these experiences have rarely been conceptualized, and as such the required training, extending from a hospital system to a domiciliary, ambulatory system, remains inadequate.

THE PHYSICIAN'S TRAINING: WHAT REQUIREMENTS FOR LONG-TERM PATIENT CARE?

Centred principally on pathophysiology of disease—on establishing a diagnosis and choosing a treatment—medical studies have not trained the student for long-term patient care. Such training will be provided only if the philosophy of medical education is changed. To the above-mentioned established themes, it is necessary to add training in strategies of treatment management, especially in long-standing illnesses.

In medical studies the student first encounters a cadaver (anatomy and dissection lectures) whereas his earliest experiences should also have been based on the ordinary live patient model. Such training would have allowed him to complete his theoretical knowledge with know-how in treatment and follow-up strategies. In this regard some recommendations can be made for the training of health personnel:

- avoid education based exclusively on factual knowledge. Promote a process of understanding by stimulating the problem-solving approach;
- enlarge the notions of pharmacological action and therapeutic indication of drugs with an understanding that promotes treatment management by the patient;
- overcome the temptation of intellectual arrogance and learn to manage ambiguity and uncertainty in diagnosis and therapy;
- be able to pass from the domain of biological thinking to the less precise but real domain of the patient's experiences and beliefs concerning his illness, health and treatment;
- complete the physician's biomedical competence with knowledge acquired in the consulting room from the realities of daily life.

It has been and it still is difficult to introduce such a change; it requires modifying certain traditions and habits of the medical profession and overcoming certain convictions. In the present context it means providing the physician with a wider education that meets the various needs of the patient, needs that far outweigh the purely biomedical dimension. It is therefore indispensable that any person looking after chronic patients should master certain elements in the following fields: a) education of the patient, b) psychology of the patient and c) organization and management of long-term follow-up.

Considered together and oriented towards clinical activity, these themes could include the following: Training in treatment education; helping the patient to manage his treatment.

PRACTICAL TRAINING FOR THE THERAPEUTIC EDUCATION OF PATIENTS

At the request of the World Health Organization's European office, a group of experts has prepared a special report (Therapeutic Patient Education: Continuing Education for Healthcare Providers in the Management of Chronic Diseases) that indicates the need of the medical community for more specific training of health care providers in the management and long-term follow-up of chronic diseases (WHO, 1998). One key concept emerged from this expert group: Patient education should be enriched and replaced by *therapeutic* patient education (Lacroix & Assal, 2003).

When health care providers teach patients, they tend to spend more time and energy speaking about the disease than providing the patient with the appropriate skills for the daily management of his or her condition. *Therapeutic patient education* therefore focuses on the skills for effective self-management of the treatment adaptation to a chronic disease and coping processes and skills, and also takes into consideration the cost to the patient and society.

Therapeutic patient education is an essential component for the efficient self-management and quality of care of all long-term diseases and conditions. However, patients with acute diseases should not be excluded from its benefit.

THE NEED FOR EDUCATIONAL PROGRAMMES IN THERAPEUTIC PATIENT EDUCATION

The World Health Organization has Defined Therapeutic Patient Education as Follows:

- Therapeutic Patient Education should enable patients to gain and maintain abilities that allow them an optimal management of life with their disease.
- Therapeutic Patient Education is therefore a continuous process, integrated in health care.
- It is patient centred; it includes organized awareness, information, self-care learning and psychosocial support activities, regarding disease, prescribed treatments, care, hospital and other health care settings, organizational information, health, and illness behaviour.
- Its aim is to help patients and their families to understand the disease and the treatment, cooperate with healthcare providers, manage their own health, and maintain and/or improve their quality of life.

Description of these various needs is beyond the scope of this chapter, but the following is a list of topics that are now part of a postgraduate and continuing education curriculum given at the Faculty of Medicine of the University of Geneva. It leads to a diploma in the field of therapeutic education of patients with chronic diseases.

- The characteristics of chronic diseases compared to the acute medical situations (how to adapt the behaviour of physicians to the specificity of chronic diseases);
- Understanding how the patient with a chronic disease functions with regard to his treatment and daily management of the control of his illness;
- Taking into account the patient's coping strategies with the diseases (Which counter-attitude do physicians develop in front of a patient who is in revolt or in the bargaining stage with his treatment?);
- Communicating with the patient and mastering the "active listening" technique (Which strategies should be used to facilitate the communication?);
- Giving therapeutic instructions to the patient (Which approach should help the physician deal with the health beliefs of the patient? How can the physician evaluate if the patient's locus of control is external or internal?);
- Assisting a patient in coping with his illness and its treatment (mastering the various barriers that interfere with the patient's adherence to the treatment, developing specific attitudes that would reinforce the process of coping);
- Integrating the patient's own experience in his therapeutic educational programme (Which educational strategies are recommended to help the patient acquire the skills for self-management?);
- Evaluating a learning process and methods used (methodologies for the evaluation of courses given to patients and the evaluation of the impact of the courses on the patients);
- Long-term follow-up of patients (Which strategies are needed to integrate patients' relapse prevention, therapeutic education, and psychosocial support into the biomedical activity of the physician?).

CONCLUSIONS

The physician's identity has been moulded during medical school and years of hospital training into a way of thinking about specific sub-systems dealing with pathology, biochemistry, and organic and laboratory diagnostic procedures. Each procedure represents a sub-system, that is, a speciality in itself, a rather "closed" entity. Management of chronic diseases forces the physician, whether he or she likes it or not, to face other sub-systems that deal with the entire person, two persons, the family, the community, and society. From this perspective, professional specialties (endocrinology, diabetology, etc.) always fall short of the need to simultaneously handle the various problems and requirements of the patient as the bearer of the disease and his family.

A professional who accepts this inter-relatedness will eventually face an identity crisis, discovering that his sub-specialty is only part of the whole. Although it is not within the scope of this chapter to address the problematic issue of professional identity, it is important here to note, at least, that this broadening of professional orientation is often initially experienced by the physician as a loss of his specialized medical power.

Medical training is slowly, but surely, improving. The fact that WHO is now strongly recommending training in therapeutic patient education and that some medical schools have already developed specific training programmes into their medical curricula is a major step forward for the quality of care. This training is also an answer to what patients and patients' associations have asked for, for so many years. These are progressive developments that fit well within the evolving dimensions of health.

Acknowledgements: I wish to thank Professor William Gunn for his valuable clinical and editorial advice and Mrs. Melodie Kaeser for her continuing secretarial assistance.

REFERENCES

Diabetes Control and Complications Trial Research Group. (1993). The effect of intensive treatment of diabetes on the development and progression of long-term complications in insulin-dependent diabetes mellitus. N Eng J Med, 329(14), 977–86.

Lacroix, A., & Assal, J. Ph. (2003). L'Education thérapeutique des patients. Nouvelles approches de la maladie chronique. 2ᵉᵐᵉ édition complétée. Editions Maloine, Paris.

Miller, L.V., & Goldstein, J. (1972). More efficient care of diabetic patients in a county hospital setting. New England Journal of Medicine, 286, 1388–91.

Reichard, P., Nilsson, B.Y., & Rosenqvist, U. (1993). The effect of long-term intensified insulin treatment on the development of microvascular complications of diabetes mellitus. N Eng J Med, 329(5), 304–9.

Wang, P.H., Lau, J., & Chalmers, T.C. (1993). Meta analysis of effects of intensive blood-glucose control on late complications of type 1 diabetes. Lancet, 341, 1306–9.

World Health Organization. Regional Office for Europe, Copenhagen. (1998). Report of a WHO Working Group. Therapeutic Patient Education. Continuing education programmes for healthcare providers in the field of prevention of chronic diseases.

Section **III**

The Dynamics

Chapter 11

The Humanitarian Imperative in Major Health Crises and Disasters

S.W.A. GUNN

All major crises that disturb nature or fray the fabric of society risk producing disasters, which, in turn, lead to health problems of considerable gravity. Likewise, major widespread diseases can lead to disastrous situations with serious environmental, economic, and social consequences. To varying degrees, no natural phenomena and no social structures can escape periodic disturbances, but wise ecological management, equitable human relationships, and basic sanitary precautions can greatly diminish their physical, social, and personal impact.

Unfortunately, however, the frequency, magnitude, and diversity of disasters are rising throughout the world, with dire consequences to man and nature. Drought, famine, war, refugees, epidemics, and technological accidents, whether happening singly or, worse, in conjunction, are events and dangers that threaten growing numbers of people. There is, at present, a "disaster belt" of earthquakes, cyclones, floods, and desertification extending over most of the non-industrialized world and affecting some 100 developing countries, few of which have the technical knowledge, planning capacity, and financial resources to cope with nature's fury, which can strike at any time. Add to these natural disasters the growing number of industrial or technological catastrophes such as Chernobyl or Bhopal and the conflict situations created by people, and the world becomes an increasingly

This chapter is based in part on the author's paper on "Disasters and Conflicts," in *Encyclopedia of Life Support Systems*, Eolss Publishers, Oxford, by kind permission.

fragile spaceship. Fragile, and lately more insecure—ideological adversities are becoming armed confrontations, millions of people are seeking asylum, traffic and road accidents are reaching epidemic proportions, violence is gaining ground, substance abuse is becoming a super-lucrative and super-destructive trade, international agreements are being down-trodden, old pandemics are returning to kill, and, to add to the sad list, otherwise available retroviral medication is being withheld from 45 million people. Disasters, in the early days of the World Health Organization, were epidemics and widespread diseases (see also chapter 12, by D. Heymann); today they are all the major crises mentioned above, and more.

DISASTERS

The notion of disaster or catastrophe is primarily sociocentric or anthropocentric, for a natural disaster that does not affect people, society, and the environment will remain a mere geological or meteorological event. Thus, humankind and human welfare are the focus of concern. A disaster, then, is the result of a vast ecological breakdown in the relations between people and their environment, a serious and sudden event (though sometimes slow, as in drought) on such a scale that the stricken community needs extraordinary efforts to cope with it, often including outside help or international assistance. Clearly, when disaster strikes, the welfare of society, the health of the people, the man-made environment, and the civic fabric are all seriously endangered, and multidisciplinary planning and multisectoral action in an interdependent manner are called for. Here, however, only the health aspects of disasters, commonly called "health disasters," will be considered, and the humanitarian imperative of the multifaceted response will be highlighted. Disaster medicine and humanitarian medicine address these issues.

A BRIEF HISTORY

Perhaps the earliest organized aid was that of hunters and warriors helping dress one another's wounds. The cave paintings of primitive Lascaux and the exquisite pottery of classical Greece are eloquent witnesses. Military medicine grew from that, and, in modern times, of course, Florence Nightingale put the stamp of feminine sensitivity on mass casualty care.

From frontline care we gradually proceed to transnational action, with the founding of the International Red Cross and the formulation of international humanitarian law, anchored in the Geneva Conventions. The national Red Cross and later Red Crescent Societies were established, and subsequently merged into a strong, worldwide federation. In all this international reorganization, the medical profession, as such, had little involvement, a pattern that has only recently begun to change. What has not changed, however, is the predominantly humanitarian core of disaster assistance, whether in natural and human-made disasters or poverty-based ill health, culminating in the International Association for Humanitarian Medicine.

World War II, like all wars and calamities, brought horrors and some beneficial consequences. Towards the end of the conflict, the United Nations Relief and Rehabilitation Administration (UNRRA) became the first disaster management enterprise on a global scale. The births of the United Nations (UN) and the World Health Organization (WHO) were the other momentous events in the aftermath of war, and their constitutions have a capital bearing on disaster management.

First of all, WHO redefined health as "a state of complete physical, mental and social well-being, and not merely the absence of disease or infirmity." The victims of disasters are thus, even in the absence of injury, lacking in well-being and deserve care. More specifically, Article 2 of the WHO Constitution states that the organization "... shall furnish appropriate technical assistance and, in emergencies, necessary aid ..." The UN Charter has similar instruments concerning people's rights to protection. It is through the moral and intellectual impetus of these global organizations that disaster studies and disaster response are gaining institutional expertise. Disaster medicine, as distinct from trauma management and clinical emergency medicine, is now enjoying an increasingly important place in overall health care delivery and development planning. The scene is now set for a new science, to which humanitarian medicine is adding a new soul.

DISASTER MEDICINE

Knowledge of wars and other conflict-caused disasters is much more advanced than our knowledge of the effects, especially health effects, of natural disasters. Military medicine, sanitary logistics, and the consequences of war have been observed and studied over several centuries, whereas disaster medicine has only recently attracted serious attention and is only now on the way to becoming an organized discipline with scientific rigour. Because of changes in the past decade or two in international relations, patterns of conflict, and regional insecurity, military medicine has had to "recycle" itself for new conditions, and military surgeons are having to readapt for non-conflict casualties and situations in collaboration with other civilian disaster managers.

The Scientific Base of Disaster Medicine

Disaster medicine is more than the age-old bandaging of wounds or providing urgent relief. It has evolved into a complex managerial system which, to be effective and efficient, must comprise all the phases and facets of the disaster cycle, including preparedness, prevention, immediate response, relief, reconstruction, rehabilitation, and development, with built-in quality control mechanisms. In this sense, disaster medicine is defined in the Gunn Dictionary as:

> *The study and collaborative application of various health disciplines, e.g., pediatrics, epidemiology, communicable diseases, nutrition, public health, trauma, emergency medicine, community care, international health, humanitarian law, to the prevention, immediate response and rehabilitation of the health problems arising from disaster, in cooperation with other disciplines involved in comprehensive disaster management.*

Disasters are always sad and destabilizing crises, and disaster response has not always been successful. More action has been undertaken with goodwill than good knowledge. To be successful, the knowledge mechanisms and action have to be based on more solid scientific and tested precepts. There are positive developments in this regard, and undeniable progress is now in process because of the increasing amount of technology involved in disaster management. However humanitarian disaster medicine may be—and it is essentially humanitarian—it must strengthen its scientific base and develop strong technical underpinnings. This applies as much to disaster medicine in the specific sense as to disaster management in the wider, multidisciplinary sense. Research and field surveys during the 1980s and 1990s shed new light on the effects of disasters and led to better ways of providing the appropriate response pro-actively as well as after the impact. From these studies and field experiences, ten principles can be enunciated for the scientific basis of disaster management:

(i) Preparedness is possible and essential. The greater the preparedness for foreseeable events or probable hazards, the more effective relief operations will be.

(ii) Prevention of many natural disasters is possible, while prevention of all human-made disasters should be possible.

(iii) No two disasters are alike, but the problems that certain categories of disaster are likely to create are quite foreseeable. Disasters have profiles and must be researched.

(iv) Based on such profiles, the disease pattern of and response to each kind of disaster can be foreseen and formulated epidemiologically.

(v) Planning and preparation on sectoral, national, and international bases are possible and essential for effective multidisciplinary response.

(vi) Mobilization of multisectoral human and material resources (in the case of health action: nurses, doctors, nutritionists, social health workers, paramedics, pharmaceuticals, medical transport, health centers, etc.) must be so organized as to be able to respond immediately when disaster strikes.

(vii) Risk assessment, evaluation of hazards, estimation of the effects of one's intervention, and a study of the post-disaster situation are essential.

(viii) The post-emergency phase offers a rare opportunity for taking steps, and, if necessary, corrective action, to mitigate the effects of a subsequent disaster. Each disaster is a lesson.

(ix) The reconstruction phase begins at once, and it is part of development.

(x) Disaster management takes into full account the stricken community, its contribution, capacities, customs. and institutions involved.

The more one provides a scientific base the more one becomes convinced that the key to truly effective disaster management is preparedness and prevention rather than a post hoc, firefighting type emergency response: Principle No. 1

For this kind of scientific approach and technical reinforcement, special studies, surveys, bench and applied research, social and natural science investigations, and managerial techniques are being applied. One particular endeavour that has proved most promising in health disasters is epidemiology. The other main thrust is the conceptualization and application of humanitarian principles.

HUMANITARIAN MEDICINE

Since the early 1980s, in line with scientific advances in emergency management and disaster medicine, the profession's and society's ways of thinking about disasters and of tackling them have undergone dramatic change, and fundamental developments are now taking place in worldwide disaster response.

- Major emergencies and disasters are no longer considered fatalistically as phenomena, but, rather, as foreseeable events that can be prevented.
- Those who provide assistance now look upon it not as a gesture of sympathy, but as a duty based on mutual aid.
- The stricken communities and nations are claiming relief not as a charity but as a right—the right to health and protection.
- Disaster assistance is being seen not as an ad hoc emergency repair episode but as an essential factor in long-term development.
- The international community now perceives emergency relief not as a magnanimous contribution but as a humanitarian obligation, with a right to intervene.
- Armed forces are now being recycled from traditional combat duties to peacekeeping and peacemaking services.
- Persecuted minority populations are being given a voice and the right to health and compensation.
- Those who conceive and create disasters and suffering are being brought to justice before the international courts.

- The medical community, which had long felt the human factor in disaster work, is now channeling disaster medicine into humanitarian medicine.
- Health is increasingly being regarded and used as a bridge to peace.

These constitute a quantum leap forward in people's scientific and humanitarian efforts to deal with emergencies and respond to disasters.

On first thought, it may be argued that according to its traditions and professional ethics all medicine is humanitarian, but let us define humanitarian medicine:

> While all medical intervention to reduce a person's sickness and suffering is in essence humanitarian, humanitarian medicine goes beyond the usual therapeutic act and promotes, provides, teaches, supports, and delivers people's health as a human right, in conformity with the ethics of Hippocratic teaching, the principles of the World Health Organization, the Charter of the United Nations, the Universal Declaration of Human Rights, the Red Cross Conventions, and other covenants and practices that ensure the most humane and best possible level of care, without any discrimination or consideration of material gain.

The Legal and Moral Base of Humanitarian Medicine

Parallel with the scientific, technical, and managerial bases of disaster medicine, the legal and moral concepts of humanitarian medicine are based on solid international instruments, ethical precepts, social values, and inalienable human rights. Out of the many declarations, treaties, principles, and obligations, five international instruments are mentioned here to underscore the legal and moral cornerstones of humanitarian medicine. Although chronologically the Universal Declaration of Human Rights was in fact signed after the ratification of the WHO Constitution, I shall take it up first.

Of the thirty articles that the Declaration contains, Art. 25 is particularly concerned with the right to health. It states:

1. Everyone has the right to a standard of living adequate for the health and well-being of himself and of his family, including food, clothing, housing, medical care, and necessary services, and the right to security in the event of unemployment, sickness, disability, widowhood, old age, or other lack of livelihood in circumstances beyond his control.

It further establishes that:

2. Motherhood and childhood are entitled to special care and assistance. All children, whether born in or out of wedlock, shall enjoy the same social protection.

1. Eight months before this Declaration was signed, the WHO Constitution had already injected new dimensions of social thinking and new concepts of health.

Its preamble states that "the enjoyment of the highest attainable standard of health is one of the fundamental rights of every human being ..." and that governments are responsible for the health of their peoples.

It further enounces the principle that health is a matter of international politics, because "the health of all peoples is fundamental to the attainment of peace and security ..."

Article 1 clearly points out the objective of WHO. This "... *shall be the attainment by all peoples of the highest possible level of health.*"

And boldly—indeed for its times iconoclastically—WHO defines *health*, not disease or infirmity. (Only later will these be formulated, in the concept of burden of disease on society.) One can easily grasp the vastness and depth of the interpretation and its implications on the provision of and access to health services everywhere.

II. Health rights begin early in life. The UN Declaration of the Rights of the Child, signed in November 1959, proclaims the following Principles:
   3. The child shall enjoy the benefits of social security. He shall be entitled to grow and develop in health: to this end special care and protection shall be provided both to him and to his mother, including adequate pre-natal and post-natal care. The child shall have the right to adequate nutrition, housing, recreation and medical services.
   4. The child shall have the right to assistance in catastrophes.

As in many other instruments, the child is also protected in the Universal Declaration on the Eradication of Hunger and Malnutrition. Endorsed in December 1974, it proclaims *"every child has the inalienable right to be free from hunger and malnutrition."* It is prohibited to entice and recruit him as soldier.

The sunken eyes of starving children seen daily on our television screens, and the constant breach of all the solemn declarations mentioned above, constitute a flagrant breach of human rights, a breach perpetrated not uncommonly by kleptocratic leaders who rob and starve the populations they are supposed to govern and protect.

III. The International Red Cross has specific principles for the protection of health.

The Geneva Conventions of 12 August, 1949, clearly protect the health and integrity of civilian populations and non-combatants as of right, and the Additional Protocols of 1977 ensure that, even in war and under combat conditions, medical personnel are protected without discrimination, so that they can perform their tasks under International Humanitarian Law.

IV. The International Association for Humanitarian Medicine Brock Chisholm continues the spirit of the Dr. Brock Chisholm Memorial Trust, founded in

1984 to perpetuate the ideals, legacy, and action of the founders of WHO. A definition of the Association describes well its philosophy, mission and humanitarian action:

A professional, non-profit, non-governmental organization that promotes and delivers health care on the principles of humanitarian medicine, named after Dr. Brock Chisholm, first Director-General of the World Health Organization. In particular it provides medical, surgical, nursing, and rehabilitation care to patients in or from developing countries deficient in the necessary specialized expertise; brings relief to victims of disasters where health aid is lacking; mobilizes hospitals and health specialists in developed countries to receive and treat such patients free of charge; promotes the concept of health as a human right and bridge to peace; and advocates humanitarian law and humanitarian principles in the practice of medicine.

Here then, are five primordial instruments, among many, that proclaim health as a human right. Naturally, these rights have to be guaranteed, safeguarded, and provided in practice; at present the universally accepted strategy to ensure health for all is through the national and international efforts in support of essential care available and accessible to all, a goal of humanitarian medicine not only in major crises or health disasters but also in on-going concern and care of the people.

HEALTH FOR ALL

"Health for All" is in fact the name of the long-term thrust pioneered by WHO and supported by all countries as a realizable social goal and human right throughout the world.

If health is a human right, and human rights are for all humans—as indeed they are—then health, too, must be for all. And that is just what the WHO strategy is about. In 1977, the World Health Assembly, drew attention to the vast health inequalities that exist throughout the world and to the inequitable distribution of resources to deal with this human tragedy, and decided that the main social target of WHO for the coming decades would be the attainment, by all citizens of the world, of a level of health that would permit them to lead socially productive lives. That is the pragmatic and, at once, also humanitarian concept of "Health for All".

The fundamental principle on which the programme and the strategy is based is that a country shall develop its own health policies in the light of its own particular health problems, its social situation, political mechanisms, and economic possibilities, within a structured programme of sustainable development. The United Nations and the World Bank have espoused the cause, and countries actively promote it.

There is no question, however, of creating a pseudo-nirvana where all disease will have been abolished. However, several things are clearly attainable: preventable illness should and can be prevented; there should and can be early diagnosis and treatment of and rehabilitation for treatable conditions; there should and can be better continuing management of incurable diseases; the burden of disease on society can and should be lightened, and an increased regard must be paid not only to the length of life but also to the quality of life. The fundamental rights of mankind demand this.

If the world's citizens, nations' statesmen, and our profession can achieve these standards and meet the old and new challenges with competence, equanimity, and humanism, then we shall have responded to at least one of the pressing global dimensions of health.

BIBLIOGRAPHY

Belanger, M. (1997). *Le Droit International de la Santé*. Presses Universitaires de France, Paris.

Boutros-Ghali, B. (2000). De l'action humanitaire. *Journal of Humanitarian Medicine, 1,* 17–18.

Clarke, B., Ehrlich, A., Gunn, S.W.A., Horner, J.S., Lee, J.M., Sharfmann, P., and von Hippel, F. (1986). *London under attack*. Report of the GLAWARS Commission. Oxford: Blackwell.

Gunn, S.W.A. (1988). Disaster medicine and emergencies. The international community's response. *J. Irish Coll. Phys. & Surgeons, 17,* 14.

Gunn, S.W.A. (1985). La médecine des catastrophes: une nouvelle discipline. *Helvetica Chirurgica Acta, 52,* 11.

Gunn, S.W.A. (1993). The effects of nuclear disaster on health. In T. Otsuka, Y. Yamamoto and N. Ninomiya (Eds.). *Further Aspects of Disaster Medicine*. Tokyo: Herusu Publications.

Gunn, S.W.A. (2000). The right to health through international co-operation. *Journal of Humanitarian Medicine, 1,* 1–3.

Gunn, S.W.A. (1990). Multilingual dictionary of disaster medicine and international relief. London, Dordrecht: Kluwer Academic Publishers.

Gunn, S.W.A. (1994). The role of the military in non-military disasters. *Prehospital and Disaster Medicine, 9*(S), 46–48.

Gunn, S.W.A. (1992). The scientific basis of disaster management. *Disaster Prevention & Management Journal, 1*(3), 16–21.

Gunn, S.W.A. (2001). Disasters and conflicts. *Encyclopedia of life support systems*. Oxford: Unesco, Eolss.

Gunn, S.W.A. (2003). The language of disasters. A brief terminology of humanitarian action. In K.M. Cahill (Ed.), *Basics of international humanitarian action*. Fordham University Press, New York.

Gunn, S.W.A. (2003). The right to health of disaster victims. *Disaster Prevention and Management, 12,* 48–51.

Mahler, H. (2003). Health for all, or hell for all? *Journal of Humanitarian Medicine, 3,* 43–45.

Masellis, M. & Gunn, S.W.A. (2002). Humanitarian medicine: A vision and action. *J. Humanitarian Med, 22,* 33–39.

Nygren-Krug, H. (2004). Health and human rights, in 25 questions and answers. *J. Humanitarian Med, 4,* 1–11.

O' Brien, E. (2003). Human rights and the making of a good doctor. In K.M. Cahill (Ed.), *Traditions, values and humanitarian action*. Fordham University Press, New York.

Pictet, J. (1983). *Développement et principes du Droit International Huimanitaire.* Institut Henry Dunant/Editions Pedone, Genève, Paris.

Silverstein, M.E. (1992). *Disasters—your right to survive.* Washington: Brassey's US Publications.

Simmonds, S., Vaughan, P., & Gunn, S.W.A. (1987). *Refugee community health care.* Oxford: Oxford University Press.

United Nations. (1988). *Human rights, a compilation of international instruments.* New York: United Nations.

Walkate, J. (2001). Freedom from fear for human well-being, *Journal of Humanitarian Medicine, 1,* 1–6.

World Health Organization. (2003). *Basic Documents.* WHO, Geneva.

World Health Organization. (2003). *International Migration, health & human rights.* WHO, Geneva.

Chapter 12

Dealing with Global Infectious Disease Emergencies

DAVID L. HEYMANN

BACKGROUND: GLOBAL INFECTIOUS DISEASE EMERGENCIES

The microbes that cause human infectious diseases are complex, dynamic, and constantly evolving. They reproduce rapidly, mutate frequently, adapt with relative ease to new environments and hosts, and frequently breach the species barrier between animals and humans. Social, economic, and environmental factors linked to a host of human populations and activities can accelerate and amplify these natural phenomena. The ability of infectious diseases to spread internationally—carried by humans, insect vectors, food and food products, and livestock—has been greatly augmented by the pressures of a crowded, closely interconnected, and highly mobile world. When they spread internationally, infectious diseases often lead to global emergencies.

The emergence of Acquired Immunodeficiency Syndrome (AIDS) and its rapid progression to endemicity demonstrates how a previously unknown pathogen can cause a worldwide emergency on a scale that threatens to destabilize social structures and economies of whole regions, leading to a potential disaster situation (Price-Smith, 2002) (see also chapter 11 by W. Gunn). Over a period of 25 years AIDS has become the most important cause of infectious disease mortality in adults, and its prevalence is predicted to continue to increase in many parts of the world (WHO/UNAIDS).

Although AIDS provides the most vivid and direct expression of the a global emergency caused by an infectious disease, the threat posed by other emerging and re-emerging infectious diseases has become increasingly difficult to ignore. These diseases affect all countries either internally, in the form of newly established or re-emerging endemic diseases, or as an external threat, in the form of internationally spreading epidemics (Heymann, 2001).

In addition to causing national or global emergencies, emerging and re-emerging infectious diseases are often highly publicized. Many are poorly understood, difficult to treat, and highly lethal as microbes from animals enter immunonaïve human populations. New infectious diseases have emerged at the rate of one per year since the mid-1970s (Woolhouse & Dye, 2001). Ebola haemorrhagic fever in Africa, hantavirus pulmonary syndrome in the USA, Nipah virus encephalitis in Southeast Asia, and severe acute respiratory syndrome (SARS) in China are just a few examples.

Over the time frame, older infectious diseases have re-emerged as well. Cholera, now in its seventh pandemic, returned to Latin American in 1991 after an absence of almost a century. Within a year, 400,000 cases and 4,000 deaths were reported from 11 countries of the Americas (Tauxe, Mintz, & Quick, 1995). Yellow Fever has threatened to cause massive urban epidemics in Africa. An urban outbreak in Côte d'Ivoire in 2001 necessitated the emergency immunization of 2.9 million persons in less than two weeks, depleting the international reserves of vaccine stocks (WHO, 2002). Yellow fever caused urban outbreaks in 2002 in Senegal that, again, required great international efforts to secure sufficient emergency vaccine supplies (Wkly Epidemiol Rec, 2002).

The 1998 epidemics of dengue and dengue haemorrhagic fever were unprecedented in geographical occurrence and numbers of cases, and the epidemics of 2002, 2003, and 2004 continued to spread internationally, causing, to mention one country, Indonesia, the Health Minister to declare a health emergency in early 2004 (WHO, 2002; WH Assembly document A55/19). A new strain of meningococcal meningitis (W135) emerged in 2002 in sub-Saharan Africa, defying emergency preparedness in the form of stockpiled vaccines against conventional strains (WHO, 2002; Wkly Epidemiol Rec, 2002). New and more severe strains of common foodborne pathogens, including E. coli O157:H7, Campylobacter, and Listeria monocytogens, have made the profile of foodborne diseases distinctly more important (Tauxe, 1997; WHO Fact sheet 124(2002); Document no. WHO/CDS/CSR/APH/2002.6). The invariably fatal variant Creutzfeldt-Jakob disease, first recognized in 1996 and probably transmitted to humans through beef or cattle products, has added considerably to this concern (Document no. WHO/CDS/CSR/EPH/2002.6). Year by year, the highly unstable influenza virus is a reminder of the ever-present threat of another lethal influenza pandemic. The avian influenza outbreaks in 2003–2004, which successfully breached the species barrier between animals and humans, are particularly worrisome because of the prospect of re-assortment and recombination (Bonn, 1997).

Disease vectors are equally resilient and adaptable. Some mosquito species that transmit malaria have developed resistance to virtually all major classes of insecticide. Others, such as the tsetse fly that transmits African sleeping sickness, have returned to areas where they had previously been well controlled. The *Aedes aegypti* mosquito that transmits both yellow fever and dengue, originally confined to tropical jungles, has adapted to breed in urban litter (Gubler, 2001; Molyneux, 2001).

The infectious diseases carried by such vectors have likewise spread to new continents or returned to former homes. Rift Valley fever is now firmly established on the Arabian Peninsula. West Nile virus, first introduced on the East coast of the USA in 1999, has now been detected in all states across the US and in provinces of Canada as well (www.cdc.gov/od/oc/media/wncount.htm).

Following the deliberate and malicious use of anthrax to incite terror in the USA in 2001, the perception of the infectious disease emergencies took on a new perspective (Knobler, Mahmoud & Pray, 2002). Preparedness for a possible bioterrorist attack has now become one of the highest profile emergencies pertaining to infectious diseases in the U.S. This risk, which has moved from a remote possibility to a distinct reality, has added to existing concerns about the threat to national and global security posed by naturally occurring infectious diseases. It has also given greater urgency to questions about the capacity of public health infrastructures to detect and contain an infectious disease threat, the best strategies for protecting populations, and the extent to which resources should be devoted to preparation for an event with low probability, yet potentially catastrophic consequences (www.who.int/emc/book_2nd_edition.htm).

Naturally occurring and deliberately caused infectious disease outbreaks have thus come to be perceived as emergencies and threats to international public health security. They have also led to the understanding of the importance of universal strengthening of public health systems as the best way to prevent or mitigate their impact. Today it is generally accepted that strengthening of public health systems for naturally occurring infectious disease outbreak detection and containment ensures better preparedness for all infectious disease outbreaks no matter how they are caused (see also chapter 1 by J. Last).

Naturally occurring outbreaks of both newly identified diseases and well-known epidemic-prone diseases occur most frequently in countries that lack the public health capacity to quickly detect them and prevent their international spread (Document no. WHO/CDS/CSR/EPH/2002.16). Just as inadequate surveillance and laboratory capacity work to the advantage of infectious diseases, strong public health systems can be viewed as a national security asset (Fidler, 2002). It is therefore in the interest of both industrialized and developing countries to strengthen public health systems in developing countries. Strengthened laboratories, well-trained health personnel, and reinvigorated public health institutions benefit developing countries by ensuring early identification and containment of outbreaks, thereby decreasing the suffering, death, and economic impact they cause. At the same time, industrialized countries benefit from the decreasing risk that these diseases will spread internationally (Document no. WHO/CDS/CSR/EPH/2002.16;

Kelley, 2000; Chyba, 2002; Kassalow, 2001). These arguments have acquired much more compelling force in light of developments including the international spread of infectious diseases such as AIDS in the early 1980s and SARS in 2003: Early detection and containment of infectious disease outbreaks can prevent their international spread and their potential to cause major emergencies (www.who.int/whr/2003/chapter5/en/).

PREVENTING THE INTERNATIONAL SPREAD OF INFECTIOUS DISEASES

Efforts to prevent or contain the international spread of infectious diseases have a long history (see chapter 1). In the 14th century, ships that were potential carriers of plague-infected rats were forcibly quarantined in the harbour of the city-state of Venice to prevent importation of plague (Howard-Jones, 1975). A series of international health agreements between the newly industrialized countries, elaborated during the 19th century, culminated in the adoption of the International Health Regulations in 1969 (International health organizations, 1969). These regulations are designed to maximize security against the international spread of infectious diseases while ensuring minimum impact on trade and travel. Administered by WHO, these are the only international regulations that require reporting of infectious diseases. Three diseases—cholera, plague and yellow fever—are targeted by the Regulations for reporting by countries. They also provide norms and standards for air and sea ports designed to prevent the spread from public conveyances of rodents or insects that may be carrying infectious diseases, and describe best practices to be used to control the spread of these diseases once they have occurred.

Concern about international capacity to detect and contain emerging and epidemic-prone diseases arose following outbreaks in the early 1990s of cholera in Latin America (1991), pneumonic plague in India (1994), and Ebola haemorrhagic fever in the Democratic Republic of the Congo (1995) (Khan, Tshioko, Heymann, et al. 1995; Tauxe, Mintz, & Quick, 1995; Wkly Epidemial Rec, 1994). While all these outbreaks caused concern throughout the world, with serious economic consequences and disruptions in travel and trade, it was the highly publicized Ebola outbreak that pointed most urgently to the need for changes in the International Health Regulations. That outbreak, which caught the international community by surprise, signaled the need for stronger infectious disease surveillance and control worldwide, for improved international preparedness to provide support when similar outbreaks occur, and for accommodating the needs of the media in providing valid information. A need for more broad-based international health regulations and electronic information systems connecting WHO with its regional and country offices also became evident, as did the realization that timely and adequate outbreak detection and response would need support from a broad coalition of partners (Heymann, Barakamfitiye, Szezeniowski, et al. 1999).

The International Health Regulations are therefore currently being revised to broaden the scope of diseases under surveillance and to serve as an up-to-date framework for global surveillance and response to internationally spreading infectious diseases in the 21st century. To support the revision process, the World Health Assembly has endorsed a series of resolutions aimed at ensuring a global surveillance and response system, operating in real time and under the framework of the International Health Regulations, that facilitates rapid disease detection and rational responses while authorizing WHO to utilize information sources about infectious diseases other than official notifications submitted by governments (World Health Assembly resolution 54.14; WHA 48.7; WHA 48.13; WH Assembly document A51/8).

THE USE OF ADVANCED INFORMATION TECHNOLOGY

Potential partners in global surveillance and outbreak response were first brought together informally by WHO in 1997, and then formally launched as the Global Outbreak Alert and Response Network (GOARN) partnership in 2000 (unpublished). Electronic communication networks and new computer applications were developed to enhance the network's power in global surveillance and response (Heymann & Rodier, 2001; unpublished). Several new mechanisms and a customized artificial intelligence engine for real-time gathering of disease information support the GOARN partnership. This tool, the Global Public Health Intelligence Network (GPHIN) maintained by Health Canada, heightens vigilance by continuously and systematically crawling web sites, news wires, local online newspapers, public health email services, and electronic discussion groups for key words that could signify outbreaks in the seven official languages of WHO (www.hcsc.gc.ca/hpb/transitn/gphin_3.pdf). In this way, the network is able to scan the world for informal news that gives cause for suspecting an unusual event.

GPHIN has brought major improvements in the speed of outbreak detection compared to traditional systems, where an alert sounds only after case reports at the local level progressively filter to the national level and are then reported to WHO.

Other sources of information linked together in the network include government and university centres, ministries of health, academic institutions, other UN agencies, networks of overseas military laboratories, and nongovernmental organizations having a strong presence in epidemic-prone countries, such as Médecins sans Frontières and the International Federation of Red Cross and Red Crescent Societies. Information from all these sources is assessed and verified on a daily basis. Validated information is made public via the WHO web site.

If international assistance is needed, as agreed upon in confidential proactive consultation with the affected country and with experts in the network, electronic communications are used to coordinate prompt assistance. To this end, global databases of professionals with expertise in specific diseases or epidemiological techniques are maintained, together with nongovernmental organizations present in countries and in a position to reach remote areas. Such mechanisms, which are further supported by the WHO network of Collaborating Centres (national laboratories and institutes throughout the world serving as international reference centres), help the world make the maximum use of expertise and resources—assets that are traditionally scarce for public health.

From July 1998 to August 2001, the network verified 578 outbreaks in 132 countries, indicating the system's broad geographical coverage. The most frequently reported outbreaks were of cholera, meningitis, haemorrhagic fever, anthrax, and viral encephalitis. During this same period, the network has launched effective international cooperative containment activities in many developing countries—Afghanistan, Bangladesh, Burkina Faso, Côte d'Ivoire, Egypt, Ethiopia, Kosovo, Sierra Leone, Sudan, Uganda, and Yemen, to name a few (Heymann & Rodier, 2001).

The work of coordinating large-scale international assistance, which involves many agencies from many nations, is facilitated by operational protocols which set out standardized procedures for the alert and verification process, communications, coordination of the response, emergency evacuation, research, monitoring, ownership of data and samples, and relations with the media. By setting out a chain of command, and bringing order to the containment response, such protocols help protect against the very real risk that samples of a lethal pathogen might be collected for later provision to or use by a terrorist group. Moreover, in building a global system for surveillance and response, the Global Outbreak Alert and Response Network has defined practical operational problems in ways that are guiding the revision and strengthening of the International Health Regulations. In early 2003, GOARN was put to the test during the SARS outbreak, and helped support a coordinated and effective global response.

GLOBAL OUTBREAK ALERT AND RESPONSE: THE SARS EXPERIENCE

Based on information collected by GOARN partners prior to 12 March 2003, the WHO had the information it needed to alert the world of the appearance of a severe respiratory illness of undetermined cause that had rapidly infected more than 40 staff at hospitals in Viet Nam and Hong Kong (www.who.int/csr/sars/archive/2003_03_12/en/). The alert also referred to two other events that raised the level of alarm: an outbreak of 305 cases, with 5 deaths, of atypical pneumonia reported in mid-February from the southern Chinese province of Guangdong, and an almost simultaneous report from Hong Kong of two confirmed cases of avian influenza A(H5N1) in family members with a recent travel history to southern China. The alert described the signs and symptoms of the unidentified illness and recommended that suspected cases be isolated, managed with barrier nursing techniques, and reported—simple measures that would provide the cornerstone for containing the outbreak as it spread within, and then outside of, Asia.

Prior to that alert, several international mechanisms for routine outbreak detection, investigation, and response had already begun to operate with a heightened sense of urgency. A new and potentially pandemic strain of the influenza virus was the first and most greatly feared suspected cause. Laboratories in the WHO Global Influenza Surveillance Network had been on alert since late November 2002, when the Global Public Health Intelligence Network (GPHIN) picked up rumours of severe "flu-like" outbreaks in Guangdong and Beijing (SARS-chronology of events, 2003). Studies conducted by Chinese scientists and confirmed by a network of influenza laboratories identified strains of influenza B virus as the cause, and concern eased. It mounted to new heights with the mid-February 2003 confirmation of avian influenza in Hong Kong, prompting WHO to activate its influenza pandemic preparedness plans (Influenza A(H5N1), 2003). To learn more about the outbreak in Guangdong, a team of experts, drawn from the WHO Global Outbreak Alert and Response Network, arrived in Beijing on 23 February, but was not granted permission to travel further. A second GOARN team began an emergency investigation in Hanoi on 28 February, two days after the first case of atypical pneumonia was admitted to hospital, and established infection control procedures and an isolation ward. Laboratories in the influenza network analysed specimens from this patient and other early cases, and conclusively ruled out influenza viruses as the cause. They also ruled out all other known causes of respiratory illness. With a new disease increasingly suspected, WHO began daily teleconferences linking its country and regional offices and response teams with headquarters operational staff. These mechanisms, too, proved to be decisive in tracking the outbreak, gathering the knowledge for recommending effective control measures, and getting support teams to countries requesting assistance.

By 15 March 2003, WHO had received reports of more than 150 new cases of atypical pneumonia of unidentified cause concentrated in the hospitals of six Asian countries and Canada (www.who.int/csr/sars/archive/2003_03_15/en/). The disease did not respond to antibiotics and antivirals known to be effective against primary atypical pneumonia and other respiratory infections. No patients, including young and previously healthy health workers, had recovered, many were in critical condition, several required mechanical ventilatory support, and four had died. Equally alarming, the disease was rapidly spreading along the routes of international air travel. The potential for further international spread was vividly demonstrated that same day when a medical doctor, who had treated the first cases of atypical pneumonia in Singapore, reported similar symptoms shortly before boarding a flight from New York to Singapore. The airline was alerted and the doctor and his wife disembarked in Frankfurt for immediate hospitalization, becoming the first cases in Europe (SARS: lessons from a new disease, 2003). Faced with these events, WHO issued a second and stronger global alert on 15 March, this time in the form of an emergency travel advisory (www.who.int/csr/sars/archive/2003_03_15/en/). The alert provided guidance for travellers, airlines and crew, set out a case definition, and gave the new disease its name: severe acute respiratory syndrome (SARS). It also launched a coordinated global outbreak response that tested a critical assumption: rapid and intense public health action could stop a new transmissible disease, of unidentified cause and unknown epidemic potential, from becoming endemic.

On 5 July 2003, the last known probable case of SARS completed a 20-day period of isolation, and WHO declared that the international outbreak had been contained (www.who.int/csr/don/2003_07_05/en/). While this achievement demonstrates the strength of classical public health measures—case detection, isolation, contact tracing and infection control—it also shows the importance of GOARN, set up at the international level, to improving global capacity to detect and respond to outbreaks of emerging and epidemic-prone diseases.

The international response to SARS—the roll-out of the mechanisms for outbreak detection and containment that had been under development through GOARN since 1997 (36)–became the first response to an internationally spreading outbreak during which regularly updated evidence-based recommendations for patient management and outbreak control could be collectively made in real-time as events unfolded around the world (unpublished). As the outbreak evolved, some of the world's most experienced laboratory experts, clinicians, and epidemiologists worked together in virtual networks, taking advantage of up-to-date communication technologies, including the internet, secure websites, and video and telephone conferencing. Laboratories in the existing influenza surveillance network formed the basis for a new virtual network to identify the causative agent, which was achieved within a month, and to develop diagnostic tests (WHO Multicentre Collaborative Network for SARS, 2003). Clinicians and field epidemiologists constituted other virtual networks, and by the end of the outbreak more than 150 experts from institutions in 17 countries had demonstrated how close collaboration and sharing of information, despite strong academic pressure to publish information in scientific journals, could serve the public health good. No estimates are available for the number of health staff who risked their lives in caring for patients, though the deaths of many have been documented.

The SARS outbreak also marked the first occasion where sufficient information became available rapidly enough to issue evidence-based international travel recommendations as a measure for preventing further international spread, particularly by air travel. As real-time evidence accumulated, further international spread was attributed to persons with SARS who continued to travel internationally by air, in some cases infecting passengers and crew during the flight (www.who.int/csr/sars/en/WHOconsensus.pdf). Daily tracking of cases also revealed that contacts of SARS patients continued to travel, becoming ill upon arrival at their destination. On 27 March, WHO therefore issued recommendations that countries with major outbreaks screen departing passengers for fever and other signs of SARS, or known contact with SARS patients (www.who.int/csr/sars/archive/2003_03_27/en/print.html). The choice of measures for putting this recommendation into effect was left to the discretion of individual countries. Some set up screening measures at international airports and border crossings with a variety of requirements, including a health declaration by each departing passenger, temperature monitoring of each passenger, and a stop list of contacts of SARS patients at immigration by which known contacts were asked not to travel.

As the outbreak progressed it became clear from information provided daily from the virtual networks, that contacts of probable SARS patients continued to travel and become ill after arrival at their destination, indicating the continuing risk of further international spread. Real time information further demonstrated that contact tracing at some sites did not fully identify chains of transmission, and that transmission was occurring outside confined settings such as the health care environment, possibly placing the general population at risk. In late March, an outbreak of 329 almost simultaneous probable cases among residents of a housing estate in Hong Kong suggested possible transmission by exposure to some factor in the environment, thus creating further opportunities for exposure in the general population (www.sars-expertcom.gov.hk/english/reports/reports.html). Additional evidence-based guidance was therefore made for the sites where contact tracing could not link all cases, understanding that if the disease were spreading in the wider community it would greatly increase the risk to travellers and the likelihood that cases would be exported to other countries. This guidance was aimed at international travellers, and recommended that they postpone all but essential travel to designated sites in order to minimize their risk of becoming infected (www.who.int/csr/don/2003_07_01/en/). Thus an important surgical congress scheduled for the summer of 2003 to be held in Bangkok, Thailand, was postponed.

The global alerts issued by WHO on 12 and 15 March provided a clear line of demarcation between areas with severe SARS outbreaks and those without. Following the SARS alerts, all areas with imported cases, with the exception of Taiwan, either prevented any further transmission or kept the number of locally transmitted cases very low (www.who.int/csr/sars/country/table2003_09_23/en/). Likewise, the travel recommendations issued by WHO appear to have been effective in helping to contain international spread of SARS. Of the 40 international flights known to have carried 37 probable SARS cases, current analysis has implicated five in transmission to passengers or crew (www.who.int/csr/sars/en/WHOconsensus.pdf). Following the 27 March recommendations for exit screening, no confirmed SARS case associated with in-flight exposure was reported to WHO. This may have been because awareness of screening procedures discouraged persons with fever from attempting to travel (Olsen, Chang, Cheung, et al. 2003).

Initial information from Hong Kong reveals that 2 probable SARS cases were identified by airport screening procedures, immediately hospitalized, and prevented from international travel (Hong Kong International Airport, personal communication). Travel recommendations also appear to have provided a benchmark for gauging the safety of international travel; when an area was declared safe from the risk of SARS transmission, traveller confidence was regained. Recommendations concerning travel were ended when epidemiological criteria indicating a low risk to travellers were met. That goal in itself became a motivation for governments and populations to collaborate in bringing the outbreaks under control. Many countries also set a second goal of removal from the list of areas with recent local transmission. The determination to attain this objective may have contributed to the speed with which the cycle of human-to-human transmission was broken globally, and confidence was restored (www.who.int/gb/EB_WHA/PDF/EB113/eeb11333.pdf). Passenger movement figures provided by the Hong Kong International Airport show a rapid rebound from the lowest number of passengers, 14,670, recorded just before 23 May when the travel recommendations for Hong Kong were removed, to 54,195 on 12 July, a month and a half later (Hong Kong International Airport, personal communication).

GLOBAL INFECTIOUS DISEASE EMERGENCIES: THE FUTURE

After the SARS outbreak had been contained, GOARN partners continued their global surveillance activities and detected and responded to isolated cases of SARS that were reported from Singapore and China (Taiwan and the mainland) (Heymann, Aylward, & Wolff, 2004). During 2004, avian influenza infections in humans were reported from Thailand and Viet Nam through GOARN partners, and responses coordinated through the GOARN partnership have been mounted (www.who.int/csr/don/2004_07_08/en/). In May 2005 the revised International Health Regulations will be reviewed by the World Health Assembly of WHO and submitted to an approval process. During this time, and for the years to come, infectious disease emergencies will continue to occur. The world will remain prepared for these emergencies through the GOARN partnership.

REFERENCES

A framework for global outbreak alert and response. (2000). Geneva: World Health Organization (unpublished document WHO/CDS/CSR/2000.2).

Bonn, D. (1997). Spared an influenza pandemic for another year? *Lancet, 349,* 36.

Chyba, C.F. (2002). Toward biological security. *Foreign Affairs, 81,* 122–136.

Communicable disease prevention and control: New, emerging, and re-emerging infectious diseases. (1995). Geneva: World Health Organization (World Health Assembly resolution WHA48.13).

Consensus document on the epidemiology of severe acute respiratory syndrome (SARS). (2003). Geneva: World Health Organization (unpublished document WHO/CDS/CSR/GAR/2003.11). Retrieved December 18, 2003, from http://www.who.int/csr/sars/en/WHOconsensus.pdf

Contagion and conflict: Health as a global security challenge. A report of the Chemical and Biological Arms Control Institute and the CSIS International Security Program. (2000). Washington DC: Center for Strategic and International Studies.

Dengue prevention and control: Report by the secretariat. (2002). Geneva: World Health Organization (World Health Assembly document A55/19).

Emerging foodborne diseases. (2002). WHO fact sheet 124.

Fidler, D.P. (2002 May 30). Public health and national security in the global age: Infectious diseases, bioterrorism, and realpolitik. Paper delivered at the London School of Hygiene and Tropical Medicine.

Global crisis—global solutions. Managing public health emergencies of international concern through the revised International Health Regulations. (2002). Geneva: World Health Organization (unpublished document WHO/CDS/CSR/AR/2002.4).

Global defence against the infectious disease threat. (2002). Geneva: World Health Organization.

Global health security: epidemic alert and response. (2001). Geneva: World Health Organization (World Health Assembly resolution WHA54.14).

Gubler, D.J. (2001). Human arbovirus infections worldwide. Annals of the New York Academy of Sciences, 951, 13–24.

Health Canada. Detecting emerging health risks around the world: GPHIN web site www.hc-sc.gc.ca/hpb/transitn/gphin_3.pdf

Heymann, D.L. (2001). The fall and rise of infectious diseases. Georgetown Journal of International Affairs, 11, 7–14.

Heymann, D.L., Aylward, R.B., & Wolff, C. (2004, May 15). Dangerous pathogens in the laboratory: from smallpox to today's SARS setbacks and tomorrow's polio-free world. Lancet, 363, 1566–1568.

Heymann, D.L., Barakamfitiye, D., Szezeniowski, M., & et al. (1999). Ebola hemorrhagic fever: Lessons from Kikwit, Democratic Republic of the Congo. Journal of Infectious Diseases, 179(Suppl 1), S283–86.

Heymann, D.L., Rodier, G.R. (2001) WHO Operational Support Team to the Global Outbreak Alert and Response Network. Hot spots in a wired world: WHO surveillance of emerging and re-emerging infectious diseases. Lancet Infectious Diseases, 1, 345–53.

Heymann, D.L., Rodier, G.R. (2001). Hot spots in a wired world. Lancet Infect Dis, 1, 345–353.

Howard-Jones, N. (1975). The scientific background of the international sanitary conferences 1851–1938. Geneva: World Health Organization.

Influenza A(H5N1), Hong Kong Special Administrative Region of China. (2003). Wkly Epidemiol Rec, 78, 49–50.

International health regulations (1969). Geneva: World Health Organization, 1983.

Kassalow, J.S. (2001). Why health is important to US foreign policy. New York: Council on Foreign Relations and Milbank Memorial Fund.

Kelley, P.W. (2000, May–June). Transnational contagion and global security. Military Review, 59–64.

Khan, A.S., Tshioko, F.K., Heymann, D.L., Le Guenno, B., Nabeth, P., Kerstiens, B., & et al. (1995). The re-emergence of Ebola hemorrhagic fever, Democratic Republic of Congo. Journal of Infectious Diseases 1999, 179(Suppl 1), S76–86.

Knobler, S.L., Mahmoud, A.A.F., & Pray, L.A., (Eds). (2002). Biological threats and terrorism: Assessing the science and response capabilities. Washington DC: National Academy Press.

Molyneux, D.H. (2001). Vector-borne infections in the tropics and health policy issues in the twenty-first century. Trans R Soc Trop Med Hyg, 95, 235–238.

Olsen, S.J., Chang, H.-L., Cheung, T.Y.-Y., Tang, A.F.-Y., Fisk, T.L., Ooi, S.P.-L. & et al. (2003). Transmission of the severe acute respiratory syndrome on aircraft. *N Engl J Med, 349*(25), 2416–22.

Plague—international team of experts, India. (1994). *Wkly Epidemiol Rec, 69,* 321–2.

Preparedness for the deliberate use of biological agents: A rational approach to the unthinkable. (2002). Geneva: World Health Organization (document no. WHO/CDS/CSR/EPH/2002.16).

Price-Smith, A.T. (2002). Pretoria's shadow: The HIV/AIDS pandemic and national security in South Africa. *CBACI health and security series*; special report 4.

Public health response to biological and chemical weapons. (2001). Geneva: World Health Organization web site www.who.int/emc/book_2nd_edition.htm

Revision and updating of the International Health Regulations. (1995). Geneva: World Health Organization (World Health Assembly resolution WHA48.7).

Revision of the International Health Regulations: Progress report. (1998). Report by the Director General. Geneva: World Health Organization (World Health Assembly document A51/8).

SARS in Hong Kong: From experience to action. Hong Kong SAR: SARS Expert Committee, 2003. Retrieved December 18, 2003, from http://www.sars-expertcom.gov.hk/english/reports/reports.html

SARS—Chronology of events. (2003). Ottawa: Health Canada, Population and Public Health Branch.

SARS: lessons from a new disease. The world health report 2003: Shaping the future. Geneva: World Health Organization.

Severe acute respiratory syndrome (SARS): report by the secretariat. (2003). Geneva: World Health Organization (Executive Board document EB113/33, 27 November 2003). Retrieved December 19, 2003, from http://www.who.int/gb/EB_WHA/PDF/EB113/eeb11333.pdf

Severe acute respiratory syndrome, update 11–WHO recommends new measures to prevent travel-related spread of SARS. Retrieved December 18, 2003, from http://www.who.int/csr/sars/archive/2003_03_27/en/print.html

Severe acute respiratory syndrome, update 92–chronology of travel recommendations, areas with local transmission. Retrieved December 18, 2003, from http://www.who.int/csr/don/2003_07_01/en/

Summary of probable SARS cases with onset of illness from 1 November 2002 to 31 July 2003 (revised 26 September 2003). Geneva: World Health Organization 2003. Retrieved December 18, 2003, from http://www.who.int/csr/sars/country/table2003_09_23/en/

Taiwan, China: SARS transmission interrupted in last outbreak area. (2003). World Health Organization SARS situation update 96, 5 July 2003. Retrieved December 18, 2003, from http://www.who.int/csr/don/2003_07_05/en/

Tauxe, R.V. (1997). Emerging foodborne diseases: An evolving public health challenge. *Emerging Infectitious Diseases, 3,* 425–434.

Tauxe, R.V., Mintz, E.D., & Quick, R.E. (1995). Epidemic cholera in the New World: Translating field epidemiology into new prevention strategies. *Emerging Infectious Diseases, 1,* 141–6.

Tauxe, R.V., Mintz, E.D., & Quick, R.E. (1995). Epidemic cholera in the new world: Translating field epidemiology into new prevention strategies. *Emerging Infectitious Diseases, 1,* 141–146.

The increasing incidence of human campylobacteriosis. Report and proceedings of a WHO consultation of experts. (2001). Geneva: World Health Organization (document no. WHO/CDS/CSR/APH 2001.7).

Understanding the BSE threat. (2002). Geneva: World Health Organization (document no. WHO/CDS/CSR/EPH/2002.6).

Urgent call for action on meningitis in Africa—vaccine price and shortage are major obstacles. (2002). *Wkly Epidemiol Rec, 77,* 330–331.

West Nile virus update: Current case count. Centers for Disease Control and Prevention web site www.cdc.gov/od/oc/media/wncount.htm

WHO Division of Emerging and Other Communicable Diseases Surveillance and Control Annual Report 1997. Geneva: World Health Organization, 1998 (unpublished document WHO/EMC/98.2).

WHO issues a global alert about cases of atypical pneumonia: Cases of severe respiratory illness may spread to hospital staff. (2003). World Health Organization press release 12 March. Retrieved December 18, 2003, from http://www.who.int/csr/sars/archive/2003_03_12/en/

Woolhouse, M.E.J., Dye, C., (Eds). (2001). Population biology of emerging and re-emerging pathogens. *Philosophical Transactions Royal Society Biological Science, 356,* 981–982.

World Health Organization issues emergency travel advisory. (2003). World Health Organization situation update 15 March. Retrieved December 18, 2003, from http://www.who.int/csr/sars/archive/2003_03_15/en/

World Health Organization Multicentre Collaborative Network for Severe Acute Respiratory Syndrome (SARS) Diagnosis. A multicentre collaboration to investigate the cause of severe acute respiratory syndrome. (2003). *Lancet, 361,* 1730–3.

World Health Organization. Avian influenza—current evaluation of risks to humans from H5N1 following recent reports, 8 July 2004. Retrieved from http://www.who.int/csr/don/ 2004_07_08/en/

World Health Report 2003. Chapter 5 SARS: Lessons learned from a new disease. http://www.who.int/whr/2003/chapter5/en/

Yellow fever, Senegal (update). (2002). *Wkly Epidemiol Rec, 77,* 373–374.

Chapter 13

Knowledge-Based Methodologies in the Health Sector

B. McA. Sayers and Juan J. Angulo

The term "knowledge," as used here, refers to information that can only be expressed directly in the form of statements rather than numerical data. In one situation discussed in this chapter, knowledge about a community is critical to describing and modelling the way an epidemic of communicable disease spreads through that community. Sometimes, the information results from a specific *post-hoc* study of a specific outbreak; but when considering how a new epidemic might spread in another community, the necessary information must be obtained from other indirect "knowledge" about the community, and this may require the aid of computational logic used as a tool for inferring the knowledge needed from that already available. The methodology for manipulating knowledge statements in this way has also other uses in the health sector. The "knowledge-based" indicator and applications to investigating "determinants of health" are discussed below. The concept should not be confused with an evidence based concept, which refers to reliance on the outcome of appropriate formal clinical trials in the design of therapeutic measures; "knowledge" is regarded as a supplement to data.

REALISTIC MODELLING OF THE SPREAD OF COMMUNICABLE DISEASE

The opportunities for global transmission of communicable disease are now considerable; new epidemics can occur in countries previously unaffected.

Understanding the spread of epidemics of communicable disease has certainly been facilitated by the use of mathematical models, but most of these models concern the situation once the epidemic is fully established. However, communicable diseases do not commonly start instantaneously in any individual country with a large number of simultaneously infected individuals. This is why understanding the way an epidemic develops is important, as well as intrinsically interesting. Achieving a realistic understanding that leads to an explanation requires a new approach.

This chapter's authors believe the fundamental components in the spread of a communicable disease are the "living elements"; this viewpoint is not commonly reflected in typical mathematical models, which tend to treat "space" and "time" as fundamental. But, at the very least, an infectious agent, an infected host, and one or more susceptible hosts in sufficient contact with the infected host, are essential components of an epidemic. So, the nature of the infective-susceptible contacts is relevant. The opportunities for contacts and their effectiveness are determined, not only by biological variables, but also by social and environmental factors. Thus, descriptions of epidemic spread that disregard the essential living elements without which an epidemic would not exist, omit a crucial determinant. As pointed out by Hudson (1972), the social structures that underlie human contacts are fundamental. If the necessary information about the social network, that is, explanations of of the social interconnections in the community, could be obtained, then it should be feasible to test the proposition, and to design more realistic models that could show what assumptions were necessary and what were sufficient. The matter of what information is needed could be clarified by the examination of epidemics that have been studied in such detail that the social network can be identified. Then, it may become clear how to collect such information in the context of any specific community, whether in order to understand *a posteriori* how an infection spread or to forecast what could happen in a community at risk from newly introduced infection.

The facts about a real epidemic would help to focus the discussion, and provide a means for demonstrating the acquisition of information and how it can be utilised in practice. But very few epidemics have been studied and reported in the (necessarily) great detail needed for an adequate demonstration. However, an outbreak of *variola minor* during 1955–56 in a Brazilian city, Bragança Paulista (State of São Paulo), is suitable for analysis because of the quite unique, detailed information gathered about this self-contained epidemic of some 514 cases that started from a single case introduced into a community free of the disease at the time. This was an epidemic of an S-I-R disease, so-called because of its characteristic sequence of events: a Susceptible, once Infected, is then Removed from the susceptible population, by reason of acquired immunity or death. The available data include extensive information about virtually every individual infected, their contacts, their households, and about the schools in the community. These records allow the progress of the epidemic to be tracked from case to case, the victims individually identified, from the onset of epidemic until its extinction. The "chain of contagion," once so determined, takes account of both intra- and inter-household spread.

The very first case, imported from another State, led to a chain of contagion linking urban households, with some intra-household cases and increasing incidence of "branching" to parallel pathways in other households. All the initial inter-household pathways finally terminated, but several had already introduced cases into the schools. This revived the progress of the epidemic, first by infection of other pupils in the class, then into their households and thence to further inter-household movement, linearly and with some branching, and, finally, to extinction. After the epidemic spread from urban areas to isolated households in rural districts, some local "mini-epidemics" did occur, but few other rural households were infected, presumably because of their social or geographical isolation.

Events in the school classrooms were apparently responsible for the ultimate extinction of the epidemic. Several factors seem to have been relevant. First, after the initial "sub-epidemic," the direct inter-household spread died out, up to the disease's introduction into the schools. Second, the rate of daily case occurrences in the school classrooms reached a maximum and started to decline before mass vaccination was started; a few days after the peak, the schools closed for the end-of-semester vacation. Perhaps as a result, the underlying pattern of daily case rate within the households that were infected through infected pupils was similar to, but delayed after, that of the post-maximum pattern in the schools. Third, a relatively small proportion of the susceptible pupils became infected.

Thus several phases can be discerned: initial inter-household spread; introduction into the schools; spread within the classrooms; transmission of the infection from the schools by pupils into their households; and subsequent inter-household spread. This is the important observation: Several substantial changes occur in the nature of the spread of infection. Without appreciating this possibility, important realities of the epidemic would be submerged. The characteristics of linear-sequential (or low-order parallel) inter-household transmission are quite different from the accelerated activity generated in the schools, and the school infection activity was influenced by the general immune situation in the classrooms. The school closures initiated a further change.

These are the realities that apply to a specific community, and it would appear that they dominate the spread of the epidemic. In short, the indications of this particular study are that the manner of spread, starting from a small number of individual cases, is greatly influenced by social networks and structures existing in that community, which also influence the timing and form of transitions as the infection moves between them. Understanding and modelling the epidemic requires that these factors be taken sufficiently into account. So the next questions are: how to identify the relevant factors likely to operate in a given community; and how to take account of these in developing a model aiming to describe the epidemic in an informative way? The answers to such questions, it is argued, would be widely applicable in public health within countries and, more generally, in global health. They could add a new dimension to the information and understanding available to investigators and planners. Further, the modelling approach based on the information so acquired would constitute a new tool for research and planning.

Firstly, it needs to be recognised that communities are not necessarily homogeneous and may only become approximately so on a very large scale. There are numerous ways in which non-stationarity (time-based changes), whether of transmission characteristics or of the susceptible population at risk at any stage, may operate. These must be community-dependent; so that they could only be identified by examining the insights generated by expert sociological observers of that community. Such insights, unstructured, perhaps, but descriptive, would emerge in the form of a series of statements about the community. Factors likely to be important to understanding an epidemic and to its modelling need to be extracted from many such statements. A few simple examples can be cited.

In this community, some households have multi-household contacts; most are known to have few, but this differs from the households infected from the schools. It has also been shown that the epidemic can be treated on a household–household basis; given the longitudinal time-course (pattern) of introductory case occurrences into households, it is possible to estimate the total pattern of subsequent cases (intra-household and all following cases) with good accuracy. Most households contain school-age children some of whom were previously vaccinated; the latter tend to be in older age groups. Schools have two "shifts" using each classroom and cases introduced into the schools could readily generate further cases; these further cases could serve as "introductory cases" into new households. But there are limiting factors. Within schools there is no mixing between classes, no mixing between two shifts using the same classroom, and pupils always occupy the same desk (i.e., physical location) in the classroom. Consequently, the presence of immune pupils would influence and inhibit the indefinite spread of infection in the classroom, particularly in those classes having age groups more likely to have been immunised. Further, the school calendar includes end-of-semester vacations, affecting the opportunities for transmission of infection. All these observations are variously relevant to understanding the several phases of the epidemic, and have been extracted from statements about the community made by expert observers.

Other factors may not be extracted so readily from expert statements because of the inevitably discursive nature and range of comments assembled without particular regard to their relevance to the current purpose. This is where computational logic may be needed: to identify significant possibilities from the many such statements about the community that could be generated by expert sociological observers. The process of identification makes use of knowledge in its technical, rather than semantic, sense: using facts, observations, beliefs, and descriptions, at least some of which are expressible only in the form of statements, not as numerical data or in quantitative relationships. Conventional numerical computing cannot help here; but computational logic based, for example, on the PROLOG computer language or its developments, could. A program can be written to generate deductions and inferences that can reasonably be drawn from an automated comparison of the various statements supplied. This process merely facilitates and automates the natural logic analysis that could be carried out by a human analyst, but also reduces the risk of overlooking anything of potential value in the confusion of information. "Knowledge-based" description and—if necessary—computational analysis about a community that is potentially susceptible to a particular communicable disease, is the first and fundamental stage of the interpretative modelling introduced here. Converted into design aspects and thus incorporated into an appropriate numerical model, the importance of the factors elucidated in this way and their sensitivity can be tested quantitatively.

The Structure of a "Knowledge-Based" Explanatory Model

The model should be probabilistic. It should generate repeated trials of the results of introducing a new source of infection into a community, in random locations, and, perhaps, at random times during the calendar year. In selecting the expected movements of the infection between households, the choice can only be statistical—on the basis of what is typical of the spread in such a community; but the precise movement cannot be known. Therefore, it should be assumed that while the contacts between households would be randomly selected, they would follow the pattern of social connectivity operating in the community. This would also be true of geographic aspects of the inter-household translations. Thus when an infection is first introduced into the model community, the contact that forwards the infection would be randomly determined, although subject to various constraints. The infection could spread within the same household or, and possibly also, to one or more other households, and perhaps to a school as well. The source of infection could be an adult, a pre-school infant, or a school-age pupil; the receptor individual could be drawn from any susceptible in these categories.

All of these considerations affect the design of the second, numerical stage of modelling. In summary, the model should draw upon probabilistic information and be subject to various powerful design constraints of sociological origin, such as those outlined above. From the data available for the specific exemplar epidemic, histograms of the relevant variables that describe the community and its inter-connections can be produced. They take account of changes, and therefore alter, as the epidemic progresses. The distributions, or rather the histograms on which they are based, are then used individually to allow the synthesis of tables of random numbers that are distributed like the corresponding histograms. Thirty-three random number tables, based on the corresponding empirical histograms, are needed to accommodate the constraints mentioned; others can be added as more design data become available. Introductory infection in a household may produce further intra-household cases and infect one or more other households; cases in these households may initiate cases in the school classrooms; these cases generate others within the classroom and some of these will in turn introduce the infection into their households, thus triggering a further inter-household spread. Thus, five sub-models are needed: an inter-household model; an intra-household model; an intra-classes model; a post-schools intra-household model; and a post-schools inter-household model. The various sub-models initiate, receive and/or forward the infection in accordance with the structure of the model, the various random number tables utilised, and the constraints that operate. As each new household or individual is infected, the relevant data for such a household or individual is collected by consulting values in the various tables of random numbers.

It can be noted that operation of the intra-classroom sub-model is subject to the two constraints already listed: because of the existence of immunes in the classrooms, and because of the impact of the school closures at the end-of-semester dates, referred to the original (randomly selected) onset calendar date, both constraints affect cases generated subsequently.

The totality of cases generated by the five sub-models constitutes the final output from the overall, probabilistic model. Each household has a specified "spatial location" and each case has an assigned "rash date" and other characteristics (e.g., adult or other family member).

Each trial (a "run") of the composite model uses individual entry points into the various random number tables for each individual case and each individual household, and would therefore be subject to statistical fluctuation. But the model can be run repeatedly; an average should yield a typical picture of the epidemic: an "epidemic curve" showing the forecast number of cases as a function of date, and the typical geographical movements of the infection. They should produce patterns of case occurrences with broadly appropriate attack patterns, maximum case rates, overall shapes of the "epidemic curve" of cases versus time, and die out, as in the real epidemic. These should acceptably match the real epidemic data on which the various random number distributions were based, but only if all factors have been fully, and correctly, taken into account.

The advantage of being able to follow in detail the way the epidemic spreads is that the role of social characteristics and structure becomes evident. Thus it may be seen that the modelling process not only explains the way the epidemic did spread from inception, but suggests possible ways in which it might have spread had the initial infection occurred in a different household or at a different time.

If the model is realistic, disregarding or altering any of the random number distributions should significantly affect the outcome. For instance, increasing slightly the proportion of susceptible infants in households immediately changes the cases within the schools and increases the growth of the epidemic. Decreasing the proportion of immune pupils in schools causes an extended growth of cases within the schools and of the households subsequently infected, so that the epidemic is sustained at a higher level and for a longer period. Disregarding the date of closure of the schools has a similar impact on the course of the epidemic—again, sustaining the epidemic for a much longer period. Enlarging the contact area for households has the effect of increasing the initial linear inter-household

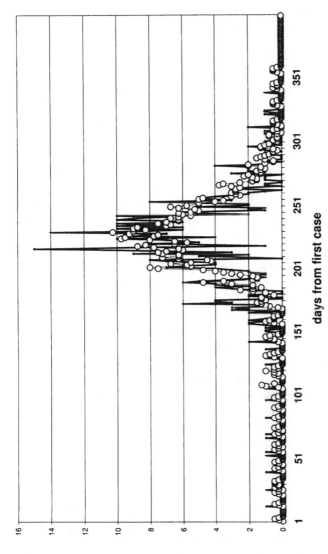

Figure 13.1. The figure for daily case occurrences (original data: solid curve; model average: circles) illustrates the match that can be achieved between the real "epidemic curve," with its remarkable pattern of growth followed by a spontaneous abatement, and the model, using the average of a number of runs (20). (The confidence interval at the peak estimate is from 9.1-11.1 cases.) In fact, three main groups of simulated "epidemic curve" emerge. The major group comprised broadly similar patterns as shown in the figure, differing mainly in the timing of the systematic acceleration of case rates attributable to households having school-age children that are thus able to introduce infection into school classrooms. Another group of patterns (some 10%) exhibited a similar pattern, but the acceleration of case rates was late and restricted, because the randomly selected households having school age children came, by chance, late in the sequence of inter-household transmission and school closures came into effect soon after. A third group (about 5%) generated few cases and no systematic pattern of case acceleration, again attributable to the nature of the households first infected.

sub-epidemic which changes the pattern of cases introduced into the schools, leading to a more rapid growth of the epidemic. The degree of "branching" (from one household to a number) is a sensitive parameter and alters as the infection spreads to households more distant from the origin. Changing, or neglecting, this alteration modifies the rate at which the epidemic develops, the way it develops, and the total cases. Such tests should be, and are, a useful guide to adequacy of the model and the utility of the approach.

As would be expected, the excellent matches between modelled and real epidemic can be achieved only when the social factors are included, which tends to confirm the importance of such factors. The model is explanatory in that it allows an understanding of how the relevant social factors—in this case, structures—influence the spread of the S-I-R infection. The proportion of susceptibles in households, the probability of infection, the existence of schools closely embedded in the community, the influence of immune and susceptible pupils in the schools, the degree of branching due to inter-household contacts both before and after the infection reached the schools, and the vacation date—all appear to be necessary factors. It appears that, while inclusion of these social factors is crucial to the success of the model, the random choice of successively infected households is acceptable. Above all, the success of this explanatory model supports the original proposition—that "living" elements are not only fundamental to the existence and spread of an epidemic but must be taken into account.

In a S-I-R disease model, the function of an infected individual is to contribute one case to the total, at the relevant rash date, and then possibly infect one or more further susceptibles, intra- or inter-household, and finally to disappear from further consideration. If however, in a different disease, the infected individual could be re-infected after, say, a latent period; this outcome could be accommodated in the model with appropriate additions. Thus, this type of model is a rich source of opportunities for further investigations. For instance, it can be used to explore the effect of different distributions of one or more parameters, such as the make-up of households, the size of school classes or the number of schools. Another option is to alter the contact pathways which alters the opportunities for multiple households or individuals to be infected from one infective, that is, the degree of branching. The probability of individual infection can be altered, even differentially as between intra-household and inter-household transmission to reflect the possibly improved mixing that could occur in the former. A transmission vector conveying the infection could be incorporated as an adjunct to or replacement of direct individual contacts. The effect of imprecise data can be investigated to help determine the likely uncertainties in forecasting epidemic spread. Equally, if the necessary parameters could be identified for any new community, a similar model could be used to explore the behaviour of an epidemic in that community. While the crucial social factors were readily identified in this case from expert insights into the community concerned, they could equally well have emerged from a computational logic analysis, had this been necessary.

Choosing parameters (the factors to be taken into account, such as the typical household contact pattern—branching—the existence of schools, the occurrence of immunes and school pupils in a typical household, and factors such as school vacations) for the model to match a different community, perhaps in a different country, depends on knowledge about that community. While such knowledge may well be available in the form of insights due to expert observers of that community, converting these insights into knowledge that can be used in model system design is not automatic. It could depend on appropriate inferences drawn from the basic information, which would themselves generally take the form of descriptive statements, for instance about the social networks in the community and linkages involving households, schools, markets, places of work, and public transport. This is where computational logic may be helpful, in supplementing the inferences that could, practicably, be made by human analysts. Automated logical inferences drawn from basic knowledge, insight or observation can be made with the aid of the technology of the "inference engine."

Computer-Based Processing of Semantic Information: An Introduction

Computational logic software typically has several key aspects, such as: clauses, objects, domains, predicates, and goals. The clauses comprise a collection of facts and rules about a specific problem situation. For instance, "This household contains school-age children," is a simply expressed fact. But: "If a household contains school-age children who attend school, then respiratory infections will be introduced into the household" is another fact, expressed as a "rule" in the form: "If . . . , Then . . . ." Objects are elements in the problem that stand in some relation, one to some other. "Household" is an object in this sense; so are "respiratory infections," and also "school-age children." Domains express the type of values that the objects can take up, such as: integer number, real number, symbol, file, character, or string of characters. Every fact or rule belongs to a predicate, which specifies the name of the relation between objects in the fact or rule, and the types of object involved.

Every program in computational logic is "declarative"; it starts with a specification of domains of the objects, predicates that specify aspects of the facts and rules, clauses expressing the facts including the known relationships between the objects, and a statement of the "goal" to which the program is aimed. A goal is expected to take the form of a logical deduction from the facts, given the rules. It is not necessary to instruct the program how to solve for the goal; programs of this type are not procedural. The program comprises, instead, the description of the problem: names and nature of objects involved in the problem; names of relations known to exist between the objects; and the facts and rules that express these relations. Finally, the chosen goal, which may involve many sub-goals, is expressed as the sought-after end result of logical operations to be performed upon the given facts and relationships; the aim of the program is to test for possibilities that would match the goal.

Expert statements of fact, observation, or belief, as well as archive information, can be made to correspond to clauses—facts and rules—taken together with objects and predicates. In this way, semantic knowledge can be represented computationally. The basic logic computation as sketched out above has now been embedded in much more sophisticated software packages that allow the introduction of knowledge and the specification of goals to be a relatively simple task, yet with the possibility of achieving highly complex logical investigations. Because the dynamic alteration of goals is feasible, very subtle procedures can be envisaged.

Utilising this technology, the inferences arising from the input information can be explored objectively and automatically. In this way, the essential social elements that are needed for a probabilistic exploratory and explanatory model are to be identified. Thus a knowledge base of expert knowledge about the community, linked to a data base of quantitative data, can be used in order to interpret a health issue—in this case, through the design of a probabilistic model that could explain how the spread of an infectious disease occurs. It illustrates a simple but important interaction between health and social sectors. Expressed this way, it raises the question: could such a development be generalised to other problems in the public health field, particularly involving other socio-economic sectors?

If so, it would provide another tool to support attempts to assess and improve the health status of communities or countries. Specifically, the approach can be generalised to the development of health- and health status- indicators and to the use of knowledge maps in studying determinants of health, in both cases with a view to guiding decisionmaking both on a national and an international scale.

FURTHER APPLICATIONS OF KNOWLEDGE-BASED TECHNOLOGY

Consider, first, the problem of assessing national or global health. Classically, various measurements are obtained to serve as the basis of assessment. But beyond health variables that can be measured, or indicators by which they may be estimated, there is another dimension of information: semantic knowledge—knowledge, for short. This is information that can only be expressed in the form of verbalised statements. The meaning conveyed by such statements is the specific contribution of this knowledge to, for example, health assessment. The reason for exploring this approach is not merely the substitution of difficult-to-get quantitative data; it is in order to take account of the influences on health that can only be represented as knowledge. Relying on quantitative data alone in health status assessment imposes constraints on understanding. It risks distorting the information sought by unavoidably accepting indirect indicators. Formal methods of knowledge processing should circumvent such difficulties.

Expert observations or judgements that constitute knowledge about aspects of health in a community are a valuable resource that has not yet been formally utilised. There are two immediate issues: to explore the meaning of the knowledge concept, and then to determine how to capitalise on the expert observation resource. It is not a trivial comment that knowledge is already a crucial, though commonly unstated, part of all measurement for health. For instance, the decision to use, say, the infant mortality rate as some measure of health in a community means that the observer has already employed a piece of knowledge, in the form of a belief that this particular measurement can be used to indicate the aspect of health that it is desired to assess. This belief is fundamental to the use of the indicator, but it is a statement not a number. Indeed, once the data are available, knowledge must result before decisions are taken. Even in the classical approach, the link between the acquisition of data and the taking of decisions in the light of these data unavoidably requires that knowledge be extracted. Thus knowledge is implicitly used in many investigations, often to focus attention on important matters rather than on the irrelevant. The present knowledge-based approach underlines, formalises and extends these simple facts.

Knowledge based information has the form of self-contained statements, each with a standard grammatical format (such as a subject; verb; object—with conditions as subordinate clauses). Knowledge comprises key information available in the form of statements of fact originating in archived sources or in observations. It may be extended to include statements of belief or perception originating in, say, expert knowledge about specific communities, provided that there is some way to establish at least, self-consistency, and preferably also the absence of bias. Taken together, such statements of fact or belief can lead to inferences , which are often important for understanding the health circumstances in, say, a particular community. However, these general inferences may be difficult to recognise without automated assistance. In this (usual) situation, it is necessary to find a way to represent the various statements that will allow computer assistance. Then it is practical to make use of computer programs employing computational logic and making use of special computer languages. When informational knowledge is acquired, or used, specifically in this way or for this purpose, the term knowledge-based is employed.

Various types of knowledge-based information can be obtained concerning health. They would include a variety of observations, which can be grouped into sections reflecting various other socio-economic sectors that impact on health. The following are illustrative, not exclusive.

Statements specifically about health: pre-existing conditions; prior exposures; historical morbidities and traumas; typical infant growth rates; availability of safe water and sewage disposal; existing "stressor" factors; and mental health.
Statements about the environment: existence of pollutants; disease vectors; and climatic stresses.Statements about education level: its influence on

employability; on hygiene; on the treatment of infant diseases within the household; on health behaviour patterns.

Statements about household circumstances: quality of housing; structure of the family; employment pattern; food preparation practices; and nutritional adequacy.

Statements about social or economic factors: stability of employment; existing debt; social structure of the community as it affects support for families and individuals; levels of social violence; individual safety; and availability of education for children.

Statements about health care provision: level of willingness to seek health care (accessibility, cost, perceived quality); quality of health care facilities as perceived by the community; co-existence of public and private health care; and availability of insurance schemes and community perceptions of them.

Statements about cultural constraints affecting health or the decision to seek health care.

It will be recognised that such statements constitute implicit propositions about inter-sectoral interactions.

"Knowledge-Based Indicators": The Knowledge-Map

Because health is a complex concept, it implies many things simultaneously. The kinds of things we mean by the health of a specific community include, in addition to the presence or absence of disease or disability: health-promoting or health-damaging behaviour patterns; historical morbidities; adequacy of nutrition; education level; cultural factors that affect health; environmental factors; adequacy of access to affordable health care and safe water; quality of housing; existence and stability of opportunities for employment; and other factors regarded as representing "quality of life." Most of these are concepts, like health itself. Each, too, can be resolved into the elements that are generally recognised as contributing to it. When these elements are examined, some will be found to be concepts also. This process of resolving concepts can be continued until elements are reached that can be either measured or described. This is the starting point from which the knowledge map of, say, the health of a community can be built up.

The essence of the knowledge-map approach is as follows: Experts familiar with a particular community develop perceptions about it that would require much difficult data gathering to identify by direct investigation—if it was possible to gather it at all. The expert is used to make these perceptions explicit: as elements, that is—measurables or observables, that is, which can be measured or described—relevant to health of the community. The next step is to assemble these elements, forming a pattern of inter-relationships and the inferences that can be drawn from these. Some of the connections in the pattern, referred to as a knowledge map, could take the form of mathematically expressed linkages. But some of the connections would certainly be statements, in the form of knowledge describing how components link. Some of the nodes (local end-points of a set of linkages) might allow translation from statements into numbers, perhaps in broadly quantised form. A couple of introductory examples will illustrate different ways of thinking about the approach.

Imagine an indicator that could be used to identify the level of peri-natal risk, during and after gestation, associated with socio-economic factors. The high-level concept (indicator): risk: is defined by a knowledge map in the following way. Risk—for the purposes of illustration in this context, it is limited to socio-economic factors—is treated as having five contributory elements, each itself being a concept. These intermediate level factors are related respectively to: quality of housing, financial support of mother, employment of mother or of partner, nature and stability of relationship, and other factors such as level of maternal education.

At a lower level still, these in turn can be decomposed into measurables or observables such as: room occupancy, accommodation facilities, employment, income, number of children supported, and so on. Some of the observables are numerical (e.g., number of children), some are category-type (e.g., income level of partner), while others are Boolean (e.g., presence or absence of facilities for washing; access to safe water). Because, at this level, all the factors are themselves no longer concepts but are all measurables or observables, no further decomposition is necessary. At this stage, the knowledge map can be reconstructed, using expert judgement to identify how the next higher level of abstraction is achieved through the relationships involved. The relationships that are perceived by expert observers to link different inputs at one level, to an output at the next level, are most frequently only expressible in semantic terms, that is, as statements of how the relationship works.

Two points can be made. First, it is possible to describe degrees of risk in different ways, for instance in ranked, or perhaps qualitative terms. Second, similar degrees of risk may arise from different causes, so it is desirable—and possible—to be able to trace downwards on the knowledge map to see how the risk arises.

The relationships constitute knowledge, which can be expressed by rules in the logic programming sense; the knowledge originates from experts familiar with the community. The application of the rule to the information available at one level results in an output at the next level, which may appear in numerical, ranked, Boolean, or semantic form. So the knowledge map in this context serves as a kind of model of the system being assessed, expressed in a rule-based form, and run in practice by making use of computational logic.

Nutritional deficiency diseases offer another illustration of a different way of thinking about knowledge-based indicators. Morbidity data—say, about nutritional cases—are descriptive; but in order to establish priorities, plan interventions,

and understand consequences, we need more insight. The kind of description, preceding decisionmaking, about the system that underlies the numbers, requires a
definition of the factors that affect the caseload, and the way they operate. One
can think of the "actions" (the term is used in a general sense) that lead from the
input to the output, that is, the caseload.

So for typical families within a community, the relevant actions are decoded
from multiple inputs and a single output:

Inputs:
availability of nutritional components of the diet
decisionmaking about use of family resources for food items:
   resources to obtain;
   understanding within the family of what a healthy diet means, and why it is
   important;
   influence of cultural practices on diet;
   influence of religious constraints on diet.
health reserve (includes health history)
nutritional history
genetic factors
Output:
potential and actual cases of nutritional deficiency diseases
The pathways:
regarded as actions that operate on the inputs to generate the output;
represented by rules

Items in italic above represent constraints: for instance, certain food items are
not acceptable—or not acceptable together. Other inputs involve the way family
priorities affect decisions. Both kinds of knowledge can only come from experts, in
the field within the community. Also, such knowledge is semantic, not numerical.
Observations are needed (e.g., nutritional history) but so is understanding (how
do families achieve decisionmaking about resources for nutrition, and how does
this affect nutritional level?). Designing questions to ask requires a special form of
domain expertise. Expressing the actions that lead from the knowledge expressed
by the answers to the output requires expert insight. Investigating the implications
is likely to require a significant amount of automated assistance. It involves the
formal construction of a knowledge map.

The Structure of a "Knowledge Map"

The map comprises the totality of the linkages that combine the basic observations, descriptions, and measurables into the next-level concepts and progressively into higher-level concepts, ultimately forming the high-level concept of
health. Linkages could also lead outside the health sector, since health issues have

a bearing on other matters such as social needs and employment. The linkages are sometimes made up of quantitative operations (adding causal effects—similar consequences of different causes—together, for instance) but many linkages take the form of semantic knowledge about how the elements combine, as derived from expert understanding or perhaps from general scientific—or even specifically sociological—knowledge. The knowledge map thus decodes how the observed inputs at the lowest level interact to form the health status concept at the highest level. And because the linkages are dependent upon semantic knowledge, the map must be constructed in the form of computer software using a computational logic language.

To summarize the proposition: It appears that much of the essence of a complex object such as the health situation can only be captured as knowledge, not as data; such knowledge is expressible only as verbalised statements of facts, observations, or expert beliefs resulting from experience within a community. A knowledge-based indicator of health would be treated as a high-level concept. The high-level concept is reconstructed from a knowledge map developed from expert knowledge about the community, its interrelations and its workings.

Analysing Determinants of Health

The knowledge-based semantic statement approach may be suited also to exploring the complex effects of the determinants of health status; this application would raise issues different from those of the previous proposals. Because of their complexity, the interactions between various determinant factors and other influences and consequences cannot be readily decoded; if such decoding is possible at all, to any realistic extent, it will require substantial technological support. Semantic statements of expert perception and judgement about individual family units in the larger social context are, in effect, the only wide-ranging source of information about determinants and how they are likely to act. Synthesising informational inputs from a variety of experts having possibly different views and experiences of health determinants in a specific community would seem to be crucial.

To summarise the concept: A knowledge-based system using expert observations and insights can be employed to construct a knowledge map of the way a selected determinant affects health and the pathways involved. The methodology is a development of a knowledge map in reverse; it, again, uses the same principles as computational logic uses. At this stage, it is not realistic to expect that all the operations required could be undertaken in a fully automatic manner. However, it is feasible to think of providing substantial automatic support to a human operator using a system based on this approach.

To pursue a simple illustration, starting with poverty as a potential determinant of health, the first question is: How is poverty manifested in the particular community? Consequences may appear in one or more of the following: nutrition; housing; physical, climatic, or social environment; exposure to disease; resistance to infection; knowledge of hygiene; exposure to trauma; employment; access to education; awareness of available social support; and other areas in which poverty manifests itself. Expert scenarios could be assembled that take account of these. Interactions could be immediately identified and expressed formally, thus leading to inferences (outputs) encapsulated in rules. For instance, the physical environment may include unsafe water and poor sanitation arrangements—there is an immediate linkage with exposures to communicable diseases or perhaps, also, to toxic chemicals. Putting these observations together with knowledge about the existing local microbiological hazards, inferences (even though obvious) start to emerge. The aim of this approach is to develop a general knowledge map that expresses as many as possible of the health consequences of the fundamental determinant. The construct depends on both expert judgement and insight, and on archival information accessible to the operator (the expert developing the knowledge map). At this stage, the general structure is complete. But there is one more, crucial, step that firms-up the knowledge map to allow application to a particular community. This step is the application of appropriate magnitude or likelihood values, wherever required, omitting those elements or pathways that are judged not to apply. In this kind of implementation of the basic scheme, the operator determines the structure—comprising rules and pathways—aided by the automated methodology outlined above, which draws attention to possible linkages.

CONCLUDING REMARKS

The key proposition of this chapter is that knowledge, in the sense used here, is an important, underused resource. It is now time to explore how best to capitalise on this resource. The usefulness of this new kind of model innovation—knowledge-based and probabilistic—which aims to describe and explain epidemic growth realistically, depends upon knowledge about the society involved, and constitutes one fully developed example showing how such knowledge can be utilised and to what effect. Extending the concept to the health sector more generally reveals new opportunities, both in creating and using knowledge maps and in studying determinants of health.

BIBLIOGRAPHY

Angulo, Juan J. (1976). Variola minor in Bragança Paulista County, 1956: Overall description of the epidemic and of its study. *International Journal of Epidemiology, 5,* 359–66.

Hudson, John C. (1972). Geographical Diffusion Theory. Studies in Geography No 19, Evanston, Illinois, Northwestern University Press.

Sayers, B. McA. Knowledge-based technology in the service of health. (1998). World Health Forum (W.H.O.), *19,* 15–20.

Chapter 14

Food Safety: A Pressing Public-Health and Economic Issue[1]

FRITZ KÄFERSTEIN

The German word for food is *Lebensmittel,* which literally translates to *substance that supports life.* Unfortunately, food is not always life supporting; if contaminated, food may acquire health damaging or even life destroying properties; one of the reasons being that food contains subtances that are not only nutritious for people but may, under certain circumstances, also support the growth of a number of pathogens. Therefore, to fulfill its role of supporting life, it is of paramount importance that food is not only available, but also nutritious and safe.

Mankind has long recognized the importance of food availability for survival and well-being: It is the concept of *food security.* Not surprisingly, this concept has been captured by the Universal Declaration of Human Rights, wherein food availability is identified as a basic human right. However, it is extremely surprising that the concept of *food safety,* that is, the absence of health and life damaging or destroying properties, has not been emphasized in the Universal Declaration of Human Rights.[2] Neither was it mentioned 30 years later in the Health for All/Primary Health Care paradigm (Primary Health Care, 1978). One of the basic

---

[1] This chapter is based on two publications: 1. Food Safety by Käferstein, F.K., Motarjemi, Y., & Moy, G., in UNESCO Encyclopedia of Life Support Systems (EOLSS); 2. The WTO Agreement on the Application of Sanitary and Phytosanitary Measures by Miyagishima, K., & Käferstein, F.K., in International Handbook of Foodborne Pathogens, edited by M.D.Milliotis & J.W. Bier. Marcel Dekker, Inc., New York & Basel, 2003.

[2] Article 25, 1948.

components of primary health care (PHC) refers explicitly to the 'promotion of food supply and proper nutrition.' The masterminds behind the PHC paradigm must have felt at the time that the notion of safe food was implicit in that component. This implicity turned out, however, to be an unfortunate omission, as will be shown later, and the correction of it had to wait yet another 14 years. The FAO/WHO International Conference on Nutrition (International Conference on Nutrition, 1992) in 1992 was the first major inter-governmental event that refered explicitly to safe food and declared the *'access to nutritionally adequate and safe food as a right of each individual.'* (Emphasis added.)

Where do we stand today? It is obvious that this human right, like so many others, is not yet enjoyed by many of our fellow citizens. However, considering the importance of food safety in health and development, as detailed below, it is obvious that its role needs to be substantially strengthened if its potential to contribute to the Millennium Development Goals (United Nations General Assembly document A56/326) is to be realized.

THE HEALTH CONSEQUENCES OF UNSAFE FOOD

In every part of the world, people wage a constant battle against food contamination, foodborne diseases, and food wastage. Efforts to reduce the survival-threatening, devastating consequences of food contamination certainly started in prehistoric times. Cooking, smoking, simple sun drying, and fermentation were probably the first methods used. Despite considerable advances in food science and technology, the safety of our food supply is, at the beginning of the third millennium, still a cause for concern.

In 1983, a group of internationally renowned experts, convened jointly by the Food and Agriculture Organization of the United Nations (FAO) and the World Health Organization (WHO), concluded that illness from contaminated food was perhaps the most widespread health problem in the contemporary world, and an important cause of reduced economic productivity (WHO, 1984). In 1992, the FAO/WHO International Conference on Nutrition recognized that hundreds of millions of people suffer from communicable diseases caused by contaminated food and drinking water. In the same year, the UN Conference on Environment and Development (United Nations Conference on Environment and Development, 1992) recognized that food was a major vehicle for the transmission of environmental contaminants, both chemical and biological, to human populations throughout the world, and urged countries to take measures to prevent or minimize these threats. In 2000, the World Health Assembly, the supreme governing body of WHO, unanimously adopted a strongly worded resolution that recognizes food safety as an essential public health function (World Health Assembly, 2000).

A wide range of biological and chemical agents (hazards) causes foodborne diseases, with varying degrees of severity ranging from mild indisposition to chronic and/or life-threatening illness.

Not only has epidemiological surveillance during the last three decades shown an increase in the prevalence of foodborne illness in many countries, there have also been devastating outbreaks of diseases such as salmonellosis, cholera, enterohaemorrhagic *Escherichia coli* (EHEC) infections, and hepatitis A, in both developed and developing countries. Furthermore, cholera and other diarrheal diseases, particularly infant diarrhea, traditionally considered to be spread by water or through person-to-person contact, were shown to be largely foodborne. In several industrialized countries, epidemiological studies showed an unexpectedly high annual prevalence of foodborne disease in 10–15% of the population. In the late 1990s, more accurate data from the US suggested that this figure may be as high as 25% (Mead, et al., 1999). While comparable data from developing countries are lacking, one can safely assume that the figure is higher and the health (and resulting economic) consequences even more severe. Infant diarrhea is probably the most important food-safety related disease in developing countries, the morbidity of which has remained virtually unchanged during the last 20 to 25 years (Kaferstein, 2003).

It is certain that contaminated food will continue to plague mankind in the twenty-first century, especially as several global trends continue to negatively influence the safety of food and drinking water. Such trends include population growth, uncontrolled urbanization, increase in international trade in food and animal feed, and other factors.

Biological contaminants, largely bacteria, viruses, and parasites, constitute the major cause of foodborne diseases. In developing countries, such contaminants are responsible for a wide range of diseases (e.g., cholera, campylobacteriosis, *Escherichia (E.) coli* gastroenteritis, salmonellosis, shigellosis, typhoid and paratyphoid fevers, brucellosis, amoebiasis, poliomyelitis, and so on). Taken together, diarrheal diseases, especially infant diarrhea, are the dominant problem and indeed one of massive proportions.

Annually, some 1.5 billion episodes of diarrhea occur in children under the age of five, resulting in some 1.8 million deaths. Whereas traditionally it was thought that contaminated water supplies were the main source of pathogens causing infant diarrhea, it is now estimated that up to 70% of diarrheal episodes may be foodborne(?). Various pathogens have been identified as a cause of diarrhea. These include bacteria such as *E. coli, Shigella spp., Salmonella spp., Vibrio cholerae O1,* and *Campylobacter jejuni;* protozoa such as *Giardia lamblia, Entamoeba histolytica,* and *Cryptosporidium spp.;* and also enteric viruses such as rotavirus, hepatitis A and E viruses, and calici viruses. Infections due to pathogenic *E. coli* are the most common cause of infant diarrhea. Complementary (weaning) food contaminated with pathogenic *E. coli* causes up to 25% of all diarrheal episodes in infants and children. Campylobacteriosis and shigellosis account for 5–15% and 10–15%, respectively, of diarrheal disease episodes in infants and children (Motarjemi, et al., 1993).

The seventh pandemic of *Vibrio cholerae O1* biotype El Tor, which started in 1961 in Indonesia, spread in 1991 to South and Central America and Mexico. In 2001, 58 countries had officially notified WHO for a total of 184,311 cases and 2,728 deaths. The actual number of cases is considered to be much higher because of poor surveillance systems and frequent underreporting, often motivated by fear of trade sanctions and lost tourism. WHO estimates that the officially reported cases represent only around 5–10% of actual cases worldwide (WHO/CDS/2003.15). Food is frequently implicated in the transmission of cholera.

Infections due to helminths are also a worldwide public health problem, and particularly affect developing countries. Examples are Trichinella spiralis, Taenia saginata, and Taenia solium, which are acquired through consumption of undercooked or uncooked meat. Ascariasis is one of the most common parasitic infections and is estimated to affect some 1, 000 millions people. Trematodes such as Clonorchis spp., Fasciola spp., Opisthorchis spp., and Paragonimus spp. infect some 40 million people, particularly in Asia, Africa, and Latin America. More than 10% of the world's population is at risk of becoming infected by these parasites, which are transmitted through the consumption of raw or inadequately processed freshwater fish, shellfish, or aquatic plants (WHO Tech. Rep. 849, 1995).

Although the situation regarding foodborne diseases is serious in developing countries, the problem is not limited to those countries. Industrialized countries have experienced a succession of major epidemics. It has been estimated that foodborne diseases in the US cause approximately 76 million illnesses, 325,000 hospitalizations, and 5,000 deaths annually (Mead, et al., 1999).

With today's improvement in standards of personal hygiene, development of basic sanitation, safe water supplies, effective vaccination programs (especially against poliomyelitis), food control infrastructure, and the wide application of food-processing technologies, many foodborne diseases (e.g. poliomyelitis, brucellosis, cholera, typhoid and paratyphoid fevers, and milkborne salmonellosis) have been either eliminated or considerably reduced in industrialized countries. Nevertheless, most countries experienced an important increase in several other foodborne diseases.

Salmonellosis is of particular importance in many countries. Raw meats, poultry, eggs, milk and dairy products, fish, shrimp, frog legs, yeast, coconut, sauces and salad dressing, cake mixes, cream-filled desserts and toppings, dried gelatin, peanut butter, cocoa, chocolate, and other foods have been identified as being contaminated with Salmonella spp, and, subsequently, as serving as vehicles for the transmission of this disease. As a result of industrialization and mass production, large outbreaks have been reported.

In 1985, a salmonellosis outbreak involving up to 197,000 people (16,000 confirmed cases) in six US states was caused by pasteurized but recontaminated milk from one Chicago dairy (Ryan, et al., 1987). Also in the US, another large salmonellosis outbreak associated with nationally distributed ice cream products occurred in 1994. While the exact number of ill people is not known, the number of persons exposed to contaminated products may have been substantial, as approximately 400,000 gallons of the implicated products were distributed throughout the US (Hennessy, et al., 1996).

In addition, many industrialized countries are experiencing outbreaks of diseases due to relatively new types of foodborne pathogens such as *Campylobacter jejuni, Listeria monocytogenes,* and *E. coli O 157:H 7*. Campylobacteriosis has increased to such an extent that it is now the leading foodborne disease in several industrialized countries. As in the case of *Salmonella*, the main vehicles for the transmission of *Campylobacter* are poultry meat and unpasteurized milk.

Listeria monocytogenes (L.m.) causes severe foodborne infections, with a high fatality rate in susceptible individuals. The fatality rate, especially in neonates and immuno-compromised adults, is in the range of 27–30%. Although diseases caused by L.m. are rare, this microorganism has been implicated in several important outbreaks involving different types of food such as milk, cheese, vegetables, and meat products (Bulletin of WHO, 1988). L.m. in hot dogs and other meat and poultry products resulted in several large product recalls in the US. At present there is no full understanding of its ecology, but it is known to be able to grow at refrigeration temperatures and at a wide range of pH; it is thus of major concern to food industries producing products that support the growth of L.m. and which have an extended shelf life, even at refrigeration temperatures.

Outbreaks of *E. coli O157: H 7* are causing concern in many countries, because the pathogen causes severe damage to health, even death, particularly in children. Outbreaks have been reported from Australia, Canada, Japan, the US, the UK, and many other European countries. In 1993, a major outbreak of *E. coli O157: H 7* infection affected some 500 people in the northwestern states of the US. Many children developed hemolytic uremic syndrome (HUS), and four died as a result. Another large outbreak caused by this pathogen occurred in Africa in 1992, affecting probably thousands of people, with an undocumented number of cases of HUS. Drinking water and cooked maize were the vehicles of transmission. In 1996, in an outbreak of *E. coli O157: H 7* in Japan, 6,309 schoolchildren and 92 school staff members were affected, resulting in two deaths. The epidemiological investigation identified fresh radish sprouts (kaiware-daikon) as the probable cause. This was the largest outbreak ever recorded from this pathogen. Another important outbreak of *E. coli O157:H 7* occurred in Scotland between November 1996 and January 1997. Some 400 people were affected, and about 20 elderly people died as a consequence. The outbreak was traced to cold cooked meat (loose or in sandwiches) bought from a local butcher (WHO/FSF/FOS/97.6).

Another emerging problem is diarrheal illness due to *Cyclospora cayetanensis*. In the US and Canada, three large outbreaks occurred in 1996, 1997, and 1998. They were attributed to the consumption of imported fresh raspberries, probably contaminated through water. The route of transmission of cyclospora needs to be further elucidated, but it is believed that the parasites may be transmitted indirectly via the fecal-oral route (Sterling & Ortega, 1999).

Hepatitis A is common all over the world: some 10 to 300 persons per 100,000 are infected annually. Shellfish grown in contaminated water have often been recognized as a source of this disease (Weekly Epidemiological Record, 1993). An epidemic of shellfish-borne hepatitis A in China in 1988 affected some 292,000 persons (with 32 fatalities), and was related to the consumption of contaminated clams (Weekly Epidemiological Record, 1988). Food contaminated by infected food handlers and not subsequently sufficiently heated may also transmit the disease. Therefore, many cases of hepatitis A are known to be restaurant associated.

Except for a few diseases, such as botulism, brucellosis, listeriosis, and typhoid fever, foodborne diseases are often viewed as mild and self-limiting. Although this may be true in a number of cases, in many other cases the health consequences are serious, even life threatening. This false perception has, in part, contributed to the lack of attention paid to the problem. Foodborne diseases vary in their health consequences depending on the disease agent, the stage of treatment, and the duration of the illness, in addition to the age and susceptibility of the individual. Acute symptoms include diarrhea, vomiting, abdominal pain, cramps, fever, and jaundice. In the case of many foodborne diseases, healthy adults recover within a few days to a few weeks from acute health effects.

Some foodborne diseases can, however, cause serious and chronic sequelae on the cardiovascular, renal, articular, respiratory, or immune systems. Examples of health complications associated with foodborne illness are reactive arthritis and rheumatoid syndromes, meningitis, endocarditis, Reiter's syndrome, Guillain-Barré syndrome, and hemolytic uremic syndrome (HUS). For example, salmonellosis has been reported to cause reactive arthritis in some subjects. In the milkborne salmonellosis outbreak that occurred in Chicago in 1985 (see above), some 2% of patients developed reactive arthritis as a result. It is estimated that up to 10% of patients with enterohemorrhagic *Escherichia coli* (including *E.coli* O 157) infection may develop HUS, with a case-fatality rate ranging from 3–5%. The manifestations of listeriosis may include septicemia, meningitis, encephalitis, osteomyelitis, and endocarditis. Infection caused by *Vibrio vulnificus* may be present as fulminate septicemia, often complicated with necrotizing cutaneous lesions. According to some studies, the case-fatality rate for patients with pre-existing liver disease is 63%, and for those without liver disease, 23%. Cysticercosis, an infection with the larval stage of *Taenia solium*, common particularly in South America, may lead to cerebral lesions. The liver flukes *Opisthorchis viverini* and *Clonorchis sinensis* cause mechanical obstruction of the biliary tract and recurrent pyogenic cholangitis, and are carcinogenic to humans.

In certain groups, for instance, the elderly, infants, young children, pregnant women, the malnourished, and immuno-compromised individuals, these health effects may be even more serious. For example, in pregnant women listeriosis can lead to abortion, stillbirth, or malformation of the fetus; the overall fatality rate is about 30%. In an outbreak of listeriosis in pregnant women in Western Australia, the fatality rate of infected fetuses was as high as 50% (WHO/FNU/FOS/97.1).

Transplacental infections with *Toxoplasma gondii* may occur in some 45% of infected pregnant women. In 10–20% of nonfatal morbidity, the infants may suffer from damage to the central nervous system and retinochoroiditis, leading to blindness. It is believed that infected but asymptomatic infants may also develop some sequelae later in life, most commonly retinochoroiditis. It is estimated that, worldwide, in about 3 out of every 1,000 pregnancies, the fetus/infant is affected by toxoplasmosis (WHO/HST/90.2). In the US, toxoplasmosis is considered the most expensive foodborne disease.

Foodborne diseases are one of the most important underlying factors for malnutrition and, indirectly, for respiratory tract infections. Repeated episodes of foodborne diseases over a period of time can lead to malnutrition, with serious impact on the growth and immune system of infants and children. An infant whose resistance is suppressed becomes more vulnerable to other diseases (including respiratory tract infections) and is subsequently caught in a vicious cycle of malnutrition and infection. Many infants and children do not survive under these circumstances.

The contamination of food by **chemical hazards** is also a public health concern worldwide. Contamination of foods may occur through environmental pollution of the air, water, and soil, as is the case with toxic metals, polychlorinated biphenyls (PCBs), and dioxins. The use of various chemicals, such as food additives, pesticides, veterinary drugs, and other agrochemicals can also pose hazards if such chemicals are not properly regulated or appropriately used. Other chemical hazards, such as naturally occurring toxicants, for instance mycotoxins, may arise at various points during food production, harvest, storage, processing, distribution, and preparation. Furthermore, accidental or intentional adulteration of food by toxic substances has resulted in serious public health incidents in both developing and industrialized countries. For example, in 1981–82 in Spain, adulterated cooking oil killed some 600 people and disabled another 20,000, many permanently. In this case, the agent responsible was never identified in spite of intensive investigations (WHO, 1992).

Over the past 50 years, the widespread introduction of chemicals in agriculture and in food processing has resulted in a more abundant food supply and considerable efforts have been undertaken to ensure its safety. At the international level, two joint FAO/WHO committees have, over a period of four decades, evaluated more than 1,500 food chemicals. The Joint FAO/WHO Expert Committee on Food Additives (JECFA) evaluates food additives, contaminants, and veterinary drug residues, and the Joint FAO/WHO Meeting on Pesticide Residues (JMPR) evaluates pesticide residues. Recommendations are made on Acceptable Daily Intake (ADI), on Maximum Residue Levels (MRLs) in the case of pesticides and animal drugs, and on Maximum Levels (MLs) in the case of food additives. In the case of contaminants, JECFA may establish a Provisional Tolerable Weekly Intake (PTWI) to protect consumers against the chronic health hazards usually associated with the long-term intake of these chemicals. JECFA and JMPR may also establish an acute reference dose (acute RfD) for a chemical that may cause adverse health effects after short-time exposure, such as one meal or one day.

Based on the recommendations of JECFA and JMPR, the Joint FAO/WHO **Codex Alimentarius Commission** (CAC), and its member governments establish international food standards, guidelines, and other recommendations. Since its inception in 1963, CAC has adopted more than 240 commodity standards, 3,500 MRLs for various pesticide and veterinary drug/commodity combinations, 780 food additive standards, and 45 codes of hygienic or technological practice. The World Trade Organization (WTO) refers to Codex standards, guidelines, and recommendations in the arbitration of trade disputes involving health and safety requirements. The Global Environment Monitoring System/Food Contamination Monitoring and Assessment Program (GEMS/Food) of WHO provides information on the levels of contaminants in food and on time trends of contamination, enabling preventive and control measures. Data from GEMS/Food and from surveys undertaken in industrialized countries suggest that the food supply in developed countries is, from the chemical viewpoint, largely safe, because of the extensive food safety infrastructure (i.e., legislation, enforcement mechanisms, surveillance, and monitoring programmes), and the cooperation of the food industry. However, data from developing countries are largely lacking. Accidental contamination or adulteration does occur in both industrialized and developing countries. Such contamination causes international concern because of extensive media coverage and the global nature of today's food supply.

Genetically modified foods (GMFs), produced with the help of modern (i.e., DNA) technology, are hotly debated in several industrialized countries. In principle, the food safety considerations of such GMFs should be basically of the same nature as those that might arise from other ways of altering the genome, such as conventional breeding, or using chemicals or radiation to induce mutations. The question is not whether GMFs are inherently less safe than foods produced by traditional genome modification techniques (e.g., animal/plant breeding, induced mutation), which they are not, but whether a country has the capacity to assess the safety of all foods, and to enact and enforce up-to-date food legislation to address all pertinent food safety questions. In countries where this is the case, such as the US, no adverse health effects related to the consumption of GMFs have been observed. However, the mere fact that many consumers in a number of countries appear to be concerned with GMFs will necessitate appropriate risk communication strategies, including consumer education.

In this context it should be noted that GMFs are of particular importance for developing countries, which look at this technology as one means of addressing the need to produce sufficient quantities of nutritionally adequate and safe food for their growing populations. In addition, this technology offers the possibility of reducing the need for certain agrochemicals, in particular pesticides, with potential health, economic, and environmental benefits.

THE DEVELOPMENTAL ASPECTS OF FOOD SAFETY

Developing countries, in order to reduce poverty and to improve the standard of living of their populations, have to develop their economies. Most of their economies are agriculturally (including fishing and aquaculture) based, although a large number of developing countries have also a sizable tourist industry or the potential to develop a tourist industry. For both industies, that is, agro-food industry and tourism, food safety is of paramount importance. The following example is illustrative of this statement: During 1991, when cholera broke out in Peru, more than US $700 million was lost because the country could no longer find buyers for its fish and fishery products. In addition, in the three months following the start of the epidemic, another US $70 million was lost due to the closure of food establishments and decrease in tourism (Motarjemi, et al., 1993).

For the **agro-food industry** to generate employment and revenues that can be 'recycled' into the national development process, primary or value-added food and/or food products have to be produced and sold in the international market. However, centuries ago, people already realized that there was a link between trade and health. In the 14th century, Italian city-states like Venice began to develop quarantine systems to guard against the importation of bubonic plague, which they believed came to them through trade (Fidler, 1997).

When the major international organizations were set up some 50 years ago, after the end of World War II, the founders recognized this linkage as well. The original General Agreement on Tariffs and Trade (GATT), which was instituted in 1947 and still remains an integral part of GATT 1994, includes provisions for countries to apply measures "necessary to protect human, animal, or plant life or health," if they do not unjustifiably discriminate between countries where similar conditions prevail, or act as a disguised restriction on international trade (UN, pp. 188–316). For its part, the World Health Assembly, back in 1949, called attention "to the need for eliminating quarantine restrictions of doubtful medical value which interfere with international trade and travel (WHA 2.15)."

Therefore, there is a reciprocal understanding that health must be protected over and above business interests, but that health protection measures should not intrude on commerce without justification (Kinnon, 1998).

Food Production—Safety First

The possible use of health protection measures to restrict trade has been a concern since the beginning of multilateral trade negotiations. However, it took nearly 50 years before trading partners concluded the Agreement on the Application of Sanitary and Phytosanitary Measures (SPS agreement, see below) in 1994. By that time, international trade in food had reached an unprecedented volume, representing some $294 billion. As the scale of international trade in food further increases (1997: $ 458 billion), there is growing threat from foodborne pathogenic microorganisms (Käferstein, et al., 1997). In addition, hazards to human health may also occur in the form of mycotoxins, pesticide residues, and other substances, the presence of which may lead to rejection or destruction of consignments by importing countries (Miyagishima & Käferstein, 1998).

Despite the risk to health related to international food trade, this trade is essential because it has at least a two-fold benefit: (i) it introduces a wider variety of foods into the diet by providing consumers in importing countries with a bigger and better choice of products, thus contributing to better nutrition; and (ii) it provides food exporting countries with foreign exchange, which is indispensable for the economic development of many countries, and thus for an improvement in the standard of living of their people.

Tariff and non-tariff barriers at the national border, however, can impede international trade in foods. Some of them are required to protect the health of consumers; others are simply detrimental to international trade. To address this concern, the Joint FAO/WHO Codex Alimentarius Commission (Codex in short) was established in 1963 to protect the health of the consumers and, at the same time, to ensure fair practices in food trade. The Codex has been working since that time and has elaborated a number of food standards, guidelines, and recommendations (see above). However, although member governments of the Codex prior to 1995 had been asked by FAO and WHO to formally accept these standards, it has been left to governments to decide whether they should or should not implement them, given that Codex texts have not been directly linked to an international trade scheme such as GATT.

What has Changed with the Establishment of the World Trade Organization in 1995?

The Uruguay Round of Multilateral Trade Negotiations was concluded in April 1994 by the signing of the Marrakech Agreement, and it gave birth to a number of multilateral trade agreements, to which all Members of the World Trade Organization (WTO)—established in January 1995—are committed (GATT, 1994).

One important outcome of the Uruguay Round was that countries agreed to reduce tariff barriers for many agricultural commodities so as to further encourage free trade. As a result, non-tariff barriers became a real concern because they could undermine the promotion of international trade if put into practice in an arbitrary or discriminatory way.

To address some of these concerns, the WTO Agreement on the Application of Sanitary and Phytosanitary Measures (SPS Agreement) was drawn up to ensure that countries apply measures to protect human and animal health (sanitary measures) and plant health (phytosanitary measures) based on the assessment of risk, or, in other words, based on science. The SPS Agreement incorporates, therefore, safety aspects of foods in trade.

It is important to mention still another WTO agreement: the Agreement on Technical Barriers to Trade (TBT Agreement). This agreement, which had been in existence as a plurilateral agreement since the Tokyo Round, was revised and converted into a multilateral agreement through the Uruguay Round. It covers all technical requirements and standards (applied to all commodities), such as labelling, which are not covered by the SPS Agreement. Therefore, the SPS and TBT Agreements can be seen as complementing each other.

One of the main objectives of the SPS Agreement is to protect human and animal health as well as the phytosanitary situation in all WTO Member countries. This is to be addressed through the establishment of a multilateral framework of rules and disciplines that will guide the development, adoption, and enforcement of sanitary and phytosanitary measures and minimize their negative effects on trade. As a natural consequence, the SPS Agreement recognized the standards and related texts of the Codex Alimentarius Commission as international points of reference. Today, the SPS Agreement is regarded as being a strong instrument which will further the goal of the Codex, that is, to harmonize food standards worldwide in order to protect human health and to facilitate international trade in food.

Likewise, international standards established by the International Office of Epizootics (OIE) and the relevant international and regional organizations operating within the framework of the International Plant Protection Convention (IPPC) have been recognized in the SPS Agreement as providing references with regard to animal and plant life or health.

In order to comply with the provisions of the SPS Agreement, it may often be necessary to strengthen national food control systems. This may require both manpower and financial investment. To address these particular difficulties, which may be encountered by many developing countries, the SPS Agreement also includes provisions for technical assistance to be provided by other countries or through international organizations. The SPS Agreement thus provides an ideal opportunity for developing countries to build modern food control and safety schemes or to upgrade existing ones. It also enables countries that don't have the financial and/or scientific resources, to develop their own risk-based food standards, by accepting Codex standards as their national standards, to comply with the food safety related WTO requirements: Codex standards and related texts are deemed necessary to protect human health. As long as a country employs these standards, its measures are presumed to be consistent with the provisions of the SPS Agreement. Harmonization with Codex will also eliminate the necessity of one country having to provide other countries with justifiable reasons as to why the measures they are applying are necessary in order to protect human health. In this way, countries are no longer subject to arbitrary measures imposed by their trading partners, but have a fair chance, as long as their foods comply with Codex recommendations, to participate in and to benefit from the international food trade. In other words, it is not any longer the 'right' of the more powerful trading partner to dictate its conditions to the less powerful one. International trade in food follows jointly elaborated risk-based rules, that is, i.e. Codex recommendations that assure health protection.

As indicated above, **tourism** is an important industry, providing employment for millions of people and playing an important part in the economy and thus in the development process of many countries. And as also has been pointed out, safe food is of paramount importance for a flourishing tourist industry. The reason being that a country or a particular company with a poor reputation regarding the safety of the food they provide to their clients (tourists) will have difficulties to attract clients.

The role of food safety in tourism is dual:

(i) People travelling to distant places are often at greater risk of foodborne illness than in their own country. Attack rates range from 10% in southern Europe to over 50% in destinations in Latin America, North Africa, India, and Nepal (Angst & Steffen, 1997).

(ii) Travellers contribute to the trans-national spread of foodborne illness and thus mitigate efforts made to prevent foodborne illness. For instance, it is estimated that a majority of cases of salmonellosis in Scandinavian countries are 'imported' by returning tourists, whereas these countries are making major efforts to prevent foodborne illness (Käferstein & Motarjemi, 2000).

On the other hand, in countries where an effort is made to improve food safety in the tourism sector, a double benefit may be expected: (i) travellers are better protected and this country will be a more attractive destination for them and (ii) the local population also benefits from the higher food safety standard. A case in point is Tunisia, whose efforts have led to a significant reduction in travellers' diarrhoea. In this country, as a result of intensive education of food handlers, the incidence of diarrheal diseases among tourists has been reduced by about one third (Cartwright & Chahed, 1997).

In summary, the role of food safety in health and development is unquestionable. However, in order for food safety to make its best possible contribution to the

Millennium Development Goals, there needs to be a paradigm shift: food should not only to be considered as an agricultural and/or trading commodity but also as a *public health issue*. Therefore, food safety has to be seen by the public health community as an *essential public health function*, as recently acknowledged by the World Health Organization (World Health Assembly, 2000). Consequently, food safety has to be integrated along the entire food chain, from *farm to table*, with the three sectors (i.e. governments, industry, and consumers) *sharing responsibility*. If the US already in 1997 conservatively estimates the medical costs and productivity losses for just 7 specific pathogens in food to be in the range of annually between US $6.5 and 35 billion (Report to the President, 1997), then time for action is overdue.

REFERENCES

Angst, F., & Steffen, R. (1997). Update of the epidemiology of travellers' diarrhea in East Africa. *Journal of Travel Medicine, 4*, 118–120.

Cartwright, R.Y., & Chahed, M. (1997). Foodborne diseases in travellers. *World Health Statistics Quarterly, 50*(1/2), 102–110.

Control of foodborne trematode infections (1995). Report of a WHO Study Group. WHO Technical Report Series Nr. 849. WHO Geneva, Switzerland.

Fidler, D.P. (1997). Trade and health: The global spread of diseases and international trade. *German Yearbook of International Law, 40*, 300–305.

Food Safety from Farm to Table: A national food safety initiative. Report to the President, May 1997.

Foodborne listeriosis. Report of a WHO Working Group, Geneva, Switzerland, February 1988. *Bulletin of the World Health Organization, 66*(4), 421–428.

Hennessy, T., et al. (1996). A national outbreak of *Salmonella enteritidis* infection from ice cream. *New England Journal of Medicine, 334*, 128.

International Conference on Nutrition (1992). World Declaration and Plan of Action, Rome, Italy, December 1992. FAO & WHO.

Käferstein, F.K. (2003). Food safety: The fourth pillar in the strategy to prevent infant diarrhoea. *Bulletin of the World Health Organization, 81*(11), 842–3.

Käferstein, F.K., et al. (1997). Foodborne disease control: A transnational challenge. *Emerging Infectious Diseases, 3*(4), 503–510.

Käferstein, F.K., & Motarjemi., Y. (2000, April). Foodborne diseases related to travellers: A public health challenge. Proceedings of the 1st NSF International Conference and Exhibition on Food Safety in Travel and Tourism, Barcelona, Spain.

Kinnon, C.M. (1998). World trade: Bringing health into the picture. *World Health Forum, 19*, 397–406.

Mead, P.S., et al. (1999). Food-related illness and death in the United States. *Emerging Infectious Diseases, 5*, 607–625.

Miyagishima, K., & Käferstein, F.K. (1998). Food safety in international trade. *World Health Forum, 19*(4), 407–411.

Motarjemi, Y., et al. (1993). Health and development aspects of food safety. Archiv für Lebensmittelhygiene, 44(2), 35–41.

Motarjemi, Y., et al. (1993). Contaminated weaning food: A major risk factor for diarrhoea and associated malnutrition. *Bulletin of the World Health Organization, 71*(1), 79–92.

Prevention and control of enterohaemorrhagic *Escherichia coli* (EHEC) infections. Report of a WHO Consultation, Geneva, Switzerland, April/May 1997. WHO/FSF/FOS/97.6.

Primary Health Care (1978). Report of the WHO/UNICEF International Conference on Primary Health Care, Alma-Ata, USSR, 6–12 September 1978. WHO Geneva, Switzerland.

Road map towards the implementation of the United Nations Millennium Declaration (2002). New York, United Nations. (United Nations General Assembly document A56/326).

Ryan, C.A., et al. (1987). Massive outbreak of antimicrobial-resistant salmonellosis traced to pasteurized milk. *JAMA, 258*, 3269.

Sterling, C.R., & Ortega, Y.R. (1999). Cyclospora: An enigma worth unraveling. *Emerging Infectious Diseases, 5*(1).

The results of the Uruguay round of multilateral trade negotiations: The legal texts. GATT, 1994.

The role of food safety in health and development. Report of a Joint FAO/WHO Expert Committee on Food Safety. Technical Report Series Nr.705. WHO Geneva, 1984.

United Nations (1947). General Agreement on tariffs and trade, article XX(b) (pp. 188–316). UN New York.

United Nations Conference on Environment and Development, Rio de Janeiro, Brazil, June 1992.

WHO (1988). Outbreak of hepatitis A—Shanghai. *Weekly Epidemiological Record, 63*, 9192.

WHO (1997). Human listeriosis. WHO Geneva, WHO/FNU/FOS/97.1.

WHO (1993). Prevention of hepatitis A. *Weekly Epidemiological Record, 68*, 25.

WHO (2003). Communicable Diseases 2002—global defense against intectious threat, edited by M.K. Kindhauser. WHO Geneva, Switzerland. WHO/CDS/2003.15.

World Health Assembly (2000, May 20). Resolution WHA53.15.

WHO (1990). Global estimates for health situation assessment and projections. WHO Geneva, Switzerland, WHO/HST/90.2.

WHO (1992). Toxic oil syndrome: Current knowledge and future perspective. WHO Copenhagen, Denmark Regional Publication, European Series Nr. 42.

WHO (1973). Handbook of resolutions and decisions of the World Health Assembly and the Executive Board, 1948–1972, Resolution WHA 2.15 (Vol. 1, p. 55). WHO Geneva, Switzerland.

Chapter 15

Future Health in an Ageing World

A. MICHAEL DAVIES

The number of elderly people is increasing by a million each month, and they will comprise almost one-fifth of the world's population within the next half-century. In some countries, one-quarter or even one-third of the population will be old. How will society adapt and what will be the impact on the health of the nation? What adjustments will need to be made in working life, pensions, living arrangements, and health services?

Two things that happened during the 20th century, and particularly during its last 50 years, have speeded up this process of demographic transformation. Fertility has fallen, so there are fewer children and a greater *proportion* of older persons. Deaths in infancy have dropped and, with them, deaths at almost every age, so that the survivors have themselves grown older. Until recent decades population aging proceeded slowly in the industrialized countries, and much slower in poorer countries. During this century, however, the process will speed up in all nations, and developing countries will provide the majority of the elderly of the world (www.un.org/popin/data.html; Kinsella & Velkoff, 2001; www.census.gov/ipc/www/idbnew.html).

Aging of populations, like health itself, is driven by many processes of social development. The health of old people is intertwined with problems of disability and loss of autonomy, so that the capacity of health-directed activities alone, simply to relieve the infirmities of old age, is limited unless complemented by the fabric of social support.

This chapter describes the aging of population groups and the interactions between the elderly and the societies of which they are a part. The increase in the number and proportion of old people in the world will be one of the most profound forces affecting the development and organization of societies for many decades to come.

THE ELDERLY: THE DEMOGRAPHIC TRANSITION

During the next half-century the world's population aged 60 and above will increase from 606 million to almost 2 billion (Kinsella & Velkoff, 2001). Already, the numbers of elderly, defined here as those aged 65 and over, are increasing at a rate of a million each month and should reach almost a billion by 2030. They will then comprise 12% of all humankind, up from 6.9% in the year 2000. This trend will vary widely by region. In Europe, the oldest continent in terms of population, the increase will be from a current 15.5% to 24.3%, in North America from 12.6% to 20.3%, in Asia from 6.0% to 12%, and in Latin America and the Caribbean from 5.5% to 11.6%. Even in SubSaharan Africa, where fertility and mortality are both very high, the proportion of those over 65, now 2.9%, is expected to rise to 3.7% (JAMA, 2003).

Elders are the survivors of the forces of mortality in their own countries who have been exposed to many environmental and social influences for 65 years or more. The result of these influences, combined with each individual genetic template, is an older individual, different in very many ways from others in his or her own cohort and, more so, from those in other cohorts. Generalizations based on age or gender or cross-country comparisons must thus be made with caution.

Aging may be defined as a progressive loss of adaptability with the passage of time so that the individual is less and less able to react adaptively to challenges from the external or internal environment (Evans & Williams, 1992). As time passes, the individual becomes progressively more frail and in need of increasing support to maintain autonomy (WHO: technical report series 1984).

The definition of old age is arbitrary. The widely used cut-off point of 65 was decided as the age of benefit in the first public social security legislation in Germany in 1873 and perpetuated in the retirement regulations of other countries that followed. There was never any physiological basis for the decision, nor for the cut-off of 60 that United Nations (UN) demographers use. Those over 65 are a very heterogeneous group, ranging from the increasingly healthy "young old" under 75, to the more frail and disabled "oldest old", aged 85 and more.

Each population group and each country proceeds along the path of *demographic transition* at its own speed, driven by the forces of social development. World fertility continues to decline, and, thus, life expectancy increases. The population of the world will age much faster in the coming decades (www.un.org/popin/data.html) and this is illustrated by the rise in the world median age from 23.6 in 1950 to 26.5 in 2000 and a predicted jump to 36.2 in 2050.

For developed countries the rise will be from 37.4 in 2000 to 46.4 in 2050 while for less developed regions the increase will be relatively much greater, from 24.3 to 35.0 during the half century. By then, the less developed regions will probably have an age structure similar to that of the more developed areas today.

Life expectancy at birth increased by 17 years during the second half of the 20th century and is projected to add a further 10 years to reach a world average of 76 by 2050. By then, there should be no country with an expectation of life less than 61.5 years and the difference between countries with the highest (Japan) and lowest (Botswana) expectations of life should decrease from 45 years in 2000 to 25 in 2050.

The aging process affects the elderly population itself, and those over 80 form the fastest growing sector, increasing globally by 3.4% each year to a projected total of 314 million by 2050. China will have 99 million inhabitants aged 80 and over, India, 48 million, the USA 30 million, and 19 other countries will have 10% of their populations in this age group. By 2050 there are predicted to be 61 million nonagenarians in the world and over 3 million centenarians. As illustration of the rapidity of growth of the very oldest group, calculations for the United Kingdom predict that there will be 36,000 centenarians in 2031 compared to 300 in 1951. For France, where the demographic transition began many decades earlier, the increase in the population over 100 will be even greater, from 200 in 1950 to 150 000 in 2050! Nearly all of them will be women.

Sex Ratios

The average woman lives 7 years, or more, than the average man, and her life expectancy is already over 80 in most of the richer nations. But the gender gap is closely linked to the status of women and is only 3–6 years in less developed countries, and 2 years or less in the very poorest nations. Women thus make up the majority of the older populations; the sex ratio decreases further in the oldest of the old. In developed countries, in the year 2000, there were 72 men for every 100 women aged 65–79 and 45 per 100 for those over 80. By the year 2030, as male survival increases, these ratios will become 81 and 57 respectively. The smaller gaps predicted in developing countries as male life expectancies improve mean that in the world of 2030 there will be 86 men per 100 women aged 65–79 and 66 per 100 for those over 80 (www.un.org/popin/data.html; Kinsella & Velkoff, 2001; www.census.gov/ipc/www/idbnew.html).

Older men are much more likely to be married and older women widowed in most countries. At age 75, two-thirds to three quarters of men were still married in the year 2000, but less than half of the women, and the discrepancies seem likely to continue for the coming decades. Thus more old women than men live, and will live, alone.

THE EPIDEMIOLOGICAL TRANSITION

The progression from mortality largely due to infectious and parasitic diseases, which characterized poor nations, to that due mainly to chronic diseases, seen in developed nations, has been noted over the past 30 years or so and termed the "epidemiological transition." Changes that took many decades in developed countries have become much accelerated all over the world. The pace of transition is particularly rapid in countries of South America and Asia where life expectancy has increased by 10 or more years within a generation and where the leading causes of death are now cardiovascular, respiratory, and cancers, although those due to infectious and parasitic agents are still common (JAMA, 2003; WHO report 2003). Because they kill slowly, chronic diseases loom large as causes of disability and, in 2002, cardiovascular, cerebrovascular, and lung diseases, together with the dementias, accounted for nearly 70% of the global burden of disease (DALYs) in the over-60 cohort (WHO: report 2003). All scenarios for change computed by Murray and Lopez (Murray & Lopez, 1997) for the years up to 2020 predict substantial shifts in mortality to older ages in every region due to a decline in the burdens of communicable diseases, maternal, peri-natal, and nutritional causes of death. In nearly all regions there will be increases in cardiovascular diseases, cancers, pulmonary, and other chronic diseases, and accidents, as causes of death, the rate of shift being slowest in subSaharan Africa.

The total burden of disability thus increases with population aging as the affliction of chronic disease is added to the frailty of old age itself. In developing countries, life is shorter but more years are lived with disability, comprising 80% of the global burden. Populations in developed countries show less disability from cardiovascular and chronic respiratory diseases and from sequelae of childhood infections and deprivations. Members of developing nations, while living longer than before, still have shorter life expectations and will spend more of their lives with disability (WHO report, 2003). In India, for instance, the average expectation of life at birth in 2002 was 61 years but 7.5 of them, 12.3%, will be lived with disability. In Japan, on the other hand, the years of expectation of healthy life (HALE) were 75 of a total of 81.9, which is a loss of 8.4% (Kinsella & Velkoff, 2001; WHO report, 2003).

There is encouraging evidence, from longitudinal studies of older populations in Sweden and the USA, of some small reduction of disability over time, although this is not supported by a study in Holland (Freedman, Martin, & Schoeni, 2002). However, in all countries, the burden remains very high, and in absolute terms will continue to grow (Kinsella & Velkoff, 2001).

Broadly, in surveys of those over 65 in established market economies, nearly half report themselves to be in good health or better, and less than a quarter report poor health. There are considerable variations, however, between countries, due in part to differences in survey method and local culture. For example, over 70% of residents of New Zealand, Canada, and the USA report good health compared to less than 30% in Japan, Italy, and Poland—and women report levels even lower (DECD indicators, 2003). In other surveys, forty percent of individuals over 65 reported an illness or a disability that limits their daily activities. Of those aged 75 and older, less than a third reported good health, and of those aged 80 and over, up to one-third could not walk outside their home unaided (Kinsella & Velkoff, 2001; WHO technical report series, 1984).

Studies of centenarians, the survivors of many vicissitudes, show them to have greater life satisfaction and fewer complaints than those 10 to 20 years younger, while preserving their cognitive functions. But they are much more limited in independence and activities of daily living (Dello, Uriciusli, & De Leo, 1998). As more individuals approach the limits of life (about 105, with only a handful of exceptions) the number of centenarians will increase greatly.

AGEING SOCIETIES

As it ages, the world population also continues to grow, albeit more slowly than in previous decades. By 2020 the working age population, defined as those aged 15–64, and comprising 60%–70% of most countries, will increase considerably in the developing world, enough to support their aging populations. In the most developed countries, however, the working populations are already down to 22% of the total and will decrease to 16% in 2020. Thus the old age dependency ratio, the ratio of persons 65 and over to working age persons aged 15–64, was, already, in 1996, three times higher in these countries than in developing countries, 20.7 compared to 7.6. By 2020, these ratios will increase considerably, to 29 and 11 respectively. The impact on the availability of human resources to meet the growing needs for support and care of the elderly is already apparent in several of the developed countries and will become a serious problem in the coming decades (DECD indicators, 2003). In the developing countries, most of the dependants will continue to be children under 15 (90% in 1996 and still 80% in 2020), so that the resource needs for elder support will be set off against those of the young.

Until recent decades, the vast majority of grandparents lived with the families of sons or daughters who cared for them when ill or frail. There were few great grandparents. Today, in developed countries, one-third to one-half of individuals over 65 may live alone, more women than men. There is also an increase in the number of households of two elderly persons, but with great differences between nations. This contrasts with an average of three-quarters of elderly in countries in Asia and South America who still live with their offspring in a wide variety of household arrangements (Kending, Hashimoto, & Coppard, 1992). However, the processes of modernization and urbanization are changing family structures and more and more elderly are living alone. This is particularly true of rural areas as young adults migrate to the cities. Another emerging phenomenon is the "sandwich generation": the daughter who traditionally cared for her aged parent is herself a grandmother who may be caring for her own grandchildren. And the devastation of the young adult populations of several countries, particularly those of sub-Saharan Africa, by AIDS, has turned grandmothers into the main child carers with no one to look after them. But even in the absence of catastrophic disease, the availability of kin to care for elderly family members is decreasing in all countries and will continue to do so (www.un.org/popin/data.html; Kinsella & Velkoff, 2001; Kending, Hashimoto, & Coppard, 1992).

Two thirds of the world's elderly in the years 2025 and beyond will live in countries in various stages of underdevelopment, the majority very poor. The main underlying cause of all ill health in most of these countries—poverty—will be relieved only very slowly and the reports of international agencies paint a grim picture for the foreseeable future (http://hdr.undp.org Human development report 2003). Poverty adversely affects morbidity and mortality rates among the elderly, women more than men, and the strength of those associations has become clearer with time. What are the chances of future improvement in poor countries? In many (but by no means in all) developing nations, the standards of living should continue to rise, with concomitant improvement in education, nutrition, and health services and increasing survival without reducing morbidity. But for many tens of millions of old persons, the disadvantages of their youth will not be overcome. From current statistics on literacy rates in the under 25s one may predict that 15% of the elders of developing countries will be illiterate in 2050, and this proportion will rise to 37.5% in the least developed nations. In the populous countries of South Asia, including India, the figure will be 31% (http://hdr.undp.org 2005). Moreover, as just one example, the frequency of maternal under-nutrition and low birth weight in most of the poor countries today (UNICEF reports) predicts higher rates of cardiovascular diseases in the decades to come (Barker, 2001).

Thus, the consequences of enhanced communications, trade, technological advances, and human mobility, which are already beginning to have an impact on economic and social development in many countries and which should affect even the least developed nations, will include increases in the populations of the old and sick. It is likely, however, if history is any guide, that the ensuing rapid change and adjustment in countries with much illiteracy and few traditions of social justice, will bring, initially, unequal advance with more marked inequalities and marginalisation of the old, the ignorant and the poor (http://hdr.undp.org 2003). But there will be increased prosperity for some and the healthier and better fed sub-populations will live longer and demand more attention and better care. Present trends indicate that the gaps between rich and poor will widen both within countries and between countries and will be a permanent feature of rapidly changing economies.

The unsettled activities that accompany social change tend to marginalize vulnerable groups, such as women and the elderly, even further. Modernization and education of the younger generations in traditional societies affect the roles and status of the elderly as heads of the family and their position in the community. The family is still the primary caregiver of the old in every society but its capacity to do so will be diminished by changing life styles and by employment of women outside the home. The continuing trends to urbanization and migration in the developing countries are likely to leave older adults unsupported in rural areas or housed under primitive conditions in the new slums, isolated from their familiar surroundings.

IMPLICATIONS FOR HEALTH AND WELFARE

Luckily the outlook is not as depressing everywhere as this scenario predicts and many countries that already have a head start along the path of demographic transition will accommodate faster. Poverty should decrease in all countries, although the rate of decline is predicted to be slower in south Asia and Latin America and minimal in Africa south of the Sahara (http://hdr.undp.org 2003). The richer among them will be able to enjoy the coming technical improvements in housing and robotic environments, the new treatments, genetic manipulation, and organ replacements that technology promises. They will have adopted healthy lifestyles and maintained their physical and mental activity in old age.

However, it must be emphasized that health in old age is by no means a dichotomy and it is almost impossible to define or measure. The Scientific Group on the Epidemiology of Ageing (WHO: technical report 1984) struggled with the application of the WHO universal definition of health and settled for the maintenance of autonomy as an operational surrogate. Moreover, diseases of organs or disorders of function are compensated for by restricting activities so that the sick individual can accommodate to a limited life style and be content. Support of family and friends and other social and intellectual activities can help maintain autonomy at a lower level so that one who is sick, medically speaking, may define himself as well. Add to these difficulties of health assessment those of the conceptualization of equity (Sen, 2000) and it will be realized that the future scenarios pictured here are often caricatures, defining the best and worst situations. Most old persons will adjust to chronic ill health and be somewhere in between the extremes.

The concept of healthy aging as a goal of lifetime health promotion requires that the elderly share the general facilities available to the population at large, but also have additional care to meet their special needs. These include the social and physical environments, the promotion of healthy lifestyles and the provision of medical and nursing care.

Equity and Social Justice

The health of the elderly is interwoven with their social vulnerability and thus with the very structure of society. The social gradient in health is influenced, inter-alia, by absolute and relative deprivation, social position and control and social participation (Marmot & Wilkinson, 1999). Ethical considerations are crucial and there is a large literature documenting frequent discrimination against the elderly in the provision of complex or costly health care, often unconsciously but frequently deliberately (Butler, 1999). As the majority of the world's elderly are women, their low status, particularly in poor countries, will continue to be a major barrier to their health The care of the elderly outside the family is and will be dependent on enlightened governments linked to regard for human rights and the democratic process (http://hdr.undp.org 2003) and countries with socio-democratic welfare regimes enjoy better health in general than those which are more 'neo-liberal' (Coburn, 2004) Chapter 18.

Social Support and Pensions

Countries advanced in their demographic transition entered the twenty-first century with long traditions of social support and with a philosophy of roles and duties of government already enshrined in legislation. Welfare nets of varying degrees exist to back up inadequate pensions. There is already a legal age of retirement and well developed old age pension plans, but the unanticipated longevity require these to be urgently revised. Moreover, for some time to come, the elderly will continue to age within a patchwork of, often independent, bureaucratic service structures of health and welfare that developed historically and will have to be rationalized (www.age2000.org.uk 1998). The needs of older populations will be greater as they live longer and their numbers grow and they will have the education and political influence to demand additional resources.

As income and educational levels improve, many developing countries become ready and able to build on traditional religious and tribal mechanisms of care for indigents and develop insurance systems of support for working and retired populations. Experience shows that pioneer schemes are first enacted for privileged groups, government officials, army officers, industrial workers, and the like and examples of selective pension schemes are already in place in many relatively poor countries (OECD, 2000). Few, however, can afford adequate old age pensions and the elderly will continue to be dependent on family support.

Voluntary support schemes, formal and informal, are expanding rapidly in countries at all stages of development to help fill the gaps in family and government support. They also offer opportunities for the active involvement of healthier older persons in helping provide care for the frail and sick and thereby contributing to their own continued health (Rowe & Kahn, 1998).

Environment

Nearly all old persons share the physical and social environments and facilities of their families and neighbours but there are emerging indications of future adaptations to their special needs. In richer societies the increase in numbers of elderly has already had considerable impact on the housing and leisure industries and on many aspects of consumption and transportation. Increasing demands for convenience and security as elders live alone and with greater purchasing capacity, yield more building of sheltered housing with supporting services. Healthy old people have the means to travel more and in comfort while their purchasing power has already led to changes in style and access to stores and supermarkets. These trends are bound to continue and urban plans will have to accommodate to the needs of the elderly population and provide open spaces, paths, public transportation and access to public places to allow for those of limited mobility.

Health Services

The chronic diseases, disability and frailty of ageing populations, place great strains on the capacity of health services to cope, at different levels, in both rich and poor countries.

Health services of poor countries face a *triple burden* of needs. To the unfinished fight against infectious and parasitic diseases must be added that against chronic diseases, cardiovascular, cerebrovascular and diabetes. This, the so-called double burden, is having added to it the care of the frail and disabled elderly. While these new needs are unlikely to have a high priority for decades to come, access to primary health care is a basic right of all ages in every country (WHO report, 2003). Older persons will share in such family and community focused schemes of primary care as are available: for most of the world's elderly this will be the only source of health care for a long time to come.

Where countries are richer and health services more developed, the primary physician is seen as the address for regular care and the gatekeeper or facilitator who will direct those patients in need of specialized care. As the population ages, nurses and doctors in primary care need more training in the special problems of the elderly. Expansion of rehabilitation and long-term care facilities in the community, together with the efforts to keep the old in their homes, is further stretching the responsibility of the primary care team in secondary and tertiary care. New systems of care in the home are leading to the development and training of new types of professional geriatric carers but there is often a shortage of personnel (Heath & Schofield, 1999).

Increasing age brings increasing episodes of disease and in developed countries persons over 65 may comprise 12%–15% of the population but use 30%–40% of the acute bed days. In several OECD countries those over 65 had a per capita health expenditure 3 to 4 times that of the under 65's while the ratio for those over 75 was 4 to 6 times higher (OECD, 2003). Public expenditure on health care of 14 European countries was calculated to be 5.3% of GDP in the year 2000 with an additional 1.3% on long term care. By the year 2050, other things being equal, the demographic shift alone will add a further 3.3% of GDP to the present average of 6.6% for both health and long term care. The increased demand for health care of the elderly has contributed greatly to total costs and to considerable turbulence in hospitalization policies. As many as 30% of elderly persons admitted to acute care hospitals in some countries need continuing care in rehabilitation or nursing facilities and these are not readily available. Individuals may thus wait in hospital and block an expensive bed needed for another, or be discharged home and require readmission within a short period. The fragmentation of different parts of the health and welfare services under different authorities is a common heritage of the industrialized countries, one they will have to reform and one that emerging countries will have to avoid (www.age2000.org.uk; Report of the Second World Assembly on Ageing, 2002).

An increasing proportion of the old, already 1%–5% in different countries, requires constant care and lives in long-term care facilities, supported by health and welfare authorities and, to varying degrees, by their families and by religious and voluntary agencies. The need reflects the increase in long-term disability and the reduction of the capacity of the family to provide adequate care. But families still maintain very many more dependent elderly at home than are admitted to institutions as long term care facilities continue to be a major unmet need (Havens, 1999; Brodsky, Habib, & Hirschfeld, 2003). As old populations grow older and needs increase, pressures mount for the creation of more and more beds in health and welfare facilities. A number of demonstration projects in different countries of Europe, North America and Japan have shown that it is possible to provide integrated services in the home and in the community to meet growing needs without excessive cost. The design of low cost service programmes appropriate to the local community is yet another part of the challenge already being taken up by several middle level developing countries (Brodsky, Habib, & Hirschfeld, 2003).

ADAPTATION TO AN AGEING SOCIETY

One can envisage three levels of reaction of a society to its own aging and the care of its elderly. The first, when no problem exists or is perceived and where social planning is in its infancy is to make no special provisions and rely on traditional family support and existing services: the situation of the poorest countries today and for the foreseeable future. The second, characteristic of countries of middle development and of industrialized countries in the past, is to accommodate to increasing numbers of elderly by expanding programs and services piecemeal and adding new ones as circumstances permit, in the manner of a patchwork quilt (America's health care safety net: Intact but endangered, 2000). The third, as in the last decade or so in many industrialized countries, is to develop new national agendas that focus on active ageing and extending the working life and which marry fiscal objectives with broad health and social goals (OECD indicators, 2003).

In this section we concentrate on health and social services. But because these are only partial answers to the needs of old persons and because of the impact of its ageing on many aspects of society, mention must be made of other facets of social planning. Essential first steps of the process in any country involve recognition of the perturbation of society by its demographic shift and the political will to meet the challenge. Freedom of access to the support and to the services necessary to facilitate health and function in old age presupposes acceptance by society of the principles of social justice and equity for health services at all ages as part of the determination of national priorities (Report of the Second World Assembly on Ageing, 2002; The Valencia report, 2002).

Rationalisation and planning of social and service support for the elderly should, ideally, start with a knowledge base of their health and welfare and their interactions with society.

Information and Research

The information available to decision makers on the state of health of their elderly populations, the need for services, and the costs and efficiency of different schemes for prevention, diagnosis and treatment is inadequate at best and frequently absent. Demographic information and measures of expectation of life and causes of death (with varying accuracy) are usually available, other than in the poorest countries. Ongoing information on morbidity patterns, when available, is often confined to a few sentinel populations so that projections that would permit an estimate of future needs for, say, rehabilitation beds or orthopedic surgeons, are frequently speculative. The information needs for planning and monitoring services for the elderly will depend on the organizational structure in place, or planned, for the combined health and social service for the elderly. They will include ongoing monitoring and surveys of health and function as well as monitoring of the quality of life of representative groups and their interaction with their environment. Involvement of old people themselves in the planning and evaluation of services is crucial. When targets have been set and strategies established, further decisions can be taken as to the information needs for planning and monitoring (Havens, 1999).

The major medical conditions that result in long-term disability are arthritis, osteoporosis, incontinence, depression, dementia, and disorders of sight and hearing. Advances in preventing or delaying the onset of these disorders and in their alleviation, could greatly increase the independence and productivity of individuals in their older years (Morley, 2004). In particular, operational research to improve the quality of care and to facilitate the application of preventive activities, as well as the new technologies, will be most cost-effective. In addition to their specific needs, elderly populations will, of course, benefit from the general advances in biomedical research and medical technology.

Operational research into improved programmes for healthy living, their availability, acceptance and impact on health is of paramount importance, both for present and for future populations of all ages. These facets of health systems research are applicable to all societies at every level of development. Should research be considered a luxury, as so often in the past, it must be realized that the poorer the nation, the less room there is for waste and the greater the need for an information base and local knowledge (Davies & Mansourian, 1992).

Pensions and Income Maintenance

While the common ages at retirement have been 65 for men and 60 for women, with a few exceptions, many countries already aim at equalizing the age to 65 for both genders in the foreseeable future, with a future rise to 67 or more. The situation is different in each country and each stage of development may require complex regulation and interactions. Raising the age of retirement will not automatically create more jobs nor are employers always eager to give preference to older and costlier workers. Markets and manufacturing will change greatly and rapidly within coming years and emphasis will have to be given to lifelong learning so that workers of all ages improve their skills and productivity (OECD, social issues 2000; Cotis, 2003).

Reforms to pension policies are crucial to the health and well being of the elderly as well as to the societies of which they form part. The rising share of older persons implies that more people will receive pensions and expensive health care at a time when a decreasing working age population will pay less taxes and social contributions. New reform agendas are emerging that marry fiscal objectives with broad social and economic policy goals and include different approaches to financing pensions, tax reform, ways to facilitate longer working life and subsidizing child care so that mothers can work and produce. The mix of policy reforms in industrialized and transition ranges from patching up deficiencies in current practice to, more and more, complete rethinking of social policies (OECD indicators 2003; Colis, 2003). The World Bank, on the other hand, has suggested that financial security for the old and economic growth would be better served if governments relied on three systems: a publicly managed system with mandatory participation and the limited goal of reducing poverty among the old, a privately managed mandatory savings system and a voluntary savings system (Averting the old age crisis; policies to protect the old and promote growth, 1994).

This impact on so many aspects of social planning again illustrates the far-reaching consequences of the demographic transition.

Education and Training

The greatest challenge in this field in the coming decades will be to spread the awareness and practice of the principles of life-long healthy living starting with adequate nutrition of pregnant women and ensuring appropriate diets of toddlers and adolescents and up the scale throughout the life span. Adequate exercise and avoidance of tobacco and obesity at every age will do much to prevent diabetes and cardiovascular diseases. One important aspect is to ensure the ready availability of reliable advice and information on health practices, disease prevention and access to professional help through the internet and popular media (www.community health.dhhs.state.nc.us/oldadult/netguide).

The education of future doctors and the vocational training of practitioners will need considerable adjustment both as a result of new knowledge, increased demand for new and expanded services by the elderly and of the differences in emphasis envisioned by the healthy aging approach. Positive approaches to the care of the elderly and the avoidance of discrimination will need to be inculcated. More specialists in geriatrics, in rehabilitation and in terminal care will be needed as well as practitioners of such sub-specialties as geriatric surgery, psycho geriatrics, gero-oncology and so on. The nursing profession has already shouldered much of the health care in old age and in all countries geriatric nursing training and curricula will be continuously modified to meet new needs. New challenges will come with the evolution of new types of training and of professional and para-professional workers capable of tackling the nursing, welfare, social, and psychological support of emerging populations (Namazi & Green, 2003, Assae).

The duty of the health professions to devise new treatments and to apply new technologies for the benefit of their patients at all levels of care is undisputed. The challenge will be to monitor their cost and effectiveness and to optimize their use. There is little evidence today for the efficacy of many of the health interventions practised in populations of any age and there is urgent need for development of medical procedures based on scientific evidence (Sackett, Strauss, Richardson, Rosenberg, & Haynes, 2000). For the elderly, some procedures in screening and in rehabilitation, to say the least, may not be cost effective. Quality control is lacking, even in countries with the most advanced care of the elderly and systematic reviews of evidence for various interventions are required (www.ahcpr.gov/consumer/qntool.htm). In particular, evaluation of low-cost interventions such as those in programmes for healthy aging and disease prevention are long overdue, particularly for developing countries.

FUTURE CHANCES

The health of older populations is part and parcel of the health of the communities to which they belong. Contemplation of the low priority given to health in global planning gives little scope for optimism for the near future (Smith, 2004) and probable scenarios are discussed in section 3 above. Nor does the emphasis on specific disease control in poor countries (WHO, report of the commission 2001, Piel) which minimizes the importance of the social and environmental context in which they are embedded (WHO report 2003; Labonte & Spiegel, 2003) So many lessons of the past have been forgotten, including Health for All (WHO report 2003; Cohen 2003.) while the advance of globalization to date shows little evidence of egalitarianism or benefit to local communities (http://hdr.undp.org).

For the majority of the next two or three generations of the world's elderly therefore, progress to health will be very slow and many, if not most, will live longer in poor health. Hopefully, there will be many exceptions to this dismal forecast.

However, as already noted (section 4), the outlook is more sanguine for the elite minority, for those in industrialized countries, which have experienced some of the impact of their ageing and are ready and willing to face the challenges. Their future elderly should continue to benefit from a continued healthy life style, to remain active in society and be able to afford and enjoy the benefits of new support and communication technologies. They will have at their disposal the advances in biomedicine for early diagnosis and treatment of disease and advanced methods of rehabilitation and long term care.

REFERENCES

Age Concern (1998). *The millennium debate of the age. Millennium paper—health and care* web site http://www.age2000.org.uk

Barker, D.J. (Ed). (2001). *Fetal origins of cardiovascular and lung disease.* New York and Basel: Marcel Dekker.

Brodsky, J., Habib, J., & Hirschfeld, M. (2003). *Key policy issues in a long-term care.* Geneva, World Health Organization, Collection on long-term care.

Butler, R. (1999). Ageing: Another form of bigotry. Gerontologist, 9, 243–6 .

Coburn, D. (2004). Beyond the income inequality hypothesis: Class, neo-liberalism and health inequalities. *Social Science and Medicine, 58,* 41–56.

Cohen, J. (2003, March 8). Worse than a crime; a mistake. Lancet, 361.

Cotis, J.P. (2003, September) *Population ageing: Facing the challenge.* OECD Observer No 239, Paris.

Davies, A.M., & Mansourian, B. (1992). *Research strategies for health.* Lewiston, N.Y., Hogrefe & Huber, on behalf of the World Health Organization.

Dello Buono, M., Uriciuoli, O., & De Leo, D. (1998). Quality of life and longevity: A study of centenarians. Age and ageing, 27, 207–216.

Division of Public Health, North Carolina Department of Health and Human Services. *Using the Internet for older adult health education and research.* Retrieved from www.communityhealth.dhhs.state.nc. us/oldadult/netguide

Evans, J.G., & Williams, T.F. (1992). *Oxford textbook of geriatric medicine.* Oxford University Press.

Freedman, V.A., Martin, L.G., & Schoeni, R.F. (2002). Recent trends in disability and functioning among older adults in the United States. A systematic review. *JAMA, 288,* 3137–3146.

Havens, B. (1999). *Home-based and long-term care. Home care issues at the approach of the 21st century from a World Health Organization perspective. An annotated bibliography.* Geneva, World Health Organization.

Heath, H., & Schofield, I. (1999). *Healthy ageing: Nursing older people.* London, Mosby.

Institute of Medicine (2000). *America's health care safety net: Intact but endangered.* Washington.

International Association of Gerontology (2002, April 1–4). *The valencia report.* A report on outcomes of a meeting of gerontological researchers, educators and providers. Valencia, Spain.

Kending, H., Hashimoto, A., & Coppard, L. (1992). *Family support for the elderly.* Oxford University Press for the World Health Organization.

Kinsella, K., & Velkoff, V.A. *An ageing world:* 2001 Washington DC, US Bureau of the Census, International population reports, 2001.

Labonte, R., & Spiegel, J. (2003, April 5). Setting global health research priorities. British Medical Journal, *326,* 722–3.

Marmot, M., & Wilkinson, R.G. (Eds). (1999). *Social determinants of health.* Oxford University Press.

Morley, J.E. (2004). The top 10 hot topics in ageing. *Journal of Gerontology, A 59,* M24–M33.

Murray, C.J.L., & Lopez, A.D. (1997). Alternative projections of mortality and disability by cause 1990–2020: Global burden of disease study. Lancet, *349,* 1498–1504.

Namazi, K.H., & Green, G. (2003). Gerontological education for allied health professionals. Journal of Allied Health, *32,* 18–26.

Organization for economic co-operation and development (2003). *Health at a glance. OECD indicators.* Paris.

Organization for Economic Co-Operation and Development (2000). *Reforms for an ageing society. Social issues.* Paris.

Rowe, J.W., & Kahn, R.L. (1998). *Successful ageing.* New York: Random House.

Sackett, D.L., Strauss, S., Richardson, W.S., Rosenberg, W., & Haynes, R.B. (2000). *Evidence-based medicine: How to practice and teach EBM* (2nd ed.). London, Churchill Livingstone.

Sen, A. (2000). Health equity: Perspectives, measurability and criteria. In: Evans, T., Whitehead, M., et al (Ed.). *Challenging inequities in health: From ethics to action* (pp. 69–75). Oxford University Press.

Smith, R. (2004). Economics first; health third, fourth, or nowhere. British Medical Journal, *328,* (31 January) (Editorial).

United Nations Population Information Network (POPIN). Data, global and regional, 2003. Retrieved from www.un.org/popin/data.html

United Nations Development Fund (UNDF). *Human development report 2003.* Retrieved from http://hdr.undp.org

United Nations Population Fund (UNFPA). *The state of world population 2003.* Retrieved from www.unfpa.org

United States Census Bureau. International Data Base (IDB) 2003. Retrieved from www.census.gov/ipc/www/ idbnew.html

US Centers for Disease Control. (2003). Public health and ageing: Trends in ageing—United States and worldwide. *JAMA, 209,* 1371–1373.

United States Senate. Committee on ageing forum. Is there a shortage of geriatricians? Discussion, May 20, 1997, Washington DC web site http://aging.senate.gov/oas/f5.htm

United Nations (2002, April 8–12). *Report of the Second World Assembly on ageing.* Madrid, New York, UN.

United States Department of Homeland Security. First gov for consumers: health. Ageing/Elder Care. Retrieved from www.ahcpr.gov/consumer/qntool.htm

World Bank. (1994). *Averting the old age crisis: Policies to protect the old and promote growth*. Oxford University Press for the World Bank.

World Health Organization. *World health report 2003*. Geneva.

World Health Organization. *The uses of epidemiology in the study of the elderly*. Report of a WHO scientific group on the epidemiology of ageing. Geneva, WHO, technical report series, 706 (1984).

World Health Organization (2001, December). *Macroeconomics and health: Investing in health for economic development. Report of the commission*, Geneva.

Section IV

The Controversies

Chapter 16

Disease and Health in the Cultural Context

ASSEN JABLENSKY

Neither disease nor health are concepts that have ever been strictly and unambiguously defined in terms of finite sets of observable referential phenomena. Medical textbooks rarely devote references to the subjects, and it seems perfectly possible for a medical professional to practice medicine and treat illnesses without possessing or using an overarching concept of disease. Yet we intuitively know that concepts of disease and health—probably originating in the earliest categorizations of the phenomenal world developed by humankind—are rooted in the culture and contain strata of rich meanings and connotations transmitted over the generations. In no culture have such meanings and connotations been entirely static; however, it is in the present technological culture that the rate of change is unprecedented. The notion of disease has accrued mutations in the course of the last two centuries by absorbing new elements in each consecutive era of social and scientific history. It is more than likely that further metamorphosis is in the making, partly as a result of current developments in the biomedical and life sciences, but perhaps more importantly as a consequence of social and cultural change.

This brief chapter focuses selectively on three aspects of the problem:

- the nature of the concept of disease explicitly or implicitly present in current medical discourse and public health;
- the impact of recent scientific advances and sociocultural change on the notions of disease and health; and
- likely future trends and their implications.

DISEASE AS A CULTURAL CATEGORY

Any discussion of the concept of disease must proceed from the recognition that the phenomena of health and disease cannot be adequately described and accounted for in terms of naturalistic concepts, as can, for example, the objects of physics or cell biology. Disease is not just "out there"; it is a generic abstraction of multiple classes of observations ranging from a variety of subjective experiences to objective measurements. Concepts of disease serve as explanatory models for a significant and existentially salient segment of "the human condition"; as such they are shared by cultures and, within cultures, particular groups (e.g., professional vs. lay public) may endorse different varieties of the concepts. Values and beliefs are, therefore, intrinsic components of disease concepts.

Recognition of the cultural roots and societal functions of the disease concept should lead to an awareness of the co-existence of different variants of the generic concept (which, insofar as anthropological research can enlighten us, is likely to be universal—Dubos, 1968). The "scientific" concept of disease, therefore, can be described and studied as *one* (a particularly influential one at that) among many such variants. The quotation marks point to the *relativity* of the term "scientific" when applied to the paradigm of disease underlying the medical enterprise. Its philosophical underpinnings can be traced to several different traditions, so that the "modern" concept of disease can be seen as a hybrid of ideas, or as an intersection of quite diverse ontological schemata.

Two major and recurrent influences, whose traces can be discerned even in present-day medical thinking, are Platonic realism and Aristotelian nominalism. Plato postulated an independent existence for the *universalia*, that is, the prototype ideas (or "forms"), of which the physical things (*res discretae*) are only partial and imperfect exemplars. Sydenham, one of the founders of the modern concept of disease, behaved as a Platonist when he wrote of "the" pox, "the" podagra, and "the" dropsy—in other words, the ideal forms of disease of which the individual and observable presentations were approximate, often blurred, copies. The art and science of diagnosis, according to this view, consisted in the ability to discern the pure form, the "idea" of the disease, amongst many variable and accidental observations, by applying a systematic search for the *signs* through which the prototype lets itself be known. In contrast to realism, nominalism attributed real existence solely to the particular "things"—abstract classes or *universalia* being only *names* (or *constructs*, in modern parlance) for similarities of properties that have no independent, real world existence. The founder of modern pathology, Virchow, defined diseases in terms of *pathological processes*, that is, observed regularities and patterns of structural changes in organs and tissues that underlie the clinical manifestations. As empirical constructs mapping a deeper reality, pathological processes, such as inflammation or neoplasia, advance knowledge beyond the clinical presentation, which was now relegated to the status of a mere appearance. The bacteriological era of medicine reinforced the emerging paradigm by adding invisible *pathogens* to the structural processes. The true nature of disease, according to this paradigm, could only be identified in the laboratory, not by the bedside.

However the successes of the laboratory-based disease model did not obliterate the mode of cognition in medicine that one might call *stylistic Platonism*—even if the relevant philosophical beliefs are no longer explicitly shared. Clinical examination performed as the art of eliciting and interpreting the symptoms and signs of disease (in search of "the" diagnosis) has not only survived but enjoys today a new lease on life with the discovery of a higher than previously expected informativeness for the clinical signs and symptoms, and the application of new methods for standardizing clinical observation and reasoning. Thus, we can find in clinical medicine today a curious undercurrent of vestigial ideas and assumptions, both Aristotelian and Platonic, which will continue to shape thinking and attitudes if left unchallenged in medical education. The true "essence" of disease today, in the minds of many medical students and practitioners, is equated with the genes, the immune system, or the cell receptors. The rest—the subjective experience, behaviour, beliefs, and social response—is often perceived as being of secondary importance, a layer of reality that obfuscates the biological facts. This belief has been termed by social scientists "the medical model of disease."

This notion, however, is simplistic. There is yet another philosophical tradition that has generated insights of at least equal importance for the disease concept. The other side of the coin: disease as a subjective experience (*dis-ease*) of pain, discomfort, impairment and anguish—often foreboding death—has been the focus of philosophical discourse, ranging from Hegel's dictum that disease is life diminished in its freedom, to Kierkagaard's preoccupation with the ways the individual confronts the dread of nothingness (Kierkagaard, 1946). Nietzsche (1977) (3), on the other hand, discussed disease and health as cultural categories and pointed out the relativity of the distinction between them: health and disease are not essentially different, they are two modes of being separated only by differences of degree ("the exaggeration, the disproportion, the lack of harmony between the normal phenomena constitute the morbid state"). Mental illness has been a natural focus for such anthropological approaches to the conceptualization of disease, because abnormal subjective experience and behaviour remain as its principal defining characteristics, notwithstanding the attempts to fit psychiatric disorders into a biological mould.

MULTIDIMENSIONAL NATURE OF THE DISEASE CONCEPT

It is unlikely that the different strata of the disease concept can be blended into a monolithic notion. The nature of the concept is best expressed as a multidimensional framework which, according to the physician and philosopher Karl Jaspers (1963) (4) should include at least four major axes:

- deviation (structural or functional) from the mean in a statistical sense;
- deviation involving reduced performance and/or a threat to survival;
- the subjective experience of illness versus health;
- the social and cultural values attached to the ideal norm and the deviations from it.

A current model which closely approximates these ideas is the triaxial concept underlying the WHO International Classification of Impairments, Disabilities and Handicaps (ICIDH), where *impairment* refers to the structural or functional lesion (deviation from the average); *disability* to the loss or reduction of the capacity to perform particular social or occupational roles; and *handicap* to the adverse social consequences of disablement. Similarly, the distinction between 'disease,' 'illness,' and 'sickness'—initially introduced by medical sociologists—has now been widely adopted as a convenient way of referring to the distinctions between objective biological data (*disease*), the subjective experience (*illness*), and the social role of being a patient (*the sick role*). Generally, the trend of the past two decades has been one towards a multidimensional or multiaxial conceptualisation of the phenomena of disease, with several relatively independent dimensions:

- clinical syndrome(s);
- structural and/or functional deviations;
- aetiology;
- co-morbidity; and
- social functioning.

Among the many examples, AIDS is a particularly useful model embodying many of the biological, social, ethical, and economic facets of a multidimensional concept of disease.

MEASUREMENT AND CLASSIFICATION

The past three decades have witnessed considerable advances in the operationalisation of diagnosis and in the clinical measurement of the manifestations of disease. The reliability of diagnosis (in terms of its reproducibility and the reduction of measurement error) has improved—including such areas as psychiatric diagnosis, which in the past was extremely sensitive to variations in subjective clinical judgement. There is a clear trend of applying decision-making theory, standard (operational) diagnostic criteria, and epidemiological databases to the clinical diagnostic process, which has resulted in the evolving new discipline of clinical epidemiology. Algorithms and decision-making flowcharts are now available for different classes of diseases and for different users and settings, including primary health care in developing countries A major need to be met in the future will be the development of population- or region-specific epidemiological databases, which would support local planning of health services and the application of new diagnostic and treatment technologies. At the population level, epidemiology now has the tools to map diseases in terms of:

- incidence and prevalence;
- lifetime risk, relative risk, and
- attributable risk; mortality; disaility-adjusted life years (DALY) and quality of life adjusted life years (QALY).

Using the advances in computing technologies, it should be possible to develop models of morbidity and mortality in specified populations by subtracting from the current picture of disease the patterns of preventable or modifiable morbidity and causes of death and thus visualising the demographic, epidemiological, and social changes that would occur.

QUALITY OF LIFE

Quality of life is usually defined as a perceived state of wellbeing that may be influenced by physical, mental, functional, social, and emotional factors. Over the years, the concept has become associated with many different meanings and its scope has broadened. For example, WHO defines quality of life as "individuals' perceptions of their position in life in the context of the culture and value systems in which they live and in relation to their goals, expectations, standards, and concerns." Such a broad definition covers the following six domains of the quality of life concept: (i) physical domain; (ii) psychological domain; (iii) level of independence; (iv) social relationships; (v) environment; and (vi) spiritual domain. Within each of these domains, there are a number of quality of life facets pertaining to that particular domain. By way of illustration, the psychological domain includes the following facets: positive feelings; thinking, learning, memory and concentration; self-esteem; body image and appearance; and negative feelings. A quality of life assessment process is based on several measurement scales concerned with the intensity, frequency, and subjective evaluation of states, behaviour, and capacities related to the above-described domains and facets.

IMPACT OF NEW SCIENTIFIC AND SOCIOCULTURAL DEVELOPMENTS ON THE CONCEPTUALISATION OF DISEASE

Current advances in several areas of biomedical research, clinical medicine and public health are likely to exert a strong influence on the ways disease and health are conceptualised by clinicians, public health professionals, health planners and politicians, and, of course, the increasing number of sectors and groups in the society at large that have financial, political, or consumer interest in such definitions. Scientists are probably the least concerned professional group in this context since it appears that their frame of reference and day-to-day work rarely involves the need for generic definitions of disease and health.

MOLECULAR BIOLOGY, MOLECULAR MEDICINE AND GENOMICS

With several thousand diseases for which a specific genetic bases has been identified, and the sequencing of the human genome already completed, molecular genetics is undoubtedly one of the most successful scientific enterprises ever launched in the life sciences. Together with advances in the molecular biology of the cell, it has a profound impact on clinical medicine, which now encompasses large areas that could be described as molecular medicine. An increasing number of diseases can be defined and classified in molecular terms, which sometimes make the elaborate clinical distinctions obsolete (e.g., within the group of neuromuscular disorders). The emergence of molecular genetic classifications of large groups of diseases, and the concomitant availability of genetic diagnostic tests, raises the possibility that the entire taxonomy of human disease may be revised in a way reflecting this new knowledge of genomics. Predictive diagnostic testing in clinically asymptomatic individuals (currently available for a limited range of disorders, e.g., Huntington's disease) will probably soon become possible in Alzheimer's disease, certain cancers and, eventually, some of the major psychiatric disorders.

Besides the serious ethical questions about the access to such information and the psychosocial repercussions of widespread testing programmes, a problem to be faced is that for large segments of society (including certain health professionals), the concept of disease may become synonymous with the carrier state for a particular set of genes. Although molecular medicine *per se* (at least in its present shape) does not seem to necessitate any change in the multidimensional concept of disease as referred to above (susceptibility genes being a particular form or level of structural and functional lesion), *genetic reductionism* may become a popular explanatory model with non-negotiable practical and ethical consequences in areas such as health insurance, the labour market, and, ultimately, human rights. Examples of such problems include:

- the genetic basis of quantitative traits and the demarcation of disease from non-disease—at which cut-off point does, for instance, short stature cease to be a normal variant and become a treatable "disease"?
- are pre-symptomatic carriers of the genetic susceptibility to disorders such as Huntington's disease (and, possibly, in the near future, Alzheimer's disease) an insurance liability?
- how will society handle the information if genes predisposing to suicide, substance abuse, and violence are eventually identified?

EPIDEMIOLOGY, PUBLIC HEALTH AND "HEALTHISM"

As a counterpart to the genetics of human disease, epidemiology has contributed substantial new knowledge on the environmental risk factors and causes of morbidity in areas such as ischaemic heart disease, cancer, nutrition, and behaviour disorders. The practical applications of such knowledge in preventive programmes in the developed countries have resulted in significant lifestyle changes for large numbers of people and in reductions in certain categories of morbidity and mortality. In a number of developing countries, the decreases in infant mortality that have occurred over the last decade are, at least in part, attributable to prevention technologies that are relatively simple at the point of delivery. By and large, the successes of preventive medicine tend to be eclipsed in the mass media by the glamour of genetic research and high-tech medicine. However, public health programmes that have been successful in lifestyle modification (smoking cessation, exercise, healthy nutrition) may be contributing to the emergence (mainly among middle-class populations in the developed countries) of a set of values and an ideology—"healthism"—endorsing a particular health/disease model. This model tends to overemphasize *indiviual* choice and autonomy while underemphasizing the collective responsibility of society for the economic and social inequities that impose upon the less privileged population groups multiple health risks that are not amenable to individual behavioural control. The risk of *attribution*, and blaming the poor and the less educated for their own health misfortunes, which at present is probably subliminal, may eventually be augmented by "the choice is yours" public education campaigns. Illness is seen as "evidence of misbehaviour" and "failures of self-care become, in a sense, crimes against society" (Fitzgerald, 1994).

COST OF MEDICAL TECHNOLOGIES AND PRESSURES OF THE HEALTH CARE MARKET

Another factor that is likely to influence the perceptions and definitions of disease and health is related to concerns about the rising share of health care in national spending, driven by a complex set of forces including, in particular, costly new diagnostic and therapeutic technologies (Leufkens *et al*, 1994; Haaijer-Ruskamp, & Bakker, 1994). Concerns about cost containment are linked, on the one hand, to the issue of cost efficiency and the introduction of market forces into the health care sector; and, on the other hand, to the prospect of rationing health care. Both issues imply measurement, valuation, and the ranking of diseases and their outcomes according to cost-benefits or cost-effectiveness in relation to various treatments. This is likely to result in an increasing influence of economic judgements in decisions about which conditions should be treated and how. Indirectly, or directly, such judgements and decisions will affect the taxonomy of disease, for instance, by defining thresholds of severity or treatability.

EVIDENCE-BASED MEDICINE AND HEALTH CONSUMERISM

The increasingly influential trend of applying the principles of decision-making theory in clinical medicine, and of explicitly basing clinical decisions on distilled evidence from controlled trials or technology evaluations, can be seen as a medical counterpart to the cost-benefit approaches in health care promoted by health economists (see also chapter 7 by J.Szczerban). While the extent of the impact of evidence-based medicine and of the so-called clinical evaluative sciences on actual clinical practice is yet uncertain, the principle itself, and much of the analysed evidence, is likely to be endorsed and widely used by the consumer groups and movements whose negotiating power is increasing. The result will be an increased transparence of medical practice and of its "grey zones" (Naylor, 1995), as well as a transfer into the public domain of much of what until now was professionally guarded specialist knowledge. The definition of what constitutes treatable disease, for which consumers and society, as a whole, would be willing to pay, will inevitably be affected.

THE CONCEPT OF DISEASE AS A SOCIAL CONTRACT

The foregoing discussion illustrates the main point stated at the outset: The generic concept of disease is a social and cultural construct. Biomedical science and clinical medicine operate with partial and specific aspects of the generic concept, such as syndromes, pathogenic mechanisms, and causes. The dimensions of disability, handicap, and sickness roles are best studied with the methods of social science. The overarching nature of the generic concepts of disease and health, however, is beyond the specific conventional concerns of the biomedical and behavioural sciences and requires a new, meta-analytical health science. The concepts of health and disease are now—more than ever—squarely placed in the domain of public discourse, societal values, and politics (Morrison & Smith, 1994). Global development and the policy trends that are apparent today suggest that in the decades to come the definitions of disease and health will be more and more the negotiated results of political and economic bargaining among different interest and power groups in society, and less and less the domain of professional medical expertise and traditional public health competence. The implications of these developments for the long-term policy and programme forecasts by the World Health Organization should be obvious: Rather than retaining an implicit, unanalysed, and probably obsolete concept of health and disease, WHO must examine critically the *philosophical* and *cultural* premises of its programmes and adjust to the realities of the 21st century.

REFERENCES

Dubos, R. (1968). *Man, medicine, and environment* (pp. 87–113). New York, Mentor Books and New American Library.

Fitzgerald, F.T. (1994). The tyranny of health. *New England Journal of Medicine, 331,* 196–198.

Jaspers, K. (1963). *General psychopathology.* Birmingham University Press.

Kierkagaard, S. (1946). The sickness unto death. In: R. Bretall (Ed.), *A Kierkagaard anthology* (pp. 339–371). New York, Modern Library.

Leufkens, H., Haaijer-Ruskamp, F., Bakker, A. & Dukes, G. (1994). Scenario analysis of the future of medicines. *British Medical Journal, 309,* 1137–1140.

Morrison, I., & Smith, R. (1994). The future of medicine. *British Medical Journal, 309,* 1099–1100.

Naylor, C.D. (1995). Grey zones of clinical practice: Some limits to evidence-based medicine. *Lancet, 345,* 840–842.

Nietzsche, F. (1977). *Umwertung aller Werte* (pp. 414–415). Munich, Deutscher Taschenbuch Verlag.

Chapter 17

Global Issues and Health Interactions

Reflexions from the South

A.P.R. ALUWIHARE

INTRODUCTION

This chapter draws attention to a range of global issues that interact, and aims to provoke thought and research on their impact on health. Initially, it deals with communication, economic issues and physician migration. Then it summarizes a wide field of mechanisms by which global forces affect health, indirectly or directly. Within this classification there has to be some overlap—for example the HIV virus causing AIDS would appear to be a direct health effect, but a shift in lifestyles that has seen an increase in the number of individuals' sexual partners—a shift that perhaps reflects a breakdown of family and religious value systems—may be the more fundamental, but indirect, cause. The view is primarily from the standpoint of developing countries, the "South," and does not eschew controversy.

COMMUNICATION

Health Effects of Communication Technology

New communications technologies have improved the speed with which the benefits or adverse effects of any new health intervention are scrutinized and spread. Difficulties in identifying infection in a poorly equipped remote centre, or performing operations in a small district hospital, and so on, are mitigated by active on-line communication. These communications remain expensive, but they are cheaper than transporting patients. The best-known example of the value of central laboratories in monitoring outbreaks of infections is the Centres for Disease Control in Atlanta, Georgia, USA.

Today in society there are new vectors that convey pathogenic influences to the mind and the body, turning them into pathological behaviour and disease, without the need for insect vectors. These are the electronic media (radio, television, the Internet) and printed matter, linked to peer pressures across nations. Subtle and sophisticated methods of communication with high-pressure presentation and advertising techniques are available, aiming to force compliant behaviour by readers and viewers, whether they are the general public, children, or potential consumers. The potential dangers of the so-called new non-communicable diseases (and of others such as diabetes, malignancy, accidental and non-accidental trauma, and family dissolution) are now recognized, as is the effect of lifestyle on them. However, the urgency that needs to pervade this subject is still missing. Even the name dulls, and perhaps the word non-communicable should be consigned to history or be entirely discarded. The term neo-communicable disease (NCD) is proposed for these conditions: this should, if only subconsciously, instil a sense of urgency.

Crime, violence, and untrammelled sexual promiscuity seem to be wholly acceptable in the media. All produce problems, and only now is television generally monitored. The Internet is still almost completely uncontrolled—and assertions about the need to protect freedom of speech are used to justify the unlimited propagation of the most sexually provocative and violent material.

However HIV may have started, its subsequent spread in humans demonstrates the consequences of an alteration in the norms of behavior. Heterosexual spread is aggravated by practices that are at variance with a holistic concept of the unitary family. In addition to technical methods of control and cure, what is more difficult to decide is whether there are relevant moral and religious arguments. The economics of the sex industry will not permit control. Human rights workers face roadblocks when they seek to inquire into the trafficking of females as sex workers and of children for war and pornography. A new dimension is the effect of web-based sexual material.

Information technology could be used better; it has yet to be exploited by the medical fraternity as a health promoting platform for marketing of preventive diets and lifestyles with the same skill, effort, and money that more harmful marketing readily achieves. It should be recognised that the psychology is important here: The opportunity to cure is more exciting than to prevent; at a global level, there is no money in prevention. Information technology could undoubtedly also be better exploited for surveillance against new and unknown diseases—for instance, in looking at changes in genes, enzymes, cell proteins, and so on.

A specific way in which the technology is actually being used, albeit inadequately—is for modelling the consequences of various health related scenarios as a diagnostic and therapeutic tool in community health, but more importantly as a method of monitoring and forecasting major health problems in terms of global perspectives and data. The capabilities of computers would be especially valuable when inter-sectoral issues need to be investigated, which is mandatory in such studies of global health.

Inappropriate Foods and Their Global 'Marketing'

Obesity is now a major problem in the United States and Britain and is increasingly so in the rest of the developed world—especially amongst children. The marketing pressures about behaviour and food that encourage this trend are now spreading to the Third World. Diabetes is now a major health problem in Asia and Africa, providing an environment for infections of skin and internal organs that have serious consequences. Levels of exercise are decreasing, and the populations and countries do not have the financial resources to prevent or manage infections effectively. Cardiovascular disease and alcohol and cirrhosis are increasing problems—with alcohol, Hepatitis B, and liver cancer being a terrible triad. These are becoming global now, with lifestyles and sexual norms changing. The poor have a triple burden of disease.

The pressures of the global-village mechanisms in food production can create other possible problems, again linked to production and marketing. Possible problems yet to be assessed include: irradiated foods; genetically modified foods (GM); the effects of processing in producing carcinogens in food; animal feeding habits like those which led to bovine spongiform encephalopathy and now the human form of that disease; packing and processing of food; and chemical post-harvest preservation.

Physical Movement

The speed of international travel and the amount of exchange of commodities mean that microorganisms can be transported into new environments in which there is almost no background resistance. Rats and mice move. Humans move. Quarantine measures are now relaxed. SARS-like outbreaks can occur in the most unexpected places.

ECONOMIC ISSUES

Poverty

Poverty is now recognized not only as a disease in itself, but also as an important cause of disease. It should be noted that the common index based on per capita income alone may not be an adequate measure of poverty in a rural area where much food is grown and living expenses are low, whether in a unitary or in an extended family. But exactly the same cash income may be inadequate if even one member of the family is in an urban area, or if the family is split up. Nevertheless, it would appear that the gap between rich and poor, in all countries, is increasing. The diseases of poverty, and diseases consequent upon poverty, are among the biggest challenges facing the international community in this new millennium.

Urbanization may increase poverty and decrease health. The importance of subsidies and of encouragement to maintain the strength of the farming community and the prospects for its young in the same profession must be recognized. Although GM foods may or may not have direct health effects, the transnational marketing of these would be harmful if farming in a country is adversely affected, leading to urbanization, breakdown of families, more cost to the government in developing cities, crime, lack of family support systems for the elderly, and so on. Unplanned urban growth is now globally epidemic. The breakdown of rural agriculture and an unwillingness to develop a strategy for industries in rural areas contribute to this problem. Independence of rural communities is also seriously at risk in this era of cheap mass production and interdependence. In this sense, multisectoral interdependance is a global threat to health.

Food Security; Subsidies

The drive towards opening markets often serves good purposes. But globalisation and World Trade Organization policies that allow food subsidies and import protection selectively in rich countries and try to forbid them in poor countries undermine food security. (The subsidy issue is currently relevant to the WTO, China, India, Brazil, USA, and EEC.) Sometimes food produced in the developed world is cheaper than food produced in the developing world, as farmers in developing countries faced with the loss of subsidies for fertiliser often price themselves out of the market (and also may incur such losses that they give up farming). Youth, who no longer wish to look after farms, become unemployed and move into towns. This can cause even more problems by undermining farming and fishing and increasing urbanisation in the developing world. Indirect effects then result from increasing urban and rural poverty. These increase disease (because of bad housing, inadequate water supply, and poor sanitation). So both food production and the economy of the country suffer disastrous consequences. A self-sustaining way of life seems to become eroded, and pockets of poverty increase. Naturally, higher productivity in developed countries is to be welcomed and emulated, but protectionism is not welcome. Other global phenomena indirectly affecting health include the development of crop predator agrochemical resistance—as this spreads across countries, international co-ordination for its control is needed.

Cost Recovery Policies

Some macroeconomic trends leading to international policies about cost recovery have distinctly negative effects, and result in ineffective and impractical policies. They cut off access to health care (and education) for the poor—as can be seen in parts of subSaharan Africa. They may also increase poverty and, therefore, indirectly negatively affect health. So the new poverty that accompanies some of the current economic policies constitutes a disappointing new threat, even though the basic policies set out originally to reduce poverty. Income disparities, as well as disparities in nutrition and education, are increasing in many countries. Poverty and unfulfilled aspirations are causes of violence. Awareness and action are needed to control this new threat; it will not disappear as part of globalisation may indeed become worse.

Funding for Health

There are huge national variations in spending on health. The low figure in Sri Lanka (of around $23 USD/capita/annum) for example, is minute compared to the 14+% of GDP the US spends on health—and the US still leaves a significant proportion of its population relatively underserved.

Corruption and Bad Governance

These remain major problems, particularly in poorer countries; it is suspected that the resources shamelessly diverted from the public sector, and especially from the budget for health and education, are a high percentage of GDP. Macro-corruption in international contracts and aid arrangements would likely be made worse by collusion and encouragement from sources in the North to the South—the poor suffer, and disease and bad treatment are the consequences. Poorer nations spend even less, and the gap is widening.

Economic Sanctions

The use of sanctions by the "morally correct," rich, and powerful nations, against those regarded as "evil," has the most devastating health effects on the innocent in a country. This has been so for a long time in Cuba, and to some extent in South Africa, and, in the relatively short term, in Iraq. To expect the "dictators" or leaders to succumb on the grounds of the suffering of the innocent is naïve! Those who impose the sanctions take a position on the moral high ground—but do they not subvert sanctions if it is convenient?

Physician Migration

Physician migration from the developing to developed areas of the world, or even within a country, occurs for financial, social, and job satisfaction reasons. This poses a real health threat. Donor developing nations experience difficulties and inequities in their health services, financial loss for the country occurs, and a loss of educated families, potential employers, and role models. The human resource for medical education is diminished. The critical mass for research and development becomes difficult to maintain. These disadvantages are not adequately compensated by increasing contacts, introduction of new ideas, or financial inflow to the donor country. Often the pull from the developed world is increased because it does not produce enough physicians of its own. The credibility of international health and educational organisations is affected because they may be thought to be trying to train more economically in the 'South' a product for the 'North.' Amelioration of this situation needs economic development and imaginative schemes in the donor countries and, ideally, ethical attitudes from recipient governments. At the very least, adequate compensation should be made to the donor country of the amount per capita that it would have cost the recipient country to produce the same product.

DIRECT EFFECTS ON HEALTH

There are many "non-medical" matters which are global, and which affect health for many reasons. Value systems are propagated by the media, travel can transport germs, marketing forces determine the spread of certain types of vehicles, and skewed distribution of resources at international and national levels to combat these problems compounds them. The rapid spread of information and knowledge can help to control and treat some diseases. Anti-smoking pressure genuinely applied to consumers and producers of tobacco (this has not happened yet) would for example, help maintain good health and save many lives and resources.

Tobacco and Alcohol

Supposedly harmless substances like tobacco and alcohol have produced enormous problems with neoplasia, cardiovascular, liver and pancreatic disease, and social disruption. The courts, for instance in the United States, have accepted many times that tobacco is addictive and harmful but the export of that same commodity to gullible consumers is allowed; the drug regulatory authority of the exporting country would be very unlikely to allow so freely the import from elsewhere of something condemned at home as roundly as tobacco. Powerful tobacco lobbies argue that "the rights of consumers" allow the export. The increase in tobacco consumption in the developing world, instigated in part by vigorous advertising and export from developed countries or their outsourced subsidiaries, will lead to huge increases in malignancies and cardiovascular disease as the twenty-first century unfolds. Alcohol abuse is similarly an increasing problem and, again, global marketing and peer pressures hinder preventive measures.

Non-accidental Injury

War, domestic, and other acts of violence are aggravated by poverty and have a direct health effect. The psychological effects on victims and family members such as children may be more severe than any direct physical injury. Affecting economic progress at national or homestead level may well amplify the immediate consequences of these factors.

Accident and Injury

Road traffic accidents are a huge and rapidly increasing problem in the Third World. The development of roads, good driving habits, law enforcement, and vehicle maintenance are inadequate. Home and work place accidents and falls (off, e.g., trees and buildings) are also an important problem.

Bacteria and Viruses

The continuing emergence of resistant organisms (bacteria, e.g., tuberculosis), new mutant bacteria and viruses, and the uncontrollable Ebola and HIV, cause huge problems. Bacteria are becoming 'cleverer' in using DNA transfer to develop resistance. The increasing sophistication of medicine also tends to disregard simple yet proven measures like washing hands between patients. The globalisation of the use of antibiotic prophylaxis may detract from the strict criteria of elegant surgery. With the increased use of animal products and xenotransplantation, it will be vital to guard also against new zoonoses.

The pharmaceutical industry is a great help in researching new drugs—but, regrettably, it tries to promote reliance on the 'latest wonder' drug. The political will not to release stocks of poliomyelitis and smallpox vaccines has to be nurtured, because if it collapses, there will be global epidemics.

Parasitic Diseases

Malaria (and other third world parasites) remains an enormous problem—the vector and parasite are clever, and the amount of money going into research may be less simply because the populations affected are not in the North. But bold global initiatives aimed at the elimination of filariasis are under way.

Environmental Toxins and Chemical Imbalances

With the increased use of pesticides and other agrochemicals and radiation, the sub-lethal exposure to agents that can damage DNA and cell function is increasing. The main effects, perhaps, remain to be seen, but they may be most evident in young persons showing tumours or infertility or impaired resistance to infection.

Drug Addiction

Drug addiction has both direct health effects and also a less direct one—AIDS and hepatitis B are spread by some methods of drug use. Additionally, the increase in violence associated with financing drugs is a cause of ill health, and the poverty that follows often addictions is the most potent and indirect factor causing ill health for families. The global nature of this terrible scourge is the kernel of the problem, because the client demand is from richer countries as well as poor, and the links between arms cartels, terrorism, money laundering, banking secrecy, and drugs constitute a tangled web which most can barely discern, let alone unravel.

Dumping Wastes and Foods

Problems occur as a result of the careless disposal and dumping of sewage, toxic industrial waste (radioactive and non radioactive), and food unfit for human consumption—Sometimes the problems originate with developing country partners of economic North multinationals. Industrial accidents, as in Bhopal, have a similar genesis. Diseases follow direct consumption of, say, the water from a poisoned river, or an animal drinks and stores the poison, humans eat the animal and fall ill (e.g., as with fish). Regulatory mechanisms either do not exist or are bought out by the money that is to be gained by noncompliance. Double standards abound; for example, after the dangers of aniline dyes and antioxidants (in the rubber industry) were recognised, these industries moved to less developed environments.

Industrial Safety

This is becoming increasingly an issue where the fear is that the developing country subsidary of a developed country's company may take a variety of short cuts as local legislation may not exist or may be easily manipulated. The adverse health consequence of the use of child labour is a variant of this. The adverse health consequences of stopping child labour on apparently "humanitarian" grounds, when the real issue is the fear that a lower price will outbid the richer country product is a sad example of deception.

Mobile Phones and Other Radiation

The mobile phone industry is now huge and global, and possible but as yet unidentified hazards from electromagnetic radiation of various kinds are emerging. Research in the use of mobile telephones may indicate some dangers to the brain. Other forms of radiation, for instance, from certain (older) computer screens, may also be hazardous.

Indirect Effects on Health

As stated, not all causes of ill health are due to direct medical effects. Indirect effects can equally be fundamental.

The Family

In all the major religions there are definitions of what is thought to constitute a stable family. All health indices are badly affected where there is no stable family structure, and particularly where the mother is not available. Family economy first, and then nutrition, education, and health are affected. The resistance to physical disease and to emotional and psychological disease resulting from peer pressure and media pressure are reduced. Value systems break down and violence is more likely.

In addition to joint and nuclear heterosexual families and single-parent families, there exist single-sex, multi-person families in which children are a commodity, for the gratification of various urges and rights of the family. This might be regarded as a form of child abuse. Abuse of a female spouse is also a problem—and there is global devaluation of women, often justified on false cultural grounds.

In all cultures' religions there are definitions of what is thought to constitute a stable family. All health indices are badly affected where there is no stable family, and particularly where the mother is not available. Family economy first, and then nutrition, education, and health are affected. The resistance to physical disease, and to emotional and psychological disease due to peer pressure and media pressure, are reduced. Value systems break down and violence is more likely. Child abuse of every kind becomes more common.

War and Violence

War and violence affect health by infrastructure destruction, displacement of persons, stultifying mental energy, breaking down discipline, retardation of economic development, and increasing poverty.

The dichotomy between the pronouncements of the evils of violence, and the marketing of it by the media, are real. The gun culture in the United States, and poorer countries like Sri Lanka, have had terrorist desertions from armed forces, and young children have grown used to guns. These generate problems that have global dimensions because of the effects of information moving from country to country. The arms industry is huge, rich, and powerful, and can be accused of affecting national policy, encouraging the distortion of intelligence, and promoting war and violence.

Here is where WHO's principle should lead: "Health as a bridge to peace."

The Pharmaceutical and Instrument Industries

The drug and instrumentation industries provide an invaluable service, for instance, biotechnology is of great global benefit. However, multinational companies want monopolies both in their base country and internationally. Openings provided by import liberalization result in the undermining of local industry. Companies with a monopoly can also control pricing and supply, irrespective of the direct or indirect health effects of such policies. These practices produce problems at a global level; however, industry in the developing world is just starting to compete more effectively. The outcome of the debates about retroviral drugs in South Africa and Brazil is a good example of the global arguments and how they can sometimes benefit the poor. But industry may also do harm, for example, by promoting disposable equipment—rather than making good reusable equipment—despite the risk that poor countries reuse what should have been discarded, with all attendant risks, because the alternative is too expensive.

The Environment

Global warming, rainfall and sea level changes, loss of forest and then water supply (which affects farming) are huge issues. Fossil fuel consumption produces greenhouse gases, and even worse, the destruction of forests provides some of the fuel. These are causes of ill health and poverty because they affect sources of income. The loss of forest cover and changes in rainfall and desertification are also alarming as they cause population shifts and displacement—with, again, poverty and disease. Recent difficulties in persuading the richer nations to cut back illustrate the real magnitude of the problem—if the Third World populations were to consume quarter the amount of fossil fuel used by the North, the world would vanish.

The terminator gene of Monsanto in wheat—now fortunately abandoned—could have been a harbinger of a global food war using gene technology. But the threat of a global health situation as a result of a GM or other strategic type substance being released as a military threat remains. There is, so far, no treaty to ban this.

Demographic Transitions

Reductions in mortality both in lower age groups and in the 50-plus group mean that more elderly but fewer economically active people generate the wealth to help the state. There are more nuclear families, also, because families are spreading themselves between town and rural areas. These changes mean greater costs for care. The world also faces the burdens of infectious, degenerative, and so-called lifestyle diseases.

CONCLUSIONS

Recognition of and response to global issues require enormous local, national, and international political will. Constructive action is even more challenging. It is disappointing that as the world advances, the forces of progress may do more harm than good; the 'Might is Right' philosophy undermines what should be a 'Right is Might' view—'Might' being negative political, military, or economic. However, if the concept of health as a positive value is to have an impact, linked to a sustainable and improving situation for all, the macro forces that are outside the control of individuals need articulation.

Therefore, new perspectives are needed:

From governments and international bodies: to bring order and civility to the behaviour of the rich and powerful.

From the health sector: to re-order disease groupings and give a sense of urgency about the double burden of disease. The term neocommunicable should be adopted.

For any sector of a country to function well, health is a prerequisite—and a basic right. It must be recognised that mismanagement and inadequacy in any one segment of society or in national and international structures has wider adverse effects on health.

Finally, a level of vigilance, conscience, and intellectual honesty is needed: to recognise the global and interrelated nature of many forces and the necessary political will to identify and act upon what may be the real 'rate limiting steps' as applied to health improvement.

BIBLIOGRAPHY

Aluwihare, A.P.R. (2003). *New and emerging health threats.* EOLSS Publications, Paris; UNESCO web site www.eolss.net

Coupland, R.M. (1999). The effect of weapons and the Solferino cycle. *British Medical Journal, 319,* 804–805.

Farmer, P. (1999). *Infections and inequalities: The modern plagues* (p. 375). Berkeley: University of California Press.

Garrett, L. (1994). *The coming plague: Newly emerging diseases in a world out of balance* (p. 750). New York: Farrar, Straus and Giroux.

Lederberg, J., Shope, R.E., & Oaks, S.C., (Eds.) (1992). *Emerging infections: Microbial threats to health in the United States* (p. 294). Washington, D.C.: National Academy Press.

Montonen, M. (1996). *Alcohol and the media.* WHO Regional Publications, European Series, No. 62. Copenhagen: WHO Regional Office for Europe.

Priya, R., & Baru, R.V. (1998). Structural adjustments and health. *World Health Forum, 19,* 2.

Editorial. Take a deep breath; stark economics mean hard choices about cigarettes (1999, March 6). *New Scientist 3.*

UNICEF (1997–1999). *Innocenti occasional papers.* Florence: UNICEF International Child Development Center.

Editorial. Violence: Developing a policy agenda (1999). *Journal of Epidemiology and Community Health, 53,* 2–3.

WHO (1998). *Manual on the prevention and control of common cancers,* WHO Regional Publications, Western Pacific Series, No. 20. Geneva: WHO.

WHO (1999). *Mobilizing NGOs and the media behind the International Framework Convention on tobacco control: Experiences from the code on marketing of breast-milk substitutes and conventions on landmines and the environment.* Prepared by INFACT (WHO Technical Briefing Series, WHO/NCD/TFI/99.3, Tobacco Control 3). Geneva: WHO.

WHO. Center for Health Development (Kobe, Japan) (1996). *Urbanization: A global health challenge.* Geneva: WHO.

WHO. Global Advisory Committee on Health Research (1998). *A research policy agenda for science and technology to support global health development.* Geneva: WHO.

Chapter 18

The Coming Storm
Health System Planning Versus
Free Market Enterprise

ANTHONY PIEL

Today, it has become an almost commonplace observation that, in the short space of barely one century—the 20th—the world has witnessed and enjoyed a most extraordinary advance in human health and development, unmatched in thousands of years of previous human history. It is generally assumed that this rate of progress, this acceleration of history, will continue in the 21st century. But will it?

Health Development Progress is a Fact

Our anecdotal sense of extraordinary progress is confirmed by current scientific studies and statistical reports by numerous national authorities as well as international organizations, such as the World Health Organization (WHO), the United Nations (UN, UNDP, UNESCO, and UNICEF), the World Bank, and other public and private institutions. Since World War II, the data show that people are living longer: average life expectancy (as a proxy for overall health status) has nearly doubled. On average, people are better fed, housed, clothed, and educated. New and better medical technologies are available. People suffer from fewer scourge diseases, many of which have been eliminated or controlled. As a result of these successes, the nature and perception of health threats, needs and priorities has shifted.

People Demand a Right to Health

When people in one country, or in one part of a country, or living "on the wrong side of the tracks," see the health, education, and social benefits that others enjoy, they seek those benefits themselves—as a matter of right. They may not expect identical or absolutely equal rights, but they do demand at least an "equitable" right to "equal opportunity" and access. Such "natural" rights have been affirmed by many of the world's leading social philosophers as well as religions. Such basic human rights are enshrined in national and international constitutions, charters, and declarations. Thus, the Constitution of the World Health Organization (signed by some 193 Member States) asserts that: "The enjoyment of the highest attainable standard of health is one of the fundamental rights of every human being." (Note that "highest attainable" standard implies that the right to health is an evolving, moving target.)

Two Critical Questions Now Confront Us

At the outset of the 21st century, we have to ask ourselves, realistically, two questions: (1) Can we keep up the rate of progress in world health development that we have enjoyed in the 20th century, and (2) if so, can we ensure that the benefits will be made equitably available to all? The answers are far from obvious, notwithstanding the fact that most of the cards at hand would seem to be stacked in favor of success. We need to take a closer look at the main factors behind our health development success to date, and then consider the main systemic constraint that may stop us in our tracks: lack of political will.

Economic and social development was, and is, one of the primordial factors in health improvement. Already in the late 19th century, well before the discovery of "germ theory" and "silver bullets" in medicine, the industrial revolution began to bring new means of production, consumer products, a wider range of foods, jobs, income, better housing, education, public water supply, heating, electricity, and new forms of enterprise and means of transportation, on land, sea and air. The industrial revolution also brought new problems—pollution, overcrowding, immigration, exploitation, and other forms of social inequity that had to be overcome. Now, the 21st century brings us a further revolution as well as opportunities in informatics, communications, automation, and new ways of commerce. These, too, bring direct benefits, jobs, income, and opportunity. So, in principle, the potential outlook for accelerated economic and social development is good.

Scientific and technological development was, and is, of critical importance to health improvement. Much of the health development success in the second half of the 20th century was directly attributable to advances in basic medical research leading to new technologies with specific applications for disease prevention, diagnosis, treatment, and cure. We owe our thanks to developers of new drugs, vaccines, pesticides, medical instruments, laboratory equipment, quality controls, and standardized hygienic practices. (A widely recognized milestone earlier on was Alexander Fleming's discovery of penicillin in 1927, although, in fact, this was a rediscovery of penicillin first used circa 1500 B.C., in Egypt, of all places.) Today, with the discovery of DNA, the sequencing of the human genome, and invention of new means of manipulation, we have the unprecedented opportunity to deal with living systems regulation, not just at the whole organ and cell levels, but at the sub-cellular level. We can draw on exciting new techniques of DNA recombination, monoclonal antibodies, stem cell transplantation and gene therapies. Some of these techniques raise serious ethical and societal issues, but they are not insurmountable. The medical benefits are enormous. So, potentially the scientific future looks bright.

Health systems development played a far greater role in 20th century health improvement than is generally realized. It was the framework that made delivery of specific technologies and services possible and accessible to a wider range of the population. But benefits do not just "happen" by themselves. Something as simple as the chlorination of community water supplies requires the cooperative planning of industry, science and technology, local government, and public and private partners. The same is true for the planning of hospitals, clinics, immunization campaigns, sanitation services, agricultural services, education, and environmental protection. This is what real democracy is about: citizens having control over what is important in their own lives, and being able to participate and collaborate in the steps that make these aspirations possible. The ballot box is only one diagnostic indicator or element of democracy. This should be fairly obvious, but there are powerful forces that would deny the full implications of true democracy. By the latter part of the 20th century, with two superpowers holding health development hostage to their overriding political aims, it was clear to those working in the international health field that a major effort was needed to put health development back at the top of the global agenda. The starting point had to be a re-birth of political will.

The "Health for All" movement, launched with passionate advocacy by Dr. Halfdan Mahler, Director-General of WHO, in the 1970s, represented a watershed in global re-commitment, moral clarity. and specificity of means, to rekindle and accelerate world health development by the end of the century. In 1977, the WHO Health Assembly and some 190 Member States resolved that the main social target of governments and WHO in the coming decades should be the attainment by all citizens of the world of "a level of health that would permit them to live a socially and economically productive life." This aspirational global target or goal of "Health for All" (HFA) was above all an *equity* principle, calling for "an acceptable level of health for all." The question then was, and it still remains: Is health for all possible? Is it operationally feasible? How is it to be done? Where to start?

Primary Health Care (PHC) was the proposed answer. In 1978 a major international conference at Alma-Ata, jointly sponsored by WHO and UNICEF, and attended by 134 Member States and some 67 organizations, reaffirmed that health is a fundamental human right, confirmed the global target of "Health for All," and declared that "Primary Health Care is the key to attaining this target." There were and are many variations and attributes of PHC, including difference in emphasis between "comprehensive" and "selective" PHC. It was recognized that every country and community is distinct, and "no one size fits all." In any event, PHC is not a standard package "delivered" to people. PHC is generated by them and for them. PHC is, in short, **democracy in health**, with the accent on **equity**.

A formal generalized definition of PHC was nevertheless adopted at Alma-Ata. It's something of a mouthful, but the words were carefully chosen: "Primary Health Care is essential health care based on practical, scientifically sound and socially acceptable methods and technology made universally accessible to individuals and families in the community through their full participation and at a cost that the community and country can afford to maintain at every stage of their development in the spirit of self-reliance and self-determination. It forms an integral part both of the country's health system, of which it is the central function and main focus, and of the overall social and economic development of the community. It is the first level of contact of individuals, the family and community with the national health system bringing health care as close as possible to where people live and work, and constitutes the first element of a continuing health care process."

Health systems research became a matter of urgent priority, with the aim to adapt principles of PHC to local conditions. WHO and UNICEF provided technical cooperation and support to more than 140 countries in this effort. For example, in one particular country, Thailand, Dr. Mahler decided to "throw the rule book out the window," to facilitate free experimentation and to ensure that WHO's internal processes did not inadvertently impede or wrongly influence cooperation within the country. This kind of effort requires a lengthy and significant investment in open communication with local citizens and interest groups. In Thailand, during the balance of the 1970s and '80s, in several hundred Thai communities, the various partners including government officials, political and business leaders, schools and universities, NGOs, WHO, UNICEF, other institutions, and, above all, thousands of ordinary Thai citizens, worked together to identify basic common needs, to seize opportunities, and to propose actions and solutions, locally and nationally.

Basic Minimum Needs (BMNs), with agreed indicators of identification and key initiating activities, gradually emerged, as a matter of local and eventual national consensus in Thailand. BMNs covered everything from adequate nutrition, safe water, and proper housing, to basic education, medical and social services, as well as security and even spiritual and cultural opportunity and freedom. These needs and intentions were arrived at *openly,* and not behind closed doors. The decisions came from Thai citizens themselves; these were not the kinds of things a

Soviet-style central bureaucracy or a "free" market corporation would be likely to imagine, let alone sponsor. An example of a BMN was the element of water within environmental health: "Every Thai family should have safe drinking water, defined as a minimum of 2 liters per person per day (of rainwater, filtered water, piped water, or pond water)." Once the BMN for water was thus defined, it became the task of community, district and national personnel, to sit down and begin to define the more specific actions, activities, programs, and costs necessary to attain at least this minimum in every household. Although starting at this basic or primary level, the Thai approach addressed the entire secondary and tertiary support network of the national health system. This was real democracy at work. The "proof of the pudding" was in the statistically measurable results: a dramatic increase in health promotion, disease prevention, health care coverage, education access and quality of life, reflected in turn in measurably improved health status indicators. The Thai approach to health systems planning was fundamentally open, democratic and self-reliant. And it worked.

The Red Queen's dilemma in health development became quite rapidly evident in Thailand and in other countries adopting the HFA/PHC/BMN approach. The very success in socioeconomic and health development meant that people lived longer, chronic diseases and new behavioral patterns came to the fore, and population overcrowding, migration, urbanization, and air and water pollution became commonplace. These emerging problems had to be addressed in new and different ways; otherwise much of the past progress would have been lost. Just as Lewis Carroll's "Red Queen" and Alice had to run faster and faster just to stay in place, the scientific, health, and development communities had to work harder and harder just to keep up.

Two Gods compete for one world. For forty-five years between 1945 and 1990, the salient feature of international relations had been the bipolar cold war—the global competition between two superpowers, armed to the teeth, championing their respective economic ideologies: Complete government-owned, centrally planned economy versus "laissez-faire" privately owned economy. WHO and Member States often had to walk a perilous tightrope between the two in matters of health development strategy, water supply, and even family planning. From the costly race for armaments to the race in space, the signs of the "Red Queen's dilemma" were omnipresent. Each superpower was forced to outspend the other, until one economy or the other collapsed. The first "God" that failed was the centrally planned Soviet-style system, for although it had shown early promise and even superiority in delivering certain technological, industrial, and military might, it failed to sense and respond to the basic human rights, needs, and aspirations of individual, ordinary citizens. It lost all sense of democracy. But the disturbing question remained: Might the other "God" fail too?

The rise of de-regulated transnational "free" market corporate capitalism, also known as *globalization,* became the salient outcome of and prize for the winning of the cold war. From 1990 onwards, "free enterprise" believed itself free of the need to counter the alleged social advantages of the Soviet system. Because capitalism had proven its superiority, it was argued, it could be safely deregulated. The underlying logic of "laissez-faire" economics, after all, was that open competition, supply and demand, "free" market pricing, and the profit motive, together made for the best arbiter of overall development and the public good. Those with capital to invest could assume leadership as a matter of right. "He who pays the piper calls the tune." On the face of it, this form of capitalism should indeed offer distinct advantages. It would seem that access to large amounts of capital and loans, and the stimulation of free competition, should lead to strengthened infrastructure, greater and more efficient industrial production, expanded markets, more jobs, more income, more revenue, and, therefore, more funding for science, education, health care, and social services. But how does deregulation work out in practice? Surely the best place to look is in the US, the home of deregulated capitalism. But here we are in for a shock. The US, with the largest GNP in the world, has the least affordable and most inequitable health system among all so-called developed or industrialized countries in the world. Why is this so? Within the US and abroad, we have to ask ourselves, why is the ideology of the deregulated free market system so often out of sync with the actual, observed facts? In science, when a theory doesn't match the evidence, the theory fails.

The burden is on the apologists for deregulation to explain why it is that in the US, over the last four years 2000–2004, several hundred major US corporations have been caught out, and have had to restate their earnings (a euphemism for papering over fraudulent accounting and financial disclosure practices)? Why is it that so many major corporations today are scurrying to destroy corporate records and prepare legal defenses to cover the illicit actions of high-ranking corporate executives who have: (a) stolen from their own companies, (b) paid themselves unconscionable remuneration, (c) misinformed and cheated their own stockholders, (d) misled the public and government officials, (e) evaded taxes, (f) gouged consumers, (g) undercut employee benefits, including pension funds and medical plans, (h) put people out of work, (i) sent jobs abroad, (j) created trade imbalances, and (k) generally did their best, out of pure self-interest, to damage the national and international economy for generations to come? The answer is simple: Capitalism is driven by self-interest. Therefore, if it isn't regulated, these are the things that happen. It comes with the territory. The problem is structural; it's part of the system. With rotten apples like this, do we really want to export the barrel?

Deregulation and privatization are being exported. Deregulated free market ideology, under the banner of globalization is actively promoted by transnational corporations as well as by international organizations, such as the International Monetary Fund (IMF), the World Bank, and the World Trade Organization

(WTO)—bodies that represent certain corporate business interests, not science, health, education, or the environment. Characteristically, decisions of vital public interest are taken by the IMF, World Bank, and WTO, with select interest groups *behind closed doors*. (This is the dead opposite of Thailand's democratic approach to PHC/BMN planning described earlier.) The World Bank's idea of development planning all too often is to decide on and dictate conditions to developing countries, especially when it comes to fee-for-service financing and privatization of countries' resources and services. The Bank's solution to most problems in diverse countries is that "one size fits all." The WTO operates on the premise that health standards are acceptable if they don't constrain trade. (This reverses the priorities of the original GATT rounds, which authorized trade decisions provided they didn't adversely affect health.) The actual participants within the WTO are businessmen, lawyers, economists, and their lobbyists. There are no participants who represent health, science, education, or the environment, even though many WTO trade decisions invade these other fields. When in the past the WTO has discussed issues ranging from dolphin-safe fishing nets to breast milk substitutes, parties representing other such interests have generally not been consulted, and are not allowed in the meeting rooms, even on request, until trade decisions have been essentially taken and are ready to be announced. An exception to this dire assessment is the fruitful collaboration between WHO, FAO, and WTO on the Codex Alimentarius dealing with food additives, and more widely and importantly on food safety. My own take on this success is that credit is due to the perseverance and professionalism of WHO and FAO programme staff. Early in the 1990s, WHO Director-General Hiroshi Nakajima drew a connection between IMF policies and cholera outbreaks in South America, because countries were not permitted to upgrade their urban water supplies until foreign bankers were paid off. The response of the IMF and World Bank was to cry foul, but Nakajima was proven right. All too often, the IMF, World Bank, and WTO have done a disservice to the world by helping to export biased ideology to other countries, and imposing solutions that don't necessarily fit local and national conditions.

Structural adjustment policies have largely failed. In all too many instances, and in all too many developing countries, IMF/World Bank "structure adjustment policies" (more recently relabeled "poverty alleviation"), as well as so-called free trade agreements, have had disastrous impacts on the countries they were supposed to help. The IMF and World Bank policies and actions in all too many cases have encouraged countries to build up extraordinary levels of debt for future generations to pay off. The resources often go to "white elephant" projects that cannot be maintained, and that put people out of jobs. The IMF and World Bank have promoted privatizing, that is to say outright taking, people's land, water, air quality, public schools, health facilities, food sources, agriculture, and oil and mineral resources, and wrecking small farms and businesses. Sometimes people just don't take this lying down. For example, recently thousands of citizens in one South American country literally had to march in the streets to force their government to buy back public water supply systems that had been taken over by foreign, transnational investors, thanks to a World Bank leveraged buyout. Does this sound like democracy? I think not. Real health planners, scientists, and informed citizens can do a better job, with the support and cooperation of a committed public and private sector. Self-interest and imposition of solutions are not going to solve the world's ills. Democratic decision-making will.

Free trade agreements are not what they seem. Ostensibly, free trade agreements are about trade. Indeed, the large print, as well as public declarations, give the impression that free trade agreements are all about lowering barriers to trade, and reducing or eliminating tariffs. But there's a Trojan horse that comes with every free trade agreement: The small print usually requires the "benefiting" country to abolish all constitutional, legal, and other barriers to transnational purchase and privatization. This means, for example, elimination of restrictions on the takeover and privatization of public hospitals and services. These are viewed as mere commodities. Free trade, in effect, condones and encourages the transnational buyout of public water supplies. The justifying theory is that that ownership of water is not a people's essential right, but merely an essential need. (WHO and the UN have long argued quite the reverse.) Health care and water share a common attribute, which makes them vulnerable. They both come in short supply. Therefore, from the investor's perspective, both health and water are inherently susceptible to monopoly. When big fish swallow little fish, monopoly is the end result. The ultimate objective is not really robust competition or fair trade. It's monopoly. That's what yields the most opportunity for maximum profit, and highest return on investment. It is said that "might makes right," but what about the citizens? Ultimately, who owns water? Whose health are we talking about? Should anyone be allowed to trade away people's rights to water and their right to health?

DOES THE THEORY OF "FREE" MARKET COMPETITION FIT REALITY IN HEALTH?

According to free market theory, consumers (in this case, patients) are free to shop the market to find the best product at lowest price. This approach works for car sales. But how realistic is free competition in health? In practice, most patients in need of treatment have nowhere to go except to their local physician, their local health care center, or their local hospital. It isn't as though there were a range of entities to choose from. With few exceptions, the patient can't price bargain with the provider. The patient has to pay the going rate, or forgo treatment. Furthermore, the scarcity of supply and the excess of demand for health care in most communities automatically generates the sort of monopoly conditions under which prices have only one way to go: up! No wonder investors want to buy up and privatize hospitals, clinics, and health maintenance organizations. They see this as a golden opportunity to corner the market. Conclusion: When it comes to provision of comprehensive health care, the theory of free market competition doesn't fit.

Privatization of hospitals is the new golden opportunity. The private purchase of hospitals is not only urged on developing countries by the World Bank, certain aid agencies and banking institutions, it is often a conditionality of grants and loans. In the homeland of this ideology—the US—it is all the rage. Typically, a big-hearted, well-heeled investor offers to buy up a struggling public hospital for, say, $20 million. Then he puts in another $10 million to upgrade facilities and better market hospital service products to customers in the market area. Thus the total investment in health reaches $30 million. Such a large sum may come as a Godsend to the hospital board or to a cash-strapped municipality. Why not let someone else take on the responsibility, and put in new investment capital too? But there's a hitch: The investor wants a return on investment of 10–15% per annum; otherwise he would have invested elsewhere, in petroleum, for instance. This means an effective drain on the hospital of some $ 3 to 4.5 million each year—an exorbitant amount that can only come out of the pockets of the patients. This is $3–4.5 million that cannot be put back in the hospital to improve services. So what has happened? Patients' suffering and patients' money have made the middleman rich. But hospital finances are not that easy to turn around, and most hospitals cannot afford to ante up the kind of return the investor wants. So then what?

What happens throughout the US, in case after case, is that after a few years of deteriorating hospital performance, the original investor sells out to a higher level of investor or holding corporation, for an augmented price of say $40–50 million, thus recouping his initial investment with a healthy capital gain on the transaction. The basic financial problem of the hospital, however, is not solved; it is merely driven upstream in the pyramid of ownership. The new owner fares no better, so typically he downsizes the hospital, cuts staff, especially nurses, eliminates low-return services for poor people, and changes the purposes of the facility. One day the local citizens, who have been kept in the dark throughout, wake up to find that they no longer have the hospital services (such as obstetrics) they thought they had, and they cannot afford to buy the hospital back. The owner may have taken tax loss deductions and disappeared into something more remunerative, such as real estate development. More than this, in the US today, there is a virtual epidemic of hospital fraud, in the billions of dollars, much of it directed against Medicare. Many hospitals actually keep a double set of inconsistent financial records, one for the public and government agencies to see, the other for the confidential use of investment insiders only. Is this exceptional? No, it seems endemic. It doesn't tend to happen so frequently in public and charitable hospitals, where the main motivation is the health of the patient; but it does tend to happen in privately owned hospitals where the principal executive-level motivation is profit.

For profit health maintenance organizations may be counterproductive. They tend to work against the patient's interest. The original idea in the US, starting with the Kaiser plan during World War II, was that by grouping employees or other identifiable clusters in a not-for-profit association, it should be possible to emphasize prevention, promote health, lower costs, and keep people healthier. With the era of deregulation in the US, however, most Health Maintenance Organisations (HMOs) have been taken over by middleman investors and converted to for-profit status. These HMOs now act not merely to ration health care; they often work to actually deny essential services to patients, because the dominant motivation is profit for the middleman investor. Unfortunately, conflict of interest appears to be inherent in the for-profit HMO approach to health care. Furthermore, for-profit HMOs have engaged in fraud and even embezzlement of hundreds of millions of dollars in the US each year, paid for by Medicare and patients. Again, this is not something that's exceptional. It's pandemic.

Prescription drug benefits have become a political football in the US. There is a curious anomaly in the current conflict. According to free market competition theory, drug prices should trend lower if markets are open. In practice, it is quite the opposite. The pharmaceutical industry in the US has made sure that there is no regulatory cap on drug prices in the US, arguing that a high profit margin is necessary to pay for research (and, we might add, advertising). As a result, the price for a typical drug in the US costs anywhere from 50% to 300% more than the very same drug manufactured in the US but purchased via neighboring Canada. Consequently, American citizens flock across the Canadian border daily to obtain medicines at fair prices. Pressured by the pharmaceutical industry, the US federal drug regulators try to outlaw this practice on the implausible and unproven grounds that drugs sold in Canada are unsafe. The latest idea in the US is to provide more affordable drugs to groups of people through purchasing associations, but if these are privatized, they will likely go the way of the for-profit HMOs.

Which way health insurance: Public or private? The US is almost alone among developed nations in denying national health insurance for all. Even Medicare, for older citizens, is at risk of partial privatization. In the US, whenever the concept of national health insurance is mentioned, a chorus of conservative voices and the well-heeled private insurance industry shout it down. Germany is criticized as a socialist state, notwithstanding that its system has worked quite well since the time of Otto von Bismarck, circa 1870. How well is health insurance doing as a component of the health care system in the US? In 2002, the independent US Academy of Science released a report declaring that the American health care system is incapable of meeting the present, let alone future, needs of the American people. The study noted that the cost of private health insurance is increasing at a rate in excess of 12% per annum.

Individuals are paying more out of pocket and receiving fewer benefits. The number of totally uninsured Americans is on the rise, and is approaching 50 million persons. For many of those who do have private health insurance, the premiums, co-pays, deductibles and outright exclusions are so high as to constitute essentially no worthwhile health insurance at all. Do these experiences in the US make a convincing argument why developing countries should prefer to adopt private health insurance in preference to public health insurance?

Should profit drive the health system of the future? Some would seem to think so. For example, the self-described "Health Care Advisory Board" of the Advisory Board Company of Washington, D.C., has put out in 2002 a report entitled "Health System of the Future." (See http://advisory.com.) The report contains a very sophisticated, polished analysis of future trends in medical technologies and facilities to deliver more advanced health care in the coming years. It represents a form of "supply side" economics. However, underlying all this is the assumption that in the optimal health system of the future, the decision whether to offer a specific health service or medical intervention will be based on its relative potential of a profit margin, as determined by free market forces, in competition with other services or interventions. Thus, profit motive will drive the decision more than relevance to the needs of citizens, especially poor persons. This will mean, and it is surely already the case in the US, that far more attention, resources, and manpower will begin to flow into higher-yielding surgical interventions, such as cosmetic surgery and "extreme makeovers." Wealthier individuals, including celebrity personalities, will be the dominant consumer group because they can pay more. The more mundane surgical and clinical interventions that serve real health needs will take a back seat because the profit margin is smaller, and ordinary persons pay less. Whether this should be the future of the health system in the US is one question. But whether it should be exported to developing countries is quite another.

Capitalism and terrorism make strange bedfellows. The triumph of deregulated, transnational corporate capitalism in the 21st century is an established fact, and it is spreading. At the same time, international terrorism is on the rise. In the US, it is politically incorrect to link the two. Basically, terrorism is a criminal reaction by the powerless to perceived irresponsible behavior and abuse of power by those who wield such power. A century ago, it was the perceived abuse of advantage by the robber barons that gave rise to extreme versions of communism, fascism, and anarchism—the terrorism of that day. Today, international terrorism is not about jealousy of failed cultures wishing to have our wealth, our freedom, or our pop culture. It is not about us being good and them being evil. It is about perceived historical, as well as recent, abuse of political, economic, and military power. It is about the exploitation of other people, their democracy, freedom, human rights, and welfare. When we fail to address people's needs, rights, and concerns, we invite crazed, desperate, but committed individuals to take up arms and commit unforgivable criminal acts of terrorism against an innocent public. International terrorism and the war against it are consuming billions of dollars that could have gone into health and social development. Human rights, freedoms and privacy are being violated in the name of security. Even the practice of scientific research and the publication of research results in sensitive areas are being curtailed. If terrorism can de-democratize society, then terrorism wins.

The export culture of violence is a phenomenon related to this social instability and terrorism. Already we witness the cultural impact of deregulated corporate globalization: displacement of local and individual self-reliance and self-determination, provoking and compounding insecurity, unsocial behavior, and violence, practically everywhere in the world. In the US today, there is a virtual corporate conspiracy of supply-side consumerism and dumbing down the citizenry through deliberate disinformation and a manufactured fascination with violence as entertainment, and as an expression of reality. This is the new imperial "Bread and Circus," designed to keep the populace apathetic, doped, obese, malleable—and violent. This culture of violence has become yet another export commodity—dehumanizing, insinuating, and destructive. When more traditional, moral cultures in other countries resist this trend, they are described as backward and as enemies of freedom and free speech. Many countries that really do face longstanding problems of insecurity, and that really do seek freedom from fear and want, are faced with a juggernaut of corporate, commercial, and political pressures and influences that can only lead to further insecurity, social unrest, and violence. Thus, deregulated capitalism is giving birth to its own Frankenstein monster, a culture of violence that will return to plague us all.

The storm is coming—can it be averted? The de-regulated free market, private enterprise, and transnational corporate system, under the banner of globalization, are on a collision course with socially responsible planning, and even with democracy itself. If the trend goes unchecked, the price could be very high for all mankind. The second "God," that of capitalism, could also fail, and for much the same reasons as the first: failure to sense and respond to ordinary citizens' rights, needs, and aspirations. What we see today as sporadic acts of protest against the WTO, IMF, and World Bank, for example, could be harbingers of things to come. When terrorists strike, we are horrified. We can target them for well-deserved retribution. But when people take to the streets en masse to retake their public water supplies, their health systems, and their democratic rights, then the handwriting is on the wall. Such protests could rapidly evolve into a generalized, unstoppable worldwide revolution. Can this storm be averted? One way is for corporate capitalism to regulate itself, but that is unlikely. A better way is for government to impose strict but fair controls on free market capitalism. In the 1930s, this was the real purpose of Franklin Roosevelt's New Deal. It was: "To save capitalism from itself." It worked. The leaders and ordinary citizens of other countries must dig in their heels to resist the juggernaut of free market transnational capitalism, and refuse the imposition of a foreign ideology that has yet to truly prove itself even in the homeland from whence it comes. The doctrine of pure self-interest is not the answer.

We must return to an older ethic, one blessed by leading philosophers and by virtually all the great religions: *"Non Sibi sed Cunctis"*—*"Not for oneself alone, but for others."*

BIBLIOGRAPHY

United Nations Charter (1945) and Universal Declaration of Human Rights (1945), re-printed 2003 by the United Nations Department of Public Information, New York, N.Y.

Constitution of the World Health Organization (1946) reprinted in Basic Documents of the World Health Organization, 2004, Geneva, Switzerland.

Declaration of Alma-Ata and Report of the International Conference on Primary Health Care, Alma-Ata, (held September 1978), published in 1978 by the World Health Organization, Geneva, Switzerland, jointly with the United Nations Children's Fund, New York, N.Y.

"National Basic Minimum Needs With Indicators," published in 1987 by the Ministry of Public Health, Bangkok, Thailand.

"From Alma-Ata to the Year 2000–Reflections at the Midpoint," report of international meeting at Riga (held May 1988), published in 1988 by the World Health Organization, Geneva, Switzerland

Ninth General Programme of Work Covering the Period 1996–2001, published in 1994 by the World Health Organization, Geneva, Switzerland.

A Research Policy Agenda for Science and Technology to Support Global Health Development–A Synopsis, published in 1997 by the World Health Organization, Geneva, Switzerland.

The World Health Report 2003–Shaping the Future, published in 2003 by the World Health Organization, Geneva, Switzerland.

"Health for All or Hell for All? The Role of Leadership in Health Equity," an address by Dr. Halfdan Mahler, Director-General Emeritus of the World Health Organization, in December 2003 and printed in the Journal of Humanitarian Medicine, Vol. III, No.4.

Chapter 19

Education, Understanding, and *Eudaemonia*
A Contrarian View on Global Health

GERHARD W. BRAUER

PROLEGOMENA

Helen Keller, a person who coped with the world while being unable either to see or hear,[1] made a profound contribution to our understanding of human capability. In her writing Keller frequently referred to various human attributes that, in her estimation, made human life good and worthwhile:

> "**Character** cannot be developed in ease and quiet. Only through experience of trial and suffering can the soul be strengthened, ambition inspired, and success achieved."

> "The most pathetic person in the world is someone who has sight but has no **vision**."

> "**Toleration** is the greatest gift of mind, it requires the same effort of the brain that it takes to balance oneself on a bicycle."

> "Science may have found a cure for most evils; but it has found no remedy for the worst of them all—the **apathy** of human beings."
>
> *Helen Keller (1880–1968).*

With the help of her teacher, Anne Sullivan, Keller overcame her handicaps to such an extent that she not only manifested the attributes mentioned in the

---

[1] Conditions that were incurred after a bout of meningitis before she was two years old.

quotations, she also achieved a degree of insight into the human condition far greater than most, less 'handicapped,' individuals. And, although these attributes are not considered to be health-related, even just two of these, intolerance and apathy, seem to be more closely and more directly associated with the burden of human suffering, degradation, and death than most conditions covered under traditional definitions of disease. Is there not something patently healthy about a human being who, like Keller's ideal, has character, vision, and tolerance, and rejects apathy? I cannot help but feel that a great tragedy is playing out on the world stage, the ironic theme of which is that the most important contributors to, and indicators of, health are ignored by extant health systems. Such neglect is due to the fact that their investigation would require serious moral and intellectual re-thinking of policy in the highest places of power in health and education.

Of course, the four traits alluded to by Keller are not the only, or even the most important, indicators of a more inclusive interpretation of health. Such a list would also have to include such qualities as compassion, courage, curiosity, diligence, generosity, gentleness, honesty, humility, imagination, intelligence, objectivity, patience, responsibility, thoughtfulness, tolerance, vision, and so on. If, in addition to these indicators of spiritual and emotional health, someone were *also* to possess physical health, this would, of course, be considered ideal. On the other hand, the presence of physical health alone, to the exclusion of any of the above traits, describes a person who lacks the essence of what we value in humanity.

Eudaemonia and *Eudaemonic* Health

It is regrettable that traditional approaches often fail to recognize adequately the importance of the human spirit or character as it pertains to health[2]. Although in an earlier paper[3] I referred to informational health, an aspect of a person's health that was related to the ability to acquire and manage information, I now eschew the terminology, considering informational health to be subsumed in a much broader conceptualization that I refer to as *eudaemonic* health. The term, which comes closer than any other to the dimension of health I wish to consider, is rooted in *eudaemonia*, a word the ancient Greeks used to signify 'a good and worthwhile life,' (Coulter and Wiens, 2002), or 'spiritual wellbeing.'[4]

---

[2] I refrain from referring to spiritual health – the use of that term has too many metaphysical connotations to be useful in this context. Having said that, it is my opinion that spirituality is the *most* important aspect of human being. But that is a personal view, and has no place in any argument, least of all one such as this.

[3] Invited keynote address to the 12th International Symposium "Computer Science for Environmental Protection" of the German Society for Informatics (GI), held in Bremen, Germany, September 15–18, 1997.

[4] http://www.wordiq.com/definition/Eudaimonia. Oxford English Dictionary mentions eudaemon or eudemon.

Eudaemonic health as an individual's state of being can be thought of as having three requirements: a) the *desire to reflect deeply* on the philosophical, the intellectual, the emotional, the sexual, the societal, and/or the political aspects of the human condition, b) the intellectual *ability* to do so, within whatever mental and physical limitations with which one is burdened, and c) the *determination to act in public*[5] according to the judgements one has made, having thusly reflected. The two phrases *deep reflection* and *action in public*, Hannah Arendt (1978) expands into *thinking*, *willing*, and *judging*. These three activities are considered by Arendt to relate directly to the human condition, which must be considered to include the health of the person, family, and community.

In order to be useful, a definition of eudaemonic health is, perforce, value-laden. In the area of global health policy, for instance, it values such characteristics as moral courage and socio-emotional maturity over physical well-being, political expediency or economic efficiency. To realize the benefits of such a shift in values will require a major shift, both philosophical and societally, in the organization of knowledge and the prioritization of expenditures. It will be very difficult, but I do not think we can afford to wait much longer before we at least try to make such changes. Recognition of eudaimonial health as critical to the human condition might be a good place to start.

Acknowledging the existence of a condition of eudaemonic health will help us recognize the importance of the philosophical, the intellectual, the emotional, the sexual, the societal[6], and the political dimensions of human health. These dimensions differ radically from physical health in that they involve intangibles: various combinations of data, information, knowledge, and understanding, and so forth. These intangible influences all are central to and underlie my argument. For the sake of simplicity, however, I will, henceforth, use the word *understanding* (in italics) to stand for the entirety of this gradient[7]. Based on this use of *understanding*, as it pertains to eudaemonic health, the question "How does *understanding* relate to health and 'a good and worthwhile life'?" becomes valid and relevant.

The Impact of Eudaemonic Disease

While the presence of eudaemonic health is illustrated by many positive moral and emotional characteristics, the presence of eudaemonic disease is revealed in serious psycho-cultural ailments, cardinal among which are such conditions as

---

[5] For an extended discussion of this idea, the reader is referred to Hannah Arendt's *The Human Condition*.

[6] Distinct from 'social,' the term 'societal' refers to the sum of human conditions and not merely to one society as a particular grouping.

[7] Data < information < knowledge < understanding < wisdom (where '<' signifies 'is less valuable than').

ambition,[8] apathy, bigotry, greed,[8] gullibility, ignorance, intolerance, moral cowardice, prejudice, pride, stupidity, and superstition. I leave it to the reader to reflect on the impact of eudaemonic disease when it is found in simple human beings, let alone when it defines the condition of those 'players' whose actions affect global events.

What interventions exist to help those with eudaemonic disease? When someone, in the developed world at least, suffers from lack of vitamins or from food poisoning, there is immediate recourse to the appropriate remedial steps[9]. If, on the other hand, an individual is suffering from a lack of understanding of, or from an inability to cope with, the world around him or her, that is, from *eudaimonial* disease, nothing is currently done. Of course, using the traditional approach to health, there is not much that *can* be done. While the problems occasioned by the failings listed above can be devastating, they are never identified as health problems. Billions have suffered and untold millions have died due to ignorance, prejudice, bigotry, and other sources of a deficiency in understanding, yet no one thinks of it as a health issue.

Eudaemonic diseases have contributed (and continue to contribute) vastly more to human misery than any medical conditions of microbial, biochemical, or degenerative origin. Mental and physical suffering, and death, when due to such factors as apathy, prejudice, greed, or a lack of thoughtfulness, are easily overlooked *as health issues* if the definition of health doesn't explicitly refer to them. Analysis of these psycho-cultural pathologies reveals that they can only be eliminated, or ameliorated, with increased knowledge, understanding, and willingness to change. More specifically, they are easily reframed in terms of deficiencies in timely, correct, and well-understood information and knowledge, and a lack of understanding of same, should it be available.

With regard to physical health, a wide range of conditions is related to the quantity and quality of nutrients consumed; it may be feasible to discuss eudaimonial disease in terms of a similar, nutritional, model. For example, in physical and eudaimonial health, the ability to identify and avoid the consumption of toxic input is of critical importance. A viable public health initiative would, in my opinion, focus on improving the public's ability to acquire, understand, and act upon information *as a nutrient*. Such abilities are the *sine qua non* of 'a good and worthwhile life' and hence of a healthy civil society, and their nurturance should be the highest responsibility of a society towards its citizens.

---

[8] The reader is referred to the writings of Max Weber and Hernando de Soto for competing ideas on ambition and greed as they relate to religion and the origin of capitalistic (acquisitive) thinking.

[9] Unless, of course, the individual is unfortunate enough to be homeless, poor, unemployed, or similarly 'untouchable.'

If we accept this reasoning, then the collective state of eudaemonic health of a population is a crucial, perhaps even defining, aspect of overall health, and relates to that aspect of the human condition that is determined by the ability to find timely and valid information, understand it, and then act in accordance with that understanding. The challenge must be to aid the respective authorities, systems, agencies, and institutions to come to understand that the biggest threat to civil society is not physical disease but eudaemonic disease—and that this threat lies not primarily in the Third or developing world but first and foremost in the highly developed nations on this globe—that is, in those nations in which the economy is well able to address any of the relevant shortcomings.

Eudaemonic health and disease could usefully be seen as the cornerstone of the public's health and education, and a critical component of the presence or absence of a general well-being. I believe that this very specific aspect of the human condition is all too often being neglected by a) the short-sighted yet ubiquitous over-emphasis on the somatic definitions of health and disease, both mental and physical, and b) the systematic crippling, by well-meaning but often ineffective institutions, of efforts to provide education based on improving our understanding of the human condition.

A thorough investigation is needed of a) what level of understanding people need, if they are to be effective citizens? and b) what intellectual skills are necessary to be able to seek out, acquire, evaluate, consume and act upon, this understanding? But that hasn't happened—the basic questions are rarely asked even in those fora where they most belong: the lecture halls and seminar rooms of higher education. It might even be suspected that there are powerful global players who are disinclined to promote high-level understanding as the key objective of the curricula available to the average citizen—it would not serve their control-oriented interests. For this reason, the establishment of a research area or discipline dealing with the topic of 'eudaemonic health and human rights' is timely—although I suspect that it will not be met with a uniformly positive response.

Topics involving health have the proclivity of evoking in people the limited idea of a fight against death, disease, disability, and discomfort. The World Health Organization (WHO) sought to ameliorate this with its constitutional (1948) definition of health as "a state of complete physical, mental, and social well-being and not merely the absence of disease or infirmity." This attempt to go beyond basic physical parameters of health does not, however, in practice, lend itself to implementation; nor, due to what it excludes, does it go far enough. I have already implied that it does not accommodate the very conspicuous and dangerous psycho-cultural ailments such as apathy, bigotry, fear, greed, gullibility, ignorance, intolerance, prejudice, stupidity, and superstition.

I suggested that such 'diseases' have in the past contributed (and continue to contribute) vastly more to human agony than any medical condition of microbial, biochemical, nutritional, neoplastic or degenerative origin. By this I mean to say that *eudaimonial* health problems such as current wars and violence were induced and are sustained by apathy, prejudice, or thoughtlessness; but they are easily overlooked *as being health related* if the definition of health doesn't explicitly include them.

The success of present-day approaches to advertising reveals a more latent eudaemonic ill health. One of the key aspects of any programme to increase the eudaemonic health of citizens will therefore be a raising of the public's awareness regarding such concepts as market creation, branding, market analysis, psycho-demographics, and opinion-shaping. Campaigns to acquaint students and the public with marketing theory and how this can be counteracted by such tactics as *adbusting*[10], would help consumers recognize that advertising, as practised today, often consists of false and foolish claims.

The situation with regard to advertising will have improved when consumers begin to use their collective power; in other words, when they recognize the impotence of the producers and their commercials in the face of discriminating purchasers *acting in concert*. The impact on the whole climate of marketing could be massive if, for instance, a critical mass of consumers, acting as a virtual community, were to resist branding and other non-critical aspects of advertising. What if consumers began purchasing only those products that are *not* falsely presented in the mass media, but that the manufacturer has submitted for objective comparative testing, and for which exhaustive descriptive material is made available on request? Having thus far depended entirely on the gullibility of the media-influenced consumer, manufacturers and advertisers would have to switch tactics dramatically.

What I believe is needed is the incorporation of the relevant critical skills of citizenship, "thinking, willing and judging,"[11] in the education of young people the world over. Only by doing this can we expect to see a generalized increase in awareness and understanding of global problems. There is no denying that much of the suffering of children in the poorest nations is being inflicted by thoughtless actions (consumption, tourism, wastage, pollution, etc.) on the part of affluent people in developed regions. Hope for the future will receive a big push as soon as an understanding of this fact begins to weigh heavily on the minds of citizens in the developed world, starting perhaps with young people. That is the group within which the requisite changes have to take a foothold, and a high level of *understanding* could be the relevant indicator of such a societal maturity.

Here it is important to make a critical observation: this is *not a plaidoyer*[12] for including, under the rubric of health, such factors as human rights and freedoms,

---

[10] Adbusters is an excellent Vancouver-based periodical in Canada dedicated to giving its readers insight into manipulative marketing practices.

[11] Hannah Arendt considers these to be key aspects of "the life of the mind."

[12] An appeal.

adequate employment, and humane living conditions. That such a broadening of mandate is indeed slowly happening is exemplified by the World Health Organization, which, as mentioned earlier, now includes 'social well-being' in its definition of health. No, what I am arguing for is the recognition that real, that is, eudaemonic, health is impossible without understanding the world in which we live; it is not a matter merely of implementing certain laws, policies, or regulations—none of which can work without an improved understanding on the part of those on whom the policies are ultimately imposed.

Sometimes one gets the feeling that there is an unspoken agreement that emotion and sentiment have no place in academic research or in corporate or political policymaking. It's nearly as if we must not allow sentiment to interfere with understanding or economic development; nor must we let education confuse the issues by revealing too much of reality. This sounds bad, but is it far from the truth? The Roman historian, Gaius Cornelius Tacitus, wrote a sharp indictment[13] (of a similar situation involving the maintenance of the Roman Empire) that I take the liberty of paraphrasing to suit *my* argument concerning the imposition and maintenance of 'free-market' imperialism:

> They pillage, plunder, and rape the earth, falsely calling it development;
> they sow ignorance, and call it education. [*pace* Tacitus]

The Barriers to Eudaemonic Health

I believe that little progress towards an improved global health picture will be made unless and until privileged leaders in education and health are willing to speak up loudly about issues of eudaimonial health such as are raised herein. But this will not be sufficient for change—even if there were the will to speak up. The commencement of an academic and public debate on eudaemonic health will not occur easily, as there exist significant barriers to critical consideration of eudaemonic health. Most prominent among these barriers is a profound degree of ignorance of, and disinterest in, history and philosophy, even among academics. Kieran Egan provides a brilliant discussion of this in his *Getting it wrong from the beginning: our progressivist inheritance from Herbert Spencer, John Dewey, and Jean Piaget*, (Egan, 2002), where, among other things, he states that:

> Today, of course, the educational establishment—almost entirely without any knowledge of what once was the backbone or staple of education and almost invariably ignorant of classical languages—takes it for granted that the classics

---

[13] Original Latin quote: *Auferre trucidare rapere falsis nominibus imperium, atque ubi solitudinem faciunt, pacem appellant.* [They plunder, pillage, and rape, falsely calling it empire; they sow desolation, and call it peace.]

should be treated as an occasional and exotic option for only a few students. (pp. 120–121)

In spite of the efforts of many dedicated and conscientious teachers, modern trends in public education have led to curricula in recent decades being most sensitive to the needs of commercial and bureaucratic interests, and rather insensitive to the needs of a civil society. This has resulted in the essential destruction, carefully described by Egan, of what used to constitute a liberal education:

> The common view of educationalists today is that this shift away from the classics marks a triumph of common sense, a democratization of education, and a recognition that schooling is properly both a preparation for the everyday life all classes of students will lead in adulthood and an expansion of their experience in the present. The less common view, held often by those with a classical education, such as Housman or, say, Michael Oakeshott, is that this shift has caused an educational catastrophe by cutting off modern generations from the great conversation of the Western tradition. The product of this move, they believe, is the condition of modern schooling in which few become educated and many become socialized—the "You've been cheated!" response. (ibid.)

The price of this break with the classics, and the concomitant loss of attention to the values mentioned above, is steep: Today, the vast majority of middle class citizens in the industrialized world, in spite of being well off financially, are self-centred, ignorant of history and philosophy, and preoccupied solely with getting good jobs and securing a comfortable retirement. Such ambivalence toward eudaemonia threatens to ring the death knell for the well-being of many future generations.

Societally, health ought to imply a preoccupation with such fundamental concepts as justice and freedom, human rights and responsibilities, honesty and truth, equity and equality, and so on, and these issues must rank highest, if the achievement of physical health is to be worth anything—that is, if 'health' is to reflect a meaningful dimension of the human condition. But, as an anthropologist and observer of the human condition, I have come to the conclusion that children, young people, and adults, around the world, are systemically being denied ready access to opportunities for achieving a sound education, and thereby cannot achieve a level of eudaimonial health conducive to the establishment and perpetuation of healthy and humane communities.

Understanding as the Key to Eudaemonic Health

It must be reiterated that this very special dimension of health depends upon *understanding*. Without going into great theoretical details as to the nature of human understanding, it is necessary to point out that the object of this complex process is, inevitably the provision of *information* in one form or another. One's state of eudaemonic health is therefore, at least to some extent, determined by the quality and amount of information one is able *to understand and act upon.*

Care must be taken to resist the notion that 'all information is simply that, information.' Much of the 'information' available via computer technology is unreliable, false, toxic or otherwise hazardous. In an excellent paper entitled "Informing Ourselves to Death," the late Neil Postman, a highly esteemed teacher and a critic of culture and technology, makes an impassioned plea to go beyond simply wanting more information in our search for solutions to societal problems:

> The message is that through more and more information, more conveniently packaged, more swiftly delivered, we will find solutions to our problems. And so all the brilliant young men and women, believing this, create ingenious things for the computer to do, hoping that in this way, we will become wiser and more decent and more noble. And who can blame them? By becoming masters of this wondrous technology, they will acquire prestige and power and some will even become famous. In a world populated by people who believe that through more and more information, paradise is attainable, the computer scientist is king. But I maintain that all of this is a monumental and dangerous waste of human talent and energy. Imagine what might be accomplished if this talent and energy were turned to philosophy, to theology, to the arts, to imaginative literature or to education? Who knows what we could learn from such people—perhaps why there are wars, and hunger, and homelessness and mental illness and anger. (Postman, 1996a)

Postman makes a very compelling argument for the need to value things *other than* information in our efforts to improve the human condition. He is, of course, quite right in this—*yet he is also quite wrong.* What Postman is saying is that *electronic* access to information will not enhance the human condition. Unfortunately, he neglects to discriminate between information as computer-based binary data streams, and information as that without which no living organism can live, let alone thrive. Given his audience, it is understandable that Postman chose to concentrate on the former, more limited, definition of information, when he states, quite correctly, that we are "informing ourselves to death." But information is absolutely necessary for health and life: it is needed to discriminate between food and poison, between friend and foe, between male and female, between homeward and away, between safety and danger. Without information there can be no health of any sort. Ironically, Postman's eloquence seems to make my job more difficult – as I argue that we are *also* in the process of "uninforming ourselves to death." But Postman would largely agree with the points I am making—a careful consideration of his writings will be helpful to an understanding of my argument.

Another issue that Postman and other critics have eloquently written on is the real and present danger of too readily accepting the ubiquitous deployment of IT in society. That applications like databases, data mining, electronic health records, and surveillance systems play a large and increasing role in human life is deplored in the writings of IT-critical authors such as Alison Armstrong (2001), Neil Postman (1971, 1993, 1996b), Clifford Stoll (1999), Theodore Roszak (2002), Jacques Vallée (2003), and Joseph Weizenbaum (1976). A drive to improve our understanding of human and societal changes, wrought by the indiscriminate deployment of information technology (IT) systems, deserves a much higher prominence.

Is Eudaemonic Health the Responsibility of Public Education?

Yes and no. In a simplistic sense, I suppose it is. On a national basis, public education has long claimed responsibility for preparing citizens who are able to function in society—this it has accomplished to a very modest, to be kind, degree. But the failure of public education to address globalization, societal homogenization, and other profit-driven evils is palpable. Without a focus on eudaemonia, education as a field of human endeavour is incapable of being bi-cultural, let alone multi- or trans-cultural. This means that traditional approaches to public education tend to perpetuate, not solve, the ubiquitous problems of 'difference.' Education systems at lower levels have become little more than expensive child-minding, and at higher levels, employment-qualification services. Are existing educational institutions and systems in a position to define and promulgate the kind of 'whole human' health envisioned herein? For the most part, I think not. While this is by no means intended to cast aspersions on those public school teachers who, although hobbled (if not crippled) by ministries and school boards, struggle mightily to be thoughtful educators, I do sense a dereliction of duty on the part of vast numbers of tenured university instructors. The latter are protected by tenure, and properly so, against wilful dismissal by the authorities who may not like what they say. There seems, however, to be a paucity of sharply critical comments.

To conclude that systems designed for education and health are failing us, one has only to examine some of the most egregious problems that plague communities: these include religious bigotry and violence, racism and tribalism, bureaucratized brutality, environmental destruction, and other tragic consequences of large scale ignorance and thoughtlessness. This suggests to me that the existing approaches to education are essentially failures. With only minimal success at fostering rudimentary social and economic intelligences, and very little success at inculcating in students the value of intellectual, emotional, sexual, and political intelligences, education systems are blocking, not promoting, the development of eudaemonic health. If one were deliberately to design a system, the long-term intentions of which were to stifle creativity, inhibit critical ideation, frustrate political and intellectual activism, foster consumerism and pollution, advocate selfishness, discourage free thought, promote race, class and gender conflict, and so on, then one might come up with an educational system much like the ones we see around us today.

We need, therefore, to see that the endemic levels of such attributes as avarice, prejudice and thoughtlessness, the socio-emotional precursors of the problems I have itemized, are refractory health issues. If we succeed in doing this, it may then be feasible to augment public education with programmes designed to provide children, young people and adults with the ways and means to a better understanding of the human condition. With that kind of health education, it may be possible to inspire an ever-increasing understanding of, and commitment to improving, the real and long-term prospects of realizing eudaemonia.

In the area of health care there are courses, diplomas, and whole programmes the purpose of which it is to train students in the analysis of the predominantly physical needs of the human body and to work towards their being understood and addressed. Eudaemonia is not yet a matter of concern, in spite of the obvious fact that human dignity, rights, freedoms, and values are at least as important as bodily functions, and any threats to rights and values occasioned by poor understanding deserve at least as much attention and funding as do other threats to physical health. Would it not be worthwhile to offer general humanities courses on "thoughtlessness and violence"[14]? Or welcome academic papers that relate internecine strife to prejudice and biased curricula? Or conduct seminars dedicated to exposing how self-centredness, gullibility, and ignorance are making people vulnerable to confidence tricksters, religious charlatans, and medical hoaxers[15]? The few books that discuss how understanding one another can reduce the risk of war are increasingly needed.

The need for a deeper understanding of the human condition is getting inadequate attention in education. My argument is that this must change. It might be argued that curricula in all fields and at all levels include, as a required part of the program, an investigation and assessment of their contribution to eudaemonic health.

Although some of the solutions are clearly to be sought in improved education, would it not be best to move the whole debate into the arena of health? We have seen the difficulties that can arise when health and education are dealt with independently of one another. An unjustifiable level of preoccupation with physical health has brought about an erosion of educational quality and the weakening of public education's ability to respond to the moral, political and environmental exigencies of our times. When, for instance, commercial interests are able to direct policy in public schools and in institutions for advanced education it ought to be clear that a significant problem exists in education.

---

[14] Hannah Arendt (1963) thought it worthwhile to dedicate part of an entire book on the topic.

[15] We need only think of the 'clergyman' in the UK who recently claimed to generate miraculous pregnancies in Africa, for women unable to have children – one woman was said to have borne 11 children in three years, none of them, miraculously, bearing her DNA.

I believe that citizens need access to a globally meaningful, moral education, because it can be demonstrated that education is the only practical tool for eudaemonic health, that is, when measured in terms of self-actualization, autonomy, and freedom. When in a state of eudaemonic health, people tend to understand the nature of information and are therefore able and willing to discriminate between useful and useless information, between credible information and propaganda, between life-enhancing and life-degrading information, between wholesome and toxic information, between stable and volatile information, between information that inspires love and spirituality and information that is conducive to hate and violence, between information needed for survival and that merely desired to enhance pleasure. They are thus in a position to choose among these options so as to increase their chances of achieving 'good and worthwhile lives,' and at the same time enhance their long-term prospects of living in freedom in a sustainable world.

Health care obviously requires more than medical, surgical, or pharmaceutical intervention. Access to clean water, sound sanitation, adequate nutrition, and humane employment have long been known to be among the most important determinants of 'whole health.' Eudaemonial health may prove to be a valid descriptor of happy, thriving individuals, families and communities, and the primary wellspring of this larger health is public education.

A person who has this kind of health will not be hard to identify: If actions are undertaken thoughtfully, with an understanding of their wider impacts, and there is a feeling of obligation to self, to others, and to the world we live in, then that goes a long way toward describing this state of being. This ideal will, however, be out of reach until the requisite thinking influences national and global policies in education, health, and the respective research fields. Of course, were this actually to happen, the implications would be staggering, and the future rich with promise.

METALEGOMENA

I would it were as easy to engender a public discussion on a broader definition of health as it is to start an argument about the comparative efficacy of the low carbohydrate and the low fat approaches to dieting for weight loss. But that is somewhat like expecting to harvest the fruits of a tree as yet unplanted. These comments are by way of a tentative invitation to help plant that tree, the eudaemon tree. It won't be easy—but then that is to be expected, given the nature of the problem. Something is surely wrong when we spend billions to save human bodies and lives, yet we spend very little on helping people achieve health by way of better *understanding* and 'a good and worthwhile life.' Something is also wrong at the other end of the system's spectrum, when a society sees fit to invest billions in preliminary research on 'terra-forming' Mars. An observer from another planetary system, say with a more sophisticated sense of societal and environmental propriety, might be forgiven for deciding that human beings are a long way from having earned the right to join the community of rational beings.

My attempts to understand this conundrum have led me to believe that the solution lies in improving education, but not in education as we conceive of it today. The education that I envisage as contributing to *understanding* and eudaemonia has very little to do with jobs, or socialization, or the search for academic facts, and everything to do with a knowledge of life support systems and understanding the human condition. The education that I see as part of the health system deals directly with such questions as: Why do seemingly intelligent people allow advanced information technology to systemically destroy their children's chances at a good and worthwhile life? Why do consumers reward those who use false, meaningless, and misleading advertising to sell products? Why do people tolerate the existence of, let alone give credence to, sensationalistic media? Why is the thoughtless despoilment of Nature accorded so little attention by affluent consumers? Why are people so reluctant to assume responsibility for the future welfare of the world that our children's children's children will have to live in?

I use the question 'why?' deliberately, in spite of its being considered unscientific, because it anticipates an answer that includes a reason, a justification for something. What are the reasons, justifications, rewards, and pay-offs that lead people to engage in greedy, thoughtless, or violent behaviour? In other words, "Why?" In seeking to answer these questions, one is forced to enter into a discussion about eudaemonic health. This could constitute the core of a form of education that leads to self-realization and spiritual growth. This, in my opinion, is what education is about, and why a dialogue on education, understanding, health and eudaemonia is urgently needed.

BIBLIOGRAPHY

Arendt, H. (1958). *The human condition.* Chicago: University of Chicago Press.

Arendt, H. (1963). *Eichmann in Jerusalem.* Viking. AU PLEASE SUPPLY LOCALE

Arendt, H. (1978). *The life of the mind.* New York: Harcourt Brace Jovanovich.

Armstrong, A., and Casement, C. (2001). *The child and the machine: How computers put our children's education at risk.* Carlton (Vic), Australia: Scribe.

Brauer, G.W. (1998). Totalitarian information technology and the age of information. Proceedings of the 12th International Symposium "Computer Science for Environmental Protection" of the German Society for Informatics; H.D. Haasis and K.C. Ranze (Eds). Vol 1, pp. 46–60. Bremen, Germany; September 15–18.

Coulter, D., & Wiens, J.R. (2002). Educational judgment: Linking the actor to the spectator. *Educational Researcher, 31*(4), 15–25.

Egan, K. (2002). *Getting it wrong from the beginning. Our progressivist inheritance from Herbert Spencer, John Dewey, and Jean Piaget.* New Haven: Yale UP.

Postman, N. (1971). *Teaching as a subversive activity.* Delta.

Postman, N. (1993). *Technopoly: The surrender of culture to technology.* Vintage.

Postman, N. (1996a). Informing ourselves to death. Keynote speech given at a meeting in Stuttgart of the German Informatics Society (Gesellschaft für Informatik) on October 11, 1990, sponsored by IBM-Germany web site http://world.std.com/~jimf/informing.html

Postman, N. (1996b). *The end of education: Redefining the value of school.* Vintage web site.

Roszak, T. (2002). *The cult of information: A neo-Luddite treatise on high tech, artificial intelligence, and the true art of thinking.* University of California Press.

Stoll, C. (1999). *High-tech heretic: Why computers don't belong in the classroom and other reflections by a computer contrarian.* New York: Doubleday.

Vallée, J. (2003). *The heart of the Internet: An insider's view of the origin and promise of the on-Line revolution.* Charlottesville, VA: Hampton Roads.

Weizenbaum, J. (1976). *Computer power and human reason: From judgment to calculation.* New York: W.H. Freeman.

Postscript: The Present and the Future of Global Health*

A. MICHAEL DAVIES

An article in Science Magazine in October 2003 listed the "Grand Challenges in Global Health," a list of 14 research objectives which were selected from more than a thousand ideas submitted by scientists in 75 countries. They call for research into complex problems of vaccine production and delivery, genetics of insect vectors, drug resistance, and so on. The last two, challenges 13 and 14, are to develop technologies for assessment of individual and population health status.

These are real problems, which demand technical fixes in facilitating the control of important diseases, and it is fitting that the efforts of scientists should be directed to applied research (Mansourian, Ch. 8). However the impact of these useful tools on the totality of the health of humankind depends on what we mean by "Global Health."

HEALTH AND GLOBAL HEALTH

The accepted concept of health as an ideal, a motivating goal, is encompassed in the definition of the World Health Organization and takes us far beyond the mere absence of disease to link to equity, life satisfaction and social justice (Manciaux

---

*Each of the chapters in this book is independent and deals with one or other aspect of Global Health in an authoritative manner. The purpose of this last chapter is to link some of the ideas expressed in a general overview of the issues.

and Fliedner, Ch. 5). But like peace, in international law, which is defined as the absence of belligerency (which is very well described) so health is assumed—and measured—in terms of absence of disease. We have no global measure of health: the World Health Report[1] provides statistics on deaths by age and cause and the burden of diseases in DALY's (disability-adjusted life years) based on extrapolations from surveys. The nearest thing to a measure of health is life expectancy and healthy life expectancy, the latter again being computed from an absence of disability.

This kind of information, which is in the grand tradition of classical public health, naturally leads to search for ways to control specific diseases and has concentrated the attention of multinational agencies on the worst offenders, to the exclusion of others. Thus HIV/AIDS, tuberculosis, and malaria are the targets of the Global Fund and priorities of the Commission on Macroeconomics and Health. The potential for saving lives is great, over 6 million persons die annually from these diseases, but the experience with former WHO attempts to eradicate malaria (Litsios, Ch. 2) should make us very aware of the limitations of vertical programs in the long term.

However, the counting of the sick and the dead is far from giving us a measure of the "complete physical, mental and social well being and not merely the absence of disease or infirmity" that the WHO definition requires. There are, of course, measures of income, of deprivation, of education, of crowding and so on, collected by many different agencies, that could fill some of the gap but it has not so far proved feasible to combine them into a composite measure of health. Sayers and Angulo (Ch. 13) provide a hint as to how this might be done in the future. Saracci[2] has claimed that this (WHO) definition is closer to happiness than to health and happiness may not be a human right. His proposal that health be defined as "a condition of well being, free of disease or infirmity." could be easier to quantify but might not satisfy some of our authors (Brauer, Ch. 19).

PROMOTERS AND DETRACTORS OF WORLD HEALTH

The classical cores of public health problems are those of the environment, physical, chemical and biological. The change in approach is the realisation that amelioration is dependent on human behaviour, both individually and collectively. All conditions of ill health are multifactorial and require plurisectoral management (Ch. 5). Both Arata (Ch. 3) and Heymann (Ch. 12) remind us that the old pestilences, which killed whole populations in the past, are very much still with us while new ones have been appearing each year since the mid-1970s. The present world plague of HIV/AIDS and the imminent threat of avian influenza and other respiratory epidemics are cited in several of the chapters.

The spread and dire effects of most of the communicable diseases are the result of poverty, ignorance and malnutrition and control demands attention to these wider aspects of the human situation as well as attention to the specific disease. Which is why former attempts to eradicate malaria failed (Ch. 3) and why the eight Millennium Development Goals[3] list eradication of extreme poverty, universal education and gender equality before reducing child mortality and improving maternal health. Combating HIV/AIDS, malaria and other diseases is seventh on the list. This realisation that health is part of general development can be said to have started, for WHO, with the concept of Health for All and the revelation that health system development is a critical part of the whole. (Ch. 18) And, principles of ethics and human rights dictate that equity of access and care be its cornerstone, even in situations of major crisis (Ch. 11). As Amartya Sen has noted, "no substantial famine has ever occurred in an independent country with a democratic form of government and a relatively free press"[4].

In 2002, infectious and parasitic diseases were estimated to account for just under a quarter of the global burden of DALYs with AIDS, tuberculosis and malaria contributing 11.1%. The 13% allocated to neuropsychiatric disorders, 12.2% to injuries and 9.9% to cardiovascular diseases (WHR 2004) are indicators of a shift in disease patterns as a result of changes in the structure, function and behaviour of society in nearly all countries. These changes are driven by very many factors, starting with demographic change and population ageing and including urbanisation, economic progress, migration, globalisation and mass communication. These forces, among others, are discussed by Davies (Ch. 15), Aluwihare (Ch. 17), Last (Ch. 1) and Manciaux and Fliedner (Ch. 5). Patterns of ill health derive more and more from chronic diseases in every country even while acute diseases remain dominant in some. The demand for medical intervention, called health care, has thus been increasing everywhere and the public health professions have become more focussed on organization and cost containment of medical services that pursue treatment rather than prevention.

As Wojtczak (Ch. 6) points out, the principles of universality, equity and public administration of health services are accepted by most developed and many developing countries although the routes to achieving them, and the measures of success, vary greatly. But public health often lacks a human rights framework and reliance on market forces and privatisation without adequate controls means that health care is confined to those who can pay. The health benefits of globalisation can be great when equitably applied[5] but may be resisted because of a perception of "Americanisation" and a belief that the health packages must incorporate restrictive policies, for instance in contraception, abortion and privatisation. (Dickens, Ch. 4).

In fact, although the many changes in societies, noted above, have been accompanied by a rise in educational level and the revolution in communication produced by the Internet, most public health planning is based on past experience, belief or religion with little attempt at scientific evaluation. Von Pettenkofer wrote in 1873 about the health conditions of his city: "As long as we have wrong ideas in our mind, we cannot find the correct answer to our problem"[6]. The convictions of donor countries or international bodies such as the World Bank[3] and the Global Fund* can and do dictate direction of development schemes and the approach to disease control in poor countries without clear measures of their results. While the techniques of impact evaluation are in their infancy it was astonishing to learn that only 2% of the projects funded by the World Bank for billions of dollars over the years have been critically appraised[7]. Thus the interactions between the many variables involved in development on those of population health remain ill understood.

One of these is the information explosion that, in the richer countries and, increasingly in the poorer ones, provides major sources of information on medical services and health behaviour. That these can bring benefit as well as be exploited unscrupulously for gain is described by Aluwihare (Ch. 17).

WHAT NEEDS TO BE DONE?

"It will not come of itself, we must do something about it" (von Pettenkofer) discussing the health of cities in 1873[6].

There can be no health without continued and sustainable development and this theme runs through many of the foregoing chapters. But sustainable development as originally propounded by the Brundtland Commission requires manageable policy objectives that encompass economic, environmental and other domains of society[8]. For the sphere of health, as, indeed for all spheres of progress, success will depend on Last's list of ingredients: awareness, understanding, capacity to control, belief that the problem is important and political will (Ch. 1).

The most difficult ingredient is political will, at local, regional and global levels. For this to happen, it appears that societies need to develop an ethics of life and health (Manciaux and Fliedner, Ch. 5) and a human rights framework to guide public health in societal analysis and response (Ch. 4). Only from this standpoint can there be balanced examination of the health needs of individuals and groups and honest decisions reached as to priorities and feasibility. This is, of course utopia and, for the majority of the human race, far in the future.

Deterrents include the great backlog in progress and the low priority given by most governments to promotion of health (however much support may be given to curative medicine). The lack of adequate progress towards the Millennium Development Goals, adopted by 14 counties, gives little expectation of any rapid movement towards global heath.[9] However, there is a glimmer of hope in that

*The Global Fund was created to finance the fight against AIDS, Tuberculosis and Malaria. www.theglobal fund.org

1.1 billion people have gained access to clean drinking water during the past 12 years, which brings global coverage to 83%. But the level of sanitation remains low. Unless there is progress in the provision of sanitary facilities 2.4 billion people will not even reach the modest goal of 75% coverage.

A major challenge to future health lies in the worldwide trend to urbanisation, to mega-cities with their loci of global poverty. Of the 3 billion or so urban dwellers in the world, almost a third live in slums and the proportion in developing regions rises to 43%, 72% in sub-Saharan Africa[10].

Global inequalities in health continue to present major political and ethical problems for the future. Healthy life expectancy for girls born in Japan is 77.7 years, in Italy 74.7 years and in most other industrialised countries more than 72 years. For a girl born in Sierra Leone it is only 29.9 years and in Zimbabwe, 33.3 years! (WHO[1]). Such discrepancies cry out for intervention.

As noted above, infectious and communicable diseases are a prominent and visible target for intervention: it is thus reasonable, and fitting, that international agencies have concentrated much of their attention to programmes for global control of AIDS, malaria, tuberculosis and others. But also as noted above, such vertical interventions need underpinning with much organisational infrastructure and social change if they are to have a permanent effect on the wider health of populations.

Many suggestions of how to further the various aspects of global health are made in the preceding chapters and it is likely that some will be adopted, albeit slowly, by more and more countries over the coming decades. But the forces that influence global progress, including health, are many, often contrary and imponderable and it would be a rash prophet who would predict change.

REFERENCES

1. Feachem R. G. A. (2001). Globalisation is good for your health, mostly. *BMJ, 323,* 504.
2. Editorial. The World Bank is finally embracing science. Lancet 2004, *364,* 731.
3. OECD Workshop (2003, May). Workshop for accounting frameworks in sustainable development. Paris, OECD, September 2004.
4. Saracci R. (1997). The World Health Organisation needs to reconsider its definition of health. *British Medical Journal, 314,* 1409.
5. Sen, A. (2000). *Development as freedom.* New Delhi, Oxford University Press.
6. UN-Habitat (2003). The challenge of slums. Global report on human settlement 2003. Nairobi, Kenya.
7. Von Pettenkofer M. (1941). *The value of health to a city. Two lectures delivered in 1873* (H. E. Sigerist, Trans.). Baltimore, Johns Hopkins.
8. World Bank (2004). The millennium development goals for health: Rising to the challenges. Washington, World Bank.
9. World Health Organization. (2004). World Health Report 2004. Geneva, WHO.
10. WHO/UNICEF. (2004). Millennium development goals. Drinking water and sanitation target. A mid term assessment of progress, Geneva, WHO.

The Contributors

A.P.R. Aluwihare is President Elect of the National Academy of Sciences of Sri Lanka. He has an Honorary Fellowship of the Bangladesh College of Physicians and Surgeons, and an Ad Hominem of the College of Surgeons of Edinburgh, the Royal College of Physicians and Surgeons of Glasgow, and an Honorary Fellow of the Royal College of Surgeons of London. He was at one time President of the Medical Section of the Sri Lanka Association for the Advancement of Science, President of the College of Surgeons of Sri Lanka, and Founder President of the South Asian Association for Regional Cooperation Surgical Care Society (the apex body for Surgery in the SAARC countries).

Juan J. Angulo is retired Head of the Exanthem-producing Viruses Section of the Instituto Adolfo Lutz, São Paulo, S.P., Saô Paulo, Brazil.

Andrew A. Arata received his Ph.D. in Biology/Ecology. He was a staff member of WHO, Research in Epidemiology and Communications Science (RECS) and Vector Biology and Control (VBC), Geneva; PAHO, Venezuela and Mexico. He was Professor of International Health and Adjunct Professor Tropical Medicine, Tulane University School of Public Health and Tropical Medicine. In addition, he has served as consultant to USAID and World Bank since 1985. He currently resides in Alexandria, Virginia, USA.

Jean-Philippe Assal is Professor at the Faculty of Medicine, University of Geneva, Switzerland. Dr. Assal is the former Chief of the Division of Therapeutic Education for Chronic Diseases at the University Hospital. Long associated with the World Health Organization, he is the Director of the WHO Collaborating Centre for Research and Development of New Educational Strategies for Patients and is currently helping various medical centers throughout the world to develop therapeutic patient education programs for the chronically ill. He is also on the Board of the International Committee of the Red Cross and Red Crescent.

Gerhard W. Brauer teaches health information science at the University of Victoria, Canada. For the past 20 years he has taught courses in epidemiology, health informatics, health care systems, and the societal and ethical implications of information technology. His academic background is in the areas of medical anthropology, epidemiology, pedagogy, philosophy, and research methodology.

A. Michael Davies is Professor of Public Health Emeritus, Hebrew University of Jerusalem. He was formerly Director of the Brookdale Institute for Gerontology, and Director, Hebrew University — Hadassah School of Public Health. Prof. Davies was also Fogarty Scholar US National Institutes of Health, a member of WHO Global Advisory Committee on Health Research, and consultant and advisor to WHO technical committees and Member Medical Councils. In addition, he was also Chief Epidemiologist, Israel Ministry of Health, Sometime Co-ordinator, National Public Health Service of Liberia.

Bernard Dickens is the Dr. William M. Scholl Professor Emeritus of Health Law and Policy at the Faculty of Law, Faculty of Medicine, and Joint Centre for Bioethics at the University of Toronto, Canada. He is a member of the English and Ontario Bars, a LL.B, LL.M., Ph.D. and LL.D. A graduate of the University of London, and a Fellow of the Royal Society of Canada, Dr. Dickens has authored or co-authored several books, many chapters of books, and over 300 articles on medical law and ethics.

T.M. Fliedner, born 1929, was one of the founding professors of the University of Ulm in 1967 and until his retirement in 1997 Director of the Department of Clinical Physiology, Occupational and Social Medicine. His scientific contributions were in the field of hematology (stem cell and cell kinetic research) as well as in occupational and social medicine. For many years, he served in important functions, first in the WHO European Regional Office (Chairman of the European Advisory Committee on Health Research, 1981–1987) and subsequently at Headquarters in Geneva as the Chairman of the Global Advisory Committee on Health Research, 1994–1998. During this time, the "Research Policy Agenda for Science and Technology to Support Global Health Development" was developed and delivered to the WHO Director-General at the end of 1998 for implementation.

S. William A. Gunn, MD, MS, FRCSC, DSc(Hon), Dr.h.c., is a surgeon and senior international health official involved in disaster management and humanitarian medicine. Formerly Head of the World Health Organization's Emergency Relief Operations, he has conducted numerous field missions, advised governments, organized academic programmes and training on complex catastrophes, services that have been recognized by two Honorary Doctorates and other humanitarian distinctions. He compiled the WHO Emergency Health Kit – supplies for the needs of 10,000 persons over three months – which is still the basis of health assistance in disasters. Among nine books, his *Dictionary of Disaster Medicine and International*

Relief is now basic reference, translated into several languages. Founding President of the WHO Medical Society and of the International Association for Humanitarian Medicine, he is editor of the Journal of Humanitarian Medicine and the Annals of Burn Disasters. Fellow of the Royal College of Surgeons of Canada and of the Royal Anthropological Institute, with several university affiliations, he is interested in the interactions between health, human rights, basic surgical needs and sustainable developmental outreach particularly to emerging societies. He is the principal editor of this book.

David L. Heymann is currently the Representative of the Director General for Polio Eradication at the World Health Organization. Prior to that, from July 1998 until July 2003, Dr Heymann was Executive Director of the WHO Communicable Diseases Cluster which includes WHO's programmes on infectious and tropical diseases, and from which the public health response to SARS was mounted in 2003. From October 1995 to July 1998 Dr Heymann was Director of the WHO Programme on Emerging and other Communicable Diseases, and prior to that was the Chief of research in the WHO Global Programme on AIDS. He is currently editor of the 18th edition of the *Control of Communicable Diseases Manual,* a joint publication of WHO and American Public Health Association publication.

Assen Jablensky graduated in medicine in Sofia (Bulgaria) and specialised in psychiatry in the UK. From 1975 to 1986 he was Senior Medical Officer with the World Health Organization in Geneva, where he was centrally involved in population studies on schizophrenia and other mental disorders. He was appointed Chair of the WHO European Advisory Committee on Health Research (1989–1992) and was elected President of the Medical Academy in Sofia, Bulgaria (1988–1991). He is currently Professor of Psychiatry and Director of the Centre for Clinical Research in Neuropsychiatry at the University of Western Australia in Perth. His main research interests are in epidemiological psychiatry, diagnosis and classification of mental disorders, and the neurobiology of schizophrenia.

Fritz Käferstein, DVM, Ph.D., graduated from the Justus von Liebig University, Giessen/Germany, in 1963. He specialised in food safety and held senior positions with the New Zealand Dept.of Agriculture (1968–72) and the German Federal Health Office, Berlin (1972–80). In 1980, he joined WHO and directed its Food Safety Programme as well as serving as WHO Joint Secretary of the Codex Alimentarius Commission. During his time with WHO, food safety developed from a marginal to a priority public health programme. At the invitation of the US Government, he served from 1998 until 2001 as Distinguished Visiting Scientist to two food safety agencies, i.e. FDA and FSIS. As of fall 2001, he works as independent International Food Safety Consultant.

Arminée Kazanjian is Professor in the Department of Health Care and Epidemiology, Faculty of Medicine, University of British Columbia, Vancouver, Canada.

Her key areas of specialty include socio-behavioral research in health services utilization, health technology assessment, factors supporting knowledge translation, and the use of research evidence in public policy decisions.

John Last is emeritus professor of epidemiology at the University of Ottawa. He is the author or editor of 16 books and about 300 articles and editorials on epidemiology and other aspects of public health sciences and practice, and has consulted in many parts of the world for the World Health Organization and other international and national agencies. He has received numerous awards and distinctions for his contributions to public health.

Socrates Litsios received his Doctorate of Science degree from MIT in 1963. He joined the World Health Organization in Geneva Switzerland in 1967 as Chief of the Operational Research Unit. When he retired in 1997, he occupied the position of Senior Scientist with the Control of Tropical Diseases Program. His publications include numerous articles on medical history plus two books: The Tomorrow of Malaria and Plague Legends: from the Miasmas of Hippocrates to the Microbes of Pasteur. Plague Legends II: in Search of Public Health (1830–1940) is with the publisher.

M. Manciaux is Emeritus Professor of social pediatrics and public health, Nancy, France. He was Medical Officer of the WHO European Office (1968–70), a Member of the WHO Expert Committee on Maternal and Child Health (1975–95), a Member and Vice Chairman of the WHO Global Advisory Committee on Health Research (1992–98), a Member of the Scientific Council of the Canadian Institute for Advanced Research (1992–98), andTechnical Advisor to the French Ministry of Health (1988–91).

Pierre B. Mansourian is a former director (ret.) of the office of research policy coordination of WHO. He holds medical degrees from the universities of Cairo and Lausanne, as well as a Ph.D. from the University of London, and is an elected member of the US Institute of Electrical and Electronics Engineers (IEEE, 1968), the Belgian Royal Academy of overseas sciences (1998) and the City and Guilds of London Institute (FCGI, 1999)

Anthony Piel is the former Legal Counsel and Director of Cabinet of the World Health Organization. Following Princeton University, Harvard Law School, M.I.T Sloan School and eight years with Citibank, he joined the WHO in 1972 in administration and finance and headquarters program planning. Piel worked in developing countries to help design comprehensive national health systems with emphasis on locally planned and implemented community-based primary health care. In 1978, he served as Secretary to the International Conference on Primary Health Care at Alma-Ata, which helped launch the global "Health for All" movement of WHO. From 1985 to 1988 Piel was based in Alexandria, Egypt as Director of Support Program of the WHO Eastern Mediterranean Region, and worked on primary health care development, particularly in Egypt, Sudan and Somalia. In 1988 Piel returned to the WHO headquarters as Director of Program Planning, Legal Counsel, Director of the Cabinet of the Director-General, and participated in the work of the WHO Advisory Committee on Health (and Medical) Research. After retirement he has continued to work with a WHO Collaborating Center at Ulm University in Germany, on radiation medicine, stem-cell research, and institutional networking. Anthony and Lizbeth Piel have two children and maintain a home in Sharon, Connecticut, US.

Bruce McA. Sayers is Emeritus Professor of Computing Applied to Medicine at Imperial College, London, UK. After a period as Biophysicist to the Baker Medical Research Institute in Melbourne Australia, he joined the academic staff of Imperial College, being elected Dean in 1984. From 1994–2000 he served on the Global Advisory Committee on Health Research, World Health Organisation.

J. Szczerban' was Chair of surgery and the department of general and liver surgery at the Warsaw Medical University and the Central University Hospital of Warsaw Poland (1979–89). Also, he was Rector of the Medical University of Warsaw (1979–82), Chairman of the Warsaw Surgical Association (1998–2004). Since 2000, he has been Chairman of the Science Council to the Ministry of Health, Poland. Also, he has been National delegate to the World Health Assemblies, a member of WHO Executive Board 1979–81, WHO Advisory Committee on Health Research (co-secretary), Chief of the Office of Research Promotion and Development WHO Headquarters 1989–1993, and member of the Advisory Committee for WHO Centre for Health Development (Kobe/Japan).

Andrzej Wojtczak MD, PhD (D.MSc) is Director of the Institute for International Medical Education in New York. Former Professor of Medicine and Dean of the School of Public Health & Social Medicine in Warsaw, Poland; he was also Director in WHO Regional Office in Copenhagen, Director of WHO Research Center in Kobe, Japan, President of the Association of Medical Education in Europe (AMEE). He has been the author of over 300 publications and editor of *Textbook of Internal Medicine*.

Index